Endocarditis: Diagnosis, Therapy and Prevention

Endocarditis: Diagnosis, Therapy and Prevention

Editor: Eric Martin

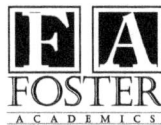

FA
FOSTER
ACADEMICS

www.fosteracademics.com

www.fosteracademics.com

FA
FOSTER
ACADEMICS

Cataloging-in-Publication Data

Endocarditis : diagnosis, therapy and prevention / edited by Eric Martin.
     p. cm.
Includes bibliographical references and index.
ISBN 978-1-63242-606-2
1. Endocarditis. 2. Endocarditis--Diagnosis. 3. Endocarditis--Treatment.
4. Endocarditis--Prevention. 5. Cardiology. I. Martin, Eric.
RC685.E5 E53 2019
616.11--dc23

Foster Academics,
118-35 Queens Blvd., Suite 400,
Forest Hills, NY 11375, USA

ISBN 978-1-63242-606-2 (Hardback)

Contents

Preface

Every book is a source of knowledge and this one is no exception. The idea that led to the conceptualization of this book was the fact that the world is advancing rapidly; which makes it crucial to document the progress in every field. I am aware that a lot of data is already available, yet, there is a lot more to learn. Hence, I accepted the responsibility of editing this book and contributing my knowledge to the community.

Endocarditis is a medical condition characterized by an inflammation of the endocardium of the heart. The inflammation occurs in the heart valves and may extend to the chordae tendineae, interventricular septum, the surfaces of intracardiac devices or the mural endocardium. Vegetations comprising of a mass of fibrin, platelets or microcolonies of scant inflammatory cells or microorganisms may occur in endocarditis. Subacute form of infective endocarditis includes a center of granulomatous tissue. Endocarditis can be infective or non-infective based on the underlying cause of the inflammation. Blood cultures and echocardiogram can aid in the diagnosis. Some common symptoms of this disease are fever, sweating or chills, weakness, anorexia, cardiac murmur, Janeway's lesions, etc. This book includes some of the vital pieces of work being conducted across the world, on various topics related to endocarditis. It provides significant information of this discipline to help develop a good understanding of the diagnosis, therapy and prevention of endocarditis. It will prove to be immensely beneficial to students and researchers in the field of cardiology.

While editing this book, I had multiple visions for it. Then I finally narrowed down to make every chapter a sole standing text explaining a particular topic, so that they can be used independently. However, the umbrella subject sinews them into a common theme. This makes the book a unique platform of knowledge.

I would like to give the major credit of this book to the experts from every corner of the world, who took the time to share their expertise with us. Also, I owe the completion of this book to the never-ending support of my family, who supported me throughout the project.

Editor

Surgical Management of Mitral Valve Endocarditis

Fabian Andres Giraldo Vallejo

Abstract

Before the antibiotic era and cardiac surgery, infective endocarditis (IE) was a predominantly fatal disease. In-hospital mortality persists relatively high despite development in medical and surgical treatment. Adequate timing and surgical management of the infected valve help prevent substantially early and late mortality. The surgical approach of mitral valve endocarditis should be based on extension of the disease and annular involvement. When the valve and annulus are severely affected, the best option is to perform a complete excision and mitral valve replacement (MVR). Only if the disease is limited to the valvular tissue, mitral valve repair is the preferred surgical option.

Keywords: infective endocarditis, epidemiology of infective endocarditis, mitral valve surgery, mitral valve repair, periannular abscess

1. Introduction

The term *infective endocarditis* (IE) refers to infection of the endocardial surface of the heart. Infection may affect heart valves mainly but may occur within a septal defect, in chordae tendinae, or in the mural endocardium. Shunt infections (e.g., arteriovenous shunts, arterioarterial shunts (patent ductus arteriosus)) or coarctation of the aorta is similar in presentation to IE. The main site of cardiac involvement is on the line of closure of a valvar surface. Most affected sites are the atrial side of the atrioventricular valves or on the ventricular surface of the semilunar valves [1].

Perhaps the most convincing hypothesis for the pathogenesis of IE has been given to Rodbar in which high velocity flows from a high-pressure source form in an orifice and enter a low-pressure sink. Bacteria are deposited through *Venturi currents* beyond the orifice to form vena contracta creating mechanical erosion and deposition of platelets and thrombin [2].

Diagnostic criteria for IE were published in 1982 by von Reyn et al. (the Beth Israel Criteria), but these criteria did not include echocardiographic findings in the case definitions [3]. Including the important role of echocardiography in the evaluation of suspected IE, new case definitions and diagnostic criteria were proposed in 1994 [4], modified in 2000 and broadly used since then [5]. The usefulness of echocardiography in the diagnosis of IE is clearly known [6]; transesophageal imaging has superior sensitivity and specificity, is cost-effective, and should be done when transthoracic approach is negative and the patient has a high clinical suspicion of IE.

Even though the infected aortic valve is difficult to repair, well-known repair techniques can be applied to patients with mitral valve endocarditis. Advantages of mitral valve repair compared with replacement are well established for noninfectious mitral valve disease and include low perioperative mortality, preserved left ventricular function, no need for long-term anticoagulation, less long-term thromboembolic complications, lower risk of IE, freedom from reoperation, and improved long-term survival [7].

2. Clinical features and diagnostic criteria

Investigators at Duke University modified the terms introduced by Jones (rheumatic fever); these criteria include major and minor signs and symptoms, echocardiographic findings, iatrogenic and nosocomial factors (indwelling catheters), and history of IV drug abuse (**Table 1**) [5]. The most common clinical manifestation of IE is fever, which can be present in 95–100% of patients. Fever may present as low grade or spiking following peak of bacteremia. It is important to draw two sets of blood cultures from different sites in any patient at risk of having IE who presents with fever of unknown origin for more than 48 h. Once blood cultures have been obtained, antibiotics should be started until proper identification of causative organism [8]. When IE is confirmed by echocardiography, surgery, or autopsy, positive blood cultures are obtained in 95% of cases when two blood specimens are obtained and are positive in 98% of cases with four blood specimens [9]. However, when dealing with prosthesis valve endocarditis (PVE), a negative-culture endocarditis can rise to about 10% of cases on most surgical series [10, 11]. The diagnosis of IE should be investigated in any patient with sepsis of unknown origin or fever associated with risk factors. Sepsis can present in a variety of forms and can range from malaise to shock depending on the virulence of the pathogen and the host immune response [12, 13]. Stroke or systemic embolism can also be present as a complication of IE. Whenever a patient presents with persistent or unexplained bacteremia, the diagnosis of IE should be ruled out. *S. aureus* bacteremia is associated with IE in 25–30% of cases, and all patients should undergo echocardiography [14, 15]. Risk factors for developing IE include previous IE, a prosthetic valve or cardiac device and valvular or congenital heart disease, indwelling intravenous lines, intravenous drug use, immunosuppression, and a recent dental or surgical procedure. Popular known signs like Osler's nodes, Janeway lesions, and Roth spots are rare; their absence does not rule out infective endocarditis. Heart failure, stroke, or metastatic infection (osteomyelitis, peripheral abscess) are much more common. Routine laboratory tests are usually nonspecific. Admission electrocardiogram is useful since new disturbances may suggest paravalvular or myocardial extension of infection [16].

Definite infective endocarditis

Pathologic criteria

- Microorganisms demonstrated by culture or histologic examination of a vegetation, a vegetation that has embolized, or an intracardiac abscess specimen
- Pathologic lesions; vegetation or intracardiac abscess confirmed by histologic examination showing active endocarditis

Clinical criteria

- Two major criteria
- One major criterion and three minor criteria
- Five minor criteria

Possible infective endocarditis

- One major criterion and one minor criterion
- Three minor criteria

Rejected

- Firm alternate diagnosis explaining evidence of IE
- Resolution of IE syndrome with antibiotic therapy for ≤4 days
- No pathologic evidence of IE at surgery or autopsy, with antibiotic therapy for ≤4 days
- Does not meet criteria for possible IE, as above

Major criteria

Blood culture positive for IE

- Typical microorganisms consistent with IE from two separate blood cultures: viridans streptococci, *Streptococcus bovis*, HACEK group, *Staphylococcus aureus*
- Community-acquired enterococci, in the absence of a primary focus
- Microorganisms consistent with IE from persistently positive blood cultures, defined as follows:
- At least two positive cultures of blood samples drawn >12 h apart
- All of three or a majority of ≥ four separate cultures of blood (with the first and last samples drawn at least 1 h apart)
- Single positive blood culture for *Coxiella burnetii* or antiphase I IgG antibody titer >1:800

Evidence of endocardial involvement

- Echocardiogram positive for IE (TEE recommended in patients with prosthetic valves, rated at least "possible IE" by clinical criteria or complicated IE [paravalvular abscess]; TTE as first test in other patients), defined as follows:
  - Oscillating intracardiac mass on valve or supporting structures, in the path of regurgitant jets, or on implanted material in the absence of an alternative anatomic explanation
  - Abscess
  - New partial dehiscence of prosthetic valve
  - New valvular regurgitation (worsening or changing of preexisting murmur not sufficient)

Minor criteria

- Predisposition, predisposing heart condition or injection drug use
- Fever, temperature > 38°C (100.4°F)
- Vascular phenomena, major arterial emboli, septic pulmonary infarcts, mycotic aneurysm, intracranial hemorrhage, conjunctival hemorrhages, and Janeway lesions
- Immunologic phenomena: glomerulonephritis, Osler's nodes, Roth's spots, and rheumatoid factor
- Microbiologic evidence: positive blood culture but does not meet a major criterion as noted above[*] or serologic evidence of active infection with organism consistent with IE
- Echocardiographic minor criteria eliminated

HACEK, *Haemophilus* spp., *Aggregatibacter* spp., *Cardiobacterium hominis*, *Eikenella corrodens*, and *Kingella* spp.; TEE, transesophageal echocardiography; TTE, transthoracic echocardiography
Modified from Li et al. [5].

Table 1. Definition of infective endocarditis (IE) according to modified Duke criteria.

Diagnosis of IE includes the sum of clinical findings, microbiological analysis, and imaging results. A definite diagnosis includes two major modified Duke criteria, one major plus three minor and five minor criteria [5]. Alternatively the diagnosis can be made by specimen culture or histology (obtained by surgery or autopsy) of the vegetation or abscess. The physicist must note that Duke criteria were devised to help in the diagnosis but never to replace the clinical judgment [17].

Infection of the mitral valve and its supporting structures is less frequent than aortic valve endocarditis but may be more indolent in its course. When *S. aureus* is the infecting organism, the mitral valve is more frequently involved (± 40% of cases) followed by the aortic valve in 36% of cases [18]. Echocardiography plays a major role in diagnosis and detection of complications. A major criterion includes the presence of valvular vegetation or abscess or new dehiscence of a prosthetic valve [19]. Besides diagnostic, echocardiography also provides information on the hemodynamic status of the valve lesion and left and right ventricular function. In native valve endocarditis (NVE), transthoracic echocardiography (TTE) has a sensitivity of 75% and specificity of >90% for detection of a vegetation. Transesophageal echocardiography (TEE) has a sensitivity >90% and should be done in a patient with a negative or equivocal TTE and high clinical likelihood of infective endocarditis [19]. As for abscess, leaflet perforation or pseudoaneurysm TEE offers better detection than TTE [20, 21]. In patients with prosthetic valves, the sensitivity of TTE is lower (36–69%), and TEE is more accurate in detecting complications and cardiac device infections [22, 23].

3. Therapy

The management of patients with IE necessitates a multidisciplinary approach where cardiologists, cardiac surgeons, and infectious disease specialists are involved. There are no clinical randomized trials that guide the management decisions nor a level A evidence in international guides [8, 24].

3.1. Antibiotics

Antibiotics should be started once blood cultures have been acquired; nevertheless if the patient is stable, the physician could wait until final report is available [25]. Empirical antibiotic regimens for the native valve endocarditis and prosthetic valve endocarditis are outlined on definite guidelines by the British Society for Antimicrobial Chemotherapy (**Table 2**) [25]. Antibiotics can be modified according to culture results, local resistance patterns, virulence, and the presence or absence of prosthetic material. Because penetration of antibiotics to vegetations is difficult, prolonged parenteral antibiotic administration is advisable. Treatment for at least 4–6 weeks is usually necessary and longer for some cases (e.g., Q fever endocarditis).

3.2. Surgery

About 40–50% of patients with IE undergo surgical therapy [26, 27]. Goals of surgery are removal of infected tissue and drainage of abscess, restoration of ventriculoarterial or atrioventricular continuity, and reversion to hemodynamic stability. In children, this process may

	Empirical antibiotic regimen and dose	Comment
Native valve endocarditis—indolent presentation	Amoxicillin (2 g, every 4 h, intravenously) + gentamicin* (optional; 1 mg/kg of actual bodyweight)	Better activity than benzylpenicillin against enterococci and many HACEK bacteria; the use of gentamicin before availability of culture results is controversial
Native valve endocarditis— severe sepsis (without risk factors for multiresistant enteric Gram-negative bacilli, Pseudomonas)	Vancomycin* (dose as per local guidelines) + gentamicin* (1 mg/kg of ideal bodyweight, every 12 h, intravenously)	Activity against staphylococci (including meticillin-resistant Staphylococcus aureus)
Native valve endocarditis—severe sepsis (with risk factors for multiresistant enteric Gram-negative bacilli, Pseudomonas)	Vancomycin* (dose as per local guidelines) + meropenem (2 g, every 8 h, intravenously)	
Prosthetic valve endocarditis—pending blood cultures or with negative blood cultures	Vancomycin* (1 g, every 12 h, intravenously) + gentamicin* (1 mg/kg, every 12 h, intravenously) + rifampicin (300–600 mg, every 12 h, orally or intravenously)	

Adapted from Gould et al. [25].
All antibiotic doses are adjusted according to renal function. HACEK=*Haemophilus* spp., *Aggregatibacter actinomycetem-comitans, Cardiobacterium hominis, Eikenella corrodens,* and *Kingella kinga.*
*Regular measurement of serum concentrations needed to monitor and adjust dosing.

Table 2. Empirical treatment for different clinical scenarios in patients with suspected infective endocarditis.

require repairing of the underlying malformation. Valve repair and replacement are options for reconstruction, and there is no evidence that favors a bioprosthetic valve over a mechanical valve. *Heart failure* caused by valvular obstruction or regurgitation is the most common indication for surgery. A dismal prognosis is ensued when refractory pulmonary edema or cardiogenic shock is present and no emergent surgery is done [28, 29].

There is limited evidence to guide clinical practice when the patient has well-tolerated severe valve regurgitation and postpone surgery until stabilization with antibiotics. *Complex or uncontrolled infection* is the second indication for surgery. The complications include abscess, pseudoaneurysm, fistula, or atrioventricular block. A pseudoaneurysm is a perivalvular cavity that communicates with the cardiac chambers (evidenced by Doppler color), whereas an abscess is a pus-filled perivalvular cavity that does not communicate [19]. If perivalvular infection progresses, a fistula can be created (usually aorto-cavitary) which can have a mortality as high as 41% even with surgery [30]. *Prevention of embolism* is the third indication for surgery. This complication can affect 25–50% of patients [31]. Stroke is the most common presentation, but embolism resulting in end-organ infarction (kidney, spleen, coronaries, mesentery, and limbs) can also be present. Most emboli occur in the first 2 weeks after diagnosis with risk decreasing rapidly after antibiotics are instituted [32, 33]. Embolism is more likely when the vegetation is large (>10 mm), highly mobile, and located in the mitral valve [34]. *Persistent or relapsing infection* and infection caused by antibiotic-resistant microorganisms (e.g., *S. aureus, S. lugdunensis, Pseudomonas,* fungi) are also indications for surgery [27].

Surgery for IE is done through partial or full median sternotomy. Suppurative pericarditis suggests a previous perforation at the aortic or mitral ring or ring abscess [35, 36]. It is recommended to use bicaval cannulation to facilitate the procedure in the presence of burrowing abscess, acquired septal perforation, unexpected right-sided valve involvement, or complex aortic root reconstruction. Intraoperative TEE plays a major role in diagnosis and treatment guidance. When left-sided IE is present, minimal manipulation of the heart is important to avoid migration of embolic material. Ample excision of infected tissue is performed with drainage of abscess and closure of defects [37]. When mitral endocarditis is present, aortic valve involvement should be considered. Although absence of echocardiographic anomalies in the aortic area argue against the presence of vegetations and inspection of the aortic valve is not necessary. Reconstruction on mitral valve area can be accomplished when the vegetation is healed or small and the tensor apparatus is mostly uncompromised. Usual sites of native valve endocarditis are drop lesion of anterior leaflet or leaflet vegetation and ring abscess of posterior portion (**Figure 1**). Small perforations may be closed using autologous pericardium or bovine pericardial patch, or otherwise the defect may be closed using continuous suture (**Figure 2**). Reconstruction of the mitral valve represents a challenge if major involvement of the valves is present. Most of the times, a replacement is considered; nevertheless, the risk for PVE is greater especially in ongoing positive blood cultures. If commissural areas are compromised by the infection, a sliding annuloplasty can be performed. Partial leaflet resection, pericardial patch replacement of mid-leaflet areas, or both may be used [37]. The remaining orifice size after reconstruction must be large enough (25 mm in an adult, z-score − 2 or greater in children) to prevent mitral stenosis [37]. Suture annuloplasty is preferable over prosthetic ring in active IE, but a biodegradable annuloplasty ring has been suggested by some authors [38]. In the absence of active IE (e.g., negative blood cultures, no inflammation), classical reconstruction techniques may be used for the mitral valve. Quadrangular resection of a portion of the posterior leaflet (**Figure 3**) or triangular resection of a portion of the anterior leaflet may be done, followed by the insertion

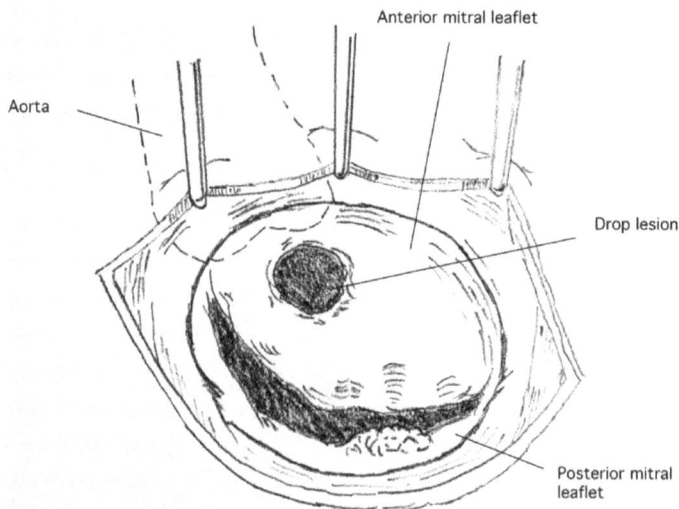

Figure 1. Drop lesion of anterior leaflet and leaflet vegetation and ring abscess of posterior leaflet.

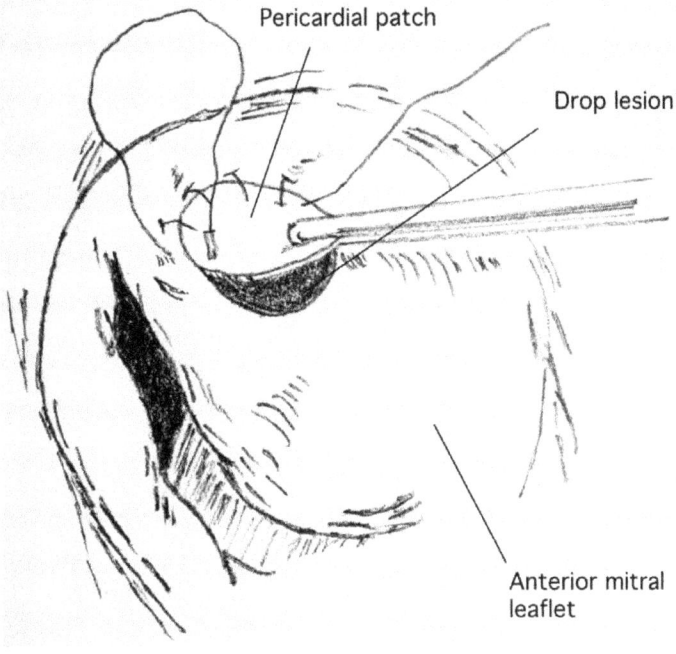

Figure 2. Pericardial patch used to close a drop lesion of the anterior leaflet.

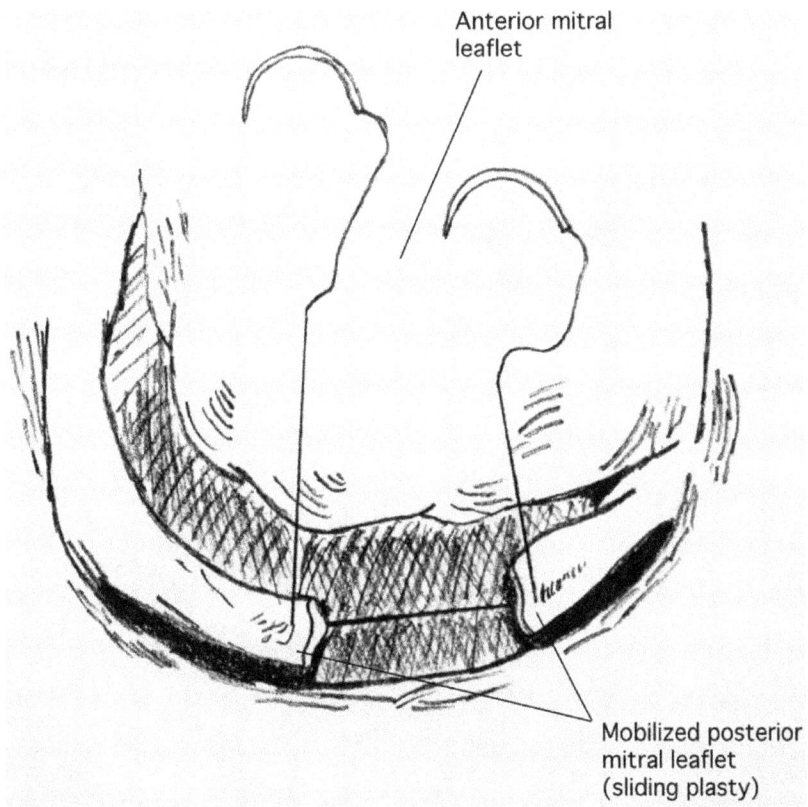

Figure 3. Limited quadrangular resection and sliding plasty of posterior leaflet.

of a partial or complete annular ring. When resecting the mitral valve, the posteroinferior zone of the mitral annulus should be inspected because myocardial ring abscess usually occurs in this location [39, 40]. When left atrioventricular discontinuity is present in mitral valve IE, a small variation of the usual valve replacement can be used. After thorough debridement of the affected tissue in the mitral ring, interrupted horizontal mattress sutures are anchored with felt or autologous pericardium pledgets to the ventricular aspect of the mitral annulus, brought up through the left atrial aspect and then through the prosthetic sewing ring. Deep bytes are performed [37]. When extensive ring abscess is present (**Figure 4**), a different approach is done. The atrioventricular discontinuity is reconstructed using an autologous or bovine pericardial patch. The ventricular aspect is anchored to the myocardium and endocardium using deep bytes of continuous 3-0 or 4-0 polypropylene suture. The superior aspect of this patch is anchored to the left atrial side with a continuous suture (**Figure 5**). The prosthesis is anchored to the ventricular aspect of the suture line using interrupted horizontal mattress sutures supported with felts pledgets (**Figure 6**) [37]. Using antibiotic, antiseptic solutions (e.g., povidone-iodine), or antifungal agents to impregnate the prosthesis and the affected area has been described to help in the management of this entity [41–43]. Mitral valve repair for IE continues to be challenging and much less commonly performed than valve replacement [44]. Repairing tissues that may be infected in the acute stages and the durability of repairing inflamed tissues are the main concerns influencing the decision [45–47]. Several studies have reported excellent results for mitral valve repair in IE [48–51].

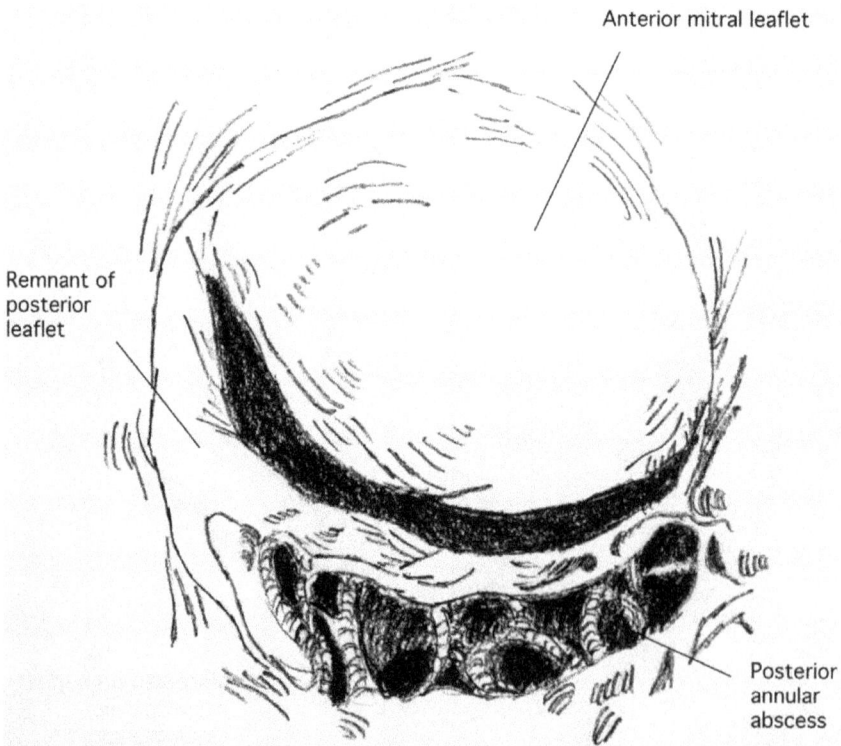

Figure 4. Infective endocarditis with ring abscess compromising the posterior leaflet of mitral valve.

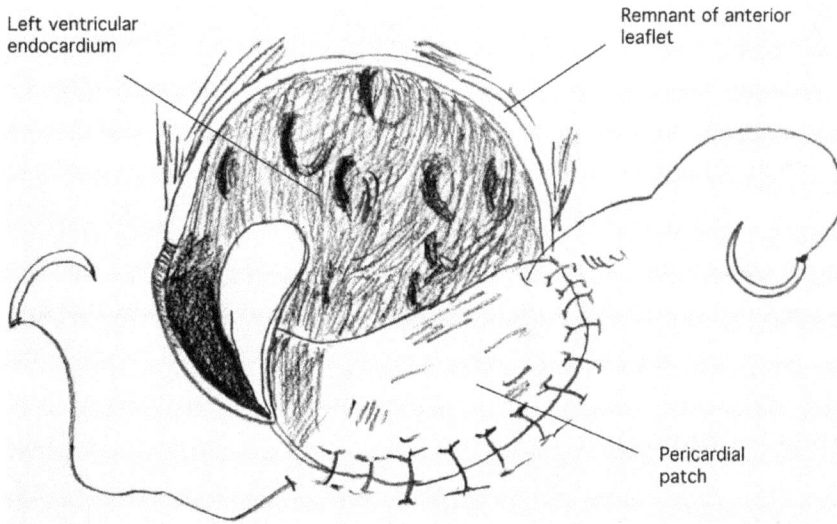

Figure 5. The defect is covered by a pericardial patch anchored within the left ventricle and extending up across the base of the posterior leaflet. Stitches then are placed to the left atrial wall.

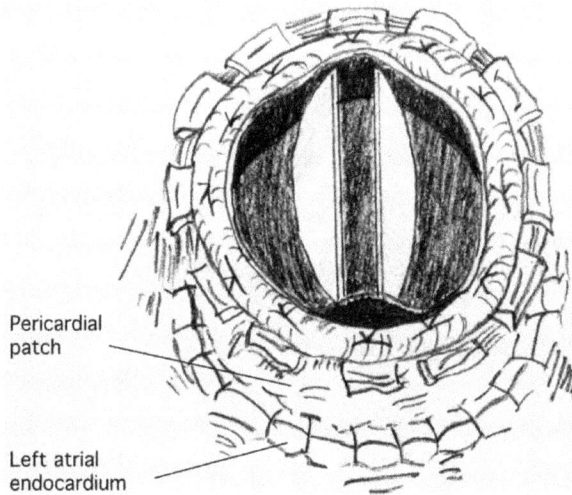

Figure 6. Prosthesis is placed in position. The posterior suture line is on the patch in this case. Eventually the prosthesis may be seated below the patch on ventricular wall.

4. Results

Hospital mortality for valve operations in patients with IE varies widely (4–30%) [52–57]. This variation can be due to several factors, especially the difference in risk between the acute phase of IE and the healed stage. A study from Richardson reported a mortality of 14% in surgically treated patients versus 44% in those medically treated. Operative mortality was affected by urgency of operation. Mortality for elective operations (next convenient day), was 5%, for urgent operations (next day), 16% and for emergent operations in patients with cardiogenic shock (immediately), 33% [58].

Freedom from reoperation is higher when the mitral valve is involved (compared with the aortic valve) probably for less annular involvement. In a series from Brigham and Women's Hospital (Boston) reporting freedom from reoperation for mitral valve IE, the results found 92 and 62% at 5 and 10 years for acute endocarditis and 94% and 84% for healed endocarditis (p = 0.7), respectively [59]. A serious complication after valve replacement for IE is a new or worsening neurologic deficit. Friable vegetation may dislodge and cause CNS deficits. Moreover, an existing CNS deficit is aggravated by operation. A study from university of Illinois found evidence of cerebral septic emboli in 42% of patients who underwent valve replacement for IE. Complications included postoperative strokes in 6%, brain abscesses in 2%, and seizures in 1% [60].

5. Indications for operation

Indications for operation are based in the hemodynamic state of the valvar lesion or defect. When active NVE is present, a lack of consensus exists about some of the specific indications for surgery [61]. General indications for operation, however, exist from both the American and European societies (**Table 3**) [8, 24]. As for timing of surgery, specific recommendations are outlined in **Table 4** [26]. However it is important to remember that no randomized controlled

---

Congestive heart failure[*]

- Congestive heart failure caused by severe aortic or mitral regurgitation or, more rarely, by valve obstruction caused by vegetations
- Severe acute aortic or mitral regurgitation with echocardiographic signs of elevated left ventricular end-diastolic pressure or significant pulmonary hypertension
- Congestive heart failure as a result of prosthetic dehiscence or obstruction

Periannular extension

- Most patients with abscess formation or fistulous tract formation

Systemic embolism[+]

- Recurrent emboli despite appropriate antibiotic therapy
- Large vegetations (10 mm) after one or more clinical or silent embolic events after initiation of antibiotic therapy
- Large vegetations and other predictors of a complicated course
- Very large vegetations (15 mm) without embolic complications, especially if valve-sparing surgery is likely (remains controversial)

Cerebrovascular complications[‡]

- Silent neurological complication or transient ischemic attack and other surgical indications
- Ischemic stroke and other surgical indications, provided that cerebral hemorrhage has been excluded and neurological complications are not severe (e.g., coma)

Persistent sepsis

- Fever or positive blood cultures persisting for >5 to 7 days despite an appropriate antibiotic regimen, assuming that vegetations or other lesions requiring surgery persist and that extracardiac sources of sepsis have been excluded
- Relapsing IE, especially when caused by organisms other than sensitive streptococci or in patients with prosthetic valves

Difficult organisms

- *S. aureus* IE involving a prosthetic valve and most cases involving a left-sided native valve
- IE caused by other aggressive organisms (*Brucella, Staphylococcus lugdunensis*)

- IE caused by multiresistant organisms (e.g., methicillin-resistant *S. aureus* or vancomycin-resistant enterococci) and rare infections caused by Gram-negative bacteria
- *Pseudomonas aeruginosa* IE
- Fungal IE
- Q fever IE and other relative indications for intervention

Prosthetic valve endocarditis

- Virtually all cases of early prosthetic valve endocarditis
- Virtually all cases of prosthetic valve endocarditis caused by *S. aureus*
- Late prosthetic valve endocarditis with heart failure caused by prosthetic dehiscence or obstruction or other indications for surgery

---

*Surgery should be performed immediately, irrespective of antibiotic therapy, in patients with persistent pulmonary edema or cardiogenic shock. If congestive heart failure disappears with medical therapy and there are no other surgical indications, intervention can be postponed to allow a period of days or weeks of antibiotic treatment under careful clinical and echocardiographic observation. In patients with well-tolerated severe valvular regurgitation or prosthetic dehiscence and no other reasons for surgery, conservative therapy under careful clinical and echocardiographic observation is recommended with consideration of deferred surgery after resolution of the infection, depending upon tolerance of the valve lesion.

†In all cases, surgery for the prevention of embolism must be performed very early since embolic risk is highest during the first days of therapy.

‡Surgery is contraindicated for at least 1 month after intracranial hemorrhage unless neurosurgical or endovascular intervention can be performed to reduce bleeding risk.

Adapted from ACC/AHA 2014 Guidelines [8].

Table 3. Indications for surgery for infective endocarditis.

Emergency surgery (within 24 h)

- Native (aortic or mitral) or prosthetic valve endocarditis and severe congestive heart failure or cardiogenic shock caused by:
    - Acute valvular regurgitation
    - Severe prosthetic dysfunction (dehiscence or obstruction)
    - Fistula into a cardiac chamber or the pericardial space

Urgent surgery (within days)

- Native valve endocarditis with persisting congestive heart failure, signs of poor hemodynamic tolerance, or abscess
- Prosthetic valve endocarditis with persisting congestive heart failure, signs of poor hemodynamic tolerance, or abscess
- Prosthetic valve endocarditis caused by staphylococci or Gram-negative organisms
- Large vegetation (10 mm) with an embolic event
- Large vegetation (10 mm) with other predictors of a complicated course
- Very large vegetation (15 mm), especially if conservative surgery is available
- Large abscess and/or periannular involvement with uncontrolled infection

Early elective surgery (during the in-hospital stay)

- Severe aortic or mitral regurgitation with congestive heart failure and good response to medical therapy
- Prosthetic valve endocarditis with valvular dehiscence or congestive heart failure and good response to medical therapy
- Presence of abscess or periannular extension
- Persisting infection when extracardiac focus has been excluded
- Fungal or other infections resistant to medical cure

Adapted from Prendergast et al. [26].

Table 4. Timing of surgery.

trials are available to guide current practice. Among the indications for surgery in IE, operation for acute heart failure provides the greatest survival benefit [62, 63].

Infective endocarditis is a serious condition associated with significant morbidity and mortality. Adequate management requires intervention of multiple specialists. Correct and timed diagnosis and antibiotics are necessary, but an important percentage of patients still require surgery. Surgical mortality is high, but long-term results continue to improve with increased number of patient undergoing valve conserving surgery.

Author details

Fabian Andres Giraldo Vallejo

Address all correspondence to: fabiangiraldomd@gmail.com

Instituto del Corazón de Bucaramanga, Bucaramanga, Colombia

References

[1] Bashore TM, Cabell C, Fowler JV. Update on infective endocarditis. Current Problems in Cardiology. 2006 Apr;**31**(4):274-352

[2] Rodbard S. Blood velocity and endocarditis. Circulation. 1963 Jan;**27**:18-28

[3] Von Reyn CF, Levy BS, Arbeit RD, Friedland G, Crumpacker CS. Infective endocarditis: An analysis based on strict case definitions. Annals of Internal Medicine. 1981 Apr;**94**(4 pt 1): 505-518

[4] Durack DT, Lukes AS, Bright DK. New criteria for diagnosis of infective endocarditis: Utilization of specific echocardiographic findings. Duke Endocarditis Service. American Journal of Medicine. 1994 Mar;**96**(3):200-209

[5] Li JS, Sexton DJ, Mick N, Nettles R, Fowler VG, Ryan T, et al. Proposed modifications to the Duke criteria for the diagnosis of infective endocarditis. Clinical Infectious Disease: An Official Publication of the Infectious Disease Society of America. 2000 Apr;**30**(4):633-638

[6] Evangelista A. Echocardiography in infective endocarditis. Heart. 2004 Jun 1;**90**(6):614-617

[7] Lawrie GM. Mitral valve repair vs replacement. Current recommendations and long-term results. Cardiology Clinics. 1998 Aug;**16**(3):437-448

[8] Nishimura RA, Otto CM, Bonow RO, Carabello BA, Erwin JP, Guyton RA, et al. 2014 AHA/ACC guideline for the Management of Patients with Valvular heart disease: A report of the American College of Cardiology/American Heart Association task force on practice guidelines. Circulation. 2014 Jun 10;**129**(23):e521-e643

[9] Bleich HL, Boro ES, Weinstein L, Schlesinger JJ. Pathoanatomic, pathophysiologic and clinical correlations in endocarditis. The New England Journal of Medicine. 1974 Oct 17; **291**(16):832-837

[10] Sandre RM, Shafran SD. Infective endocarditis: Review of 135 cases over 9 years. Clinical infectious diseases : an official publication of the Infectious Diseases Society of America. 1996 Feb;**22**(2):276-286

[11] Hoen B, Selton-Suty C, Lacassin F, Etienne J, Briançon S, Leport C, et al. Infective endocarditis in patients with negative blood cultures: Analysis of 88 cases from a one-year nationwide survey in France. Clinical infectious diseases : an official publication of the Infectious Diseases Society of America. 1995 Mar;**20**(3):501-506

[12] Werdan K, Dietz S, Löffler B, Niemann S, Bushnaq H, Silber R-E, et al. Mechanisms of infective endocarditis: Pathogen–host interaction and risk states. Nature Reviews. Cardiology. 2013 Nov 19;**11**(1):35-50

[13] Olmos C, Vilacosta I, Fernandez C, Lopez J, Sarria C, Ferrera C, et al. Contemporary epidemiology and prognosis of septic shock in infective endocarditis. European Heart Journal. 2013 Jul 2;**34**(26):1999-2006

[14] Fowler VG, Li J, Corey GR, Boley J, Marr KA, Gopal AK, et al. Role of echocardiography in evaluation of patients with *Staphylococcus aureus* bacteremia: Experience in 103 patients. Journal of the American College of Cardiology. 1997 Oct;**30**(4):1072-1078

[15] Joseph JP, Meddows TR, Webster DP, Newton JD, Myerson SG, Prendergast B, et al. Prioritizing echocardiography in *Staphylococcus aureus* bacteraemia. The Journal of Antimicrobial Chemotherapy. 2013 Feb 1;**68**(2):444-449

[16] Meine TJ, Nettles RE, Anderson DJ, Cabell CH, Corey GR, Sexton DJ, et al. Cardiac conduction abnormalities in endocarditis defined by the Duke criteria. American Heart Journal. 2001 Aug;**142**(2):280-285

[17] Prendergast BD. Diagnostic criteria and problems in infective endocarditis. Heart. 2004 Jun 1;**90**(6):611-613

[18] Miro JM, Anguera I, Cabell CH, Chen AY, Stafford JA, Corey GR, et al. *Staphylococcus aureus* native valve infective endocarditis: Report of 566 episodes from the international collaboration on endocarditis merged database. Clinical Infectious Diseases. 2005 Aug 15; **41**(4):507-514

[19] Habib G, Badano L, Tribouilloy C, et al. recommendations for the practice of echocardiography in infective endocarditis. European Journal of Echocardiography. 2010 Mar 1; **11**(2):202-219

[20] De Castro S, Cartoni D, d'Amati G, Beni S, Yao J, Fiorelli M, et al. Diagnostic accuracy of transthoracic and multiplane transesophageal echocardiography for valvular perforation in acute infective endocarditis: Correlation with anatomic findings. Clinical Infectious Diseases. 2000 May 1;**30**(5):825-826

[21] Daniel WG, Mügge A, Martin RP, Lindert O, Hausmann D, Nonnast-Daniel B, et al. Improvement in the diagnosis of abscesses associated with endocarditis by transesophageal echocardiography. The New England Journal of Medicine. 1991 Mar 21;324(12): 795-800

[22] Victor F, De Place C, Camus C, Le Breton H, Leclercq C, Pavin D, et al. Pacemaker lead infection: Echocardiographic features, management, and outcome. Heart. 1999 Jan;81(1, 1): 82-87

[23] Dundar C, Tigen K, Tanalp C, Izgi A, Karaahmet T, Cevik C, et al. The prevalence of echocardiographic accretions on the leads of patients with permanent pacemakers. Journal of the American Society of Echocardiography. 2011 Jul;24(7):803-807

[24] Endorsed by the European Society of Clinical Microbiology and Infectious Diseases (ESCMID) and by the International Society of Chemotherapy (ISC) for Infection and Cancer, Authors/Task Force Members, Habib G, Hoen B, Tornos P, Thuny F, et al. Guidelines on the prevention, diagnosis, and treatment of infective endocarditis (new version 2009): The task force on the prevention, diagnosis, and treatment of infective endocarditis of the European Society of Cardiology (ESC). European Heart Journal. 2009 Oct 1;30(19):2369-2413

[25] Gould FK, Denning DW, Elliott TSJ, Foweraker J, Perry JD, Prendergast BD, et al. Guidelines for the diagnosis and antibiotic treatment of endocarditis in adults: A report of the working Party of the British Society for antimicrobial chemotherapy. The Journal of Antimicrobial Chemotherapy. 2012 Feb 1;67(2):269-289

[26] Prendergast BD, Tornos P. Surgery for infective endocarditis: Who and when? Circulation. 2010 Mar;121(9, 9):1141-1152

[27] Malhotra A, Rayner J, Williams TM, Prendergast B. Infective endocarditis: Therapeutic options and indications for surgery. Current Cardiology Report [Internet]. 2014 Apr [cited 2017 Dec 22];16(4) Available from: http://link.springer.com/10.1007/s11886-014-0464-9

[28] Richardson JV, Karp RB, Kirklin JW, Dismukes WE. Treatment of infective endocarditis: A 10-year comparative analysis. Circulation. 1978 Oct;58(4):589-597

[29] Croft CH, Woodward W, Elliott A, Commerford PJ, Barnard CN, Beck W. Analysis of surgical versus medical therapy in active complicated native valve infective endocarditis. The American Journal of Cardiology. 1983 Jun;51(10):1650-1655

[30] Anguera I, Miro JM, Vilacosta I, Almirante B, Anguita M, Muñoz P, et al. Aorto-cavitary fistulous tract formation in infective endocarditis: Clinical and echocardiographic features of 76 cases and risk factors for mortality. European Heart Journal. 2005 Feb 1;26(3):288-297

[31] Thuny F. Risk of embolism and death in infective endocarditis: Prognostic value of echocardiography: A prospective multicenter study. Circulation. 2005 Jun 27;112(1):69-75

[32] Vilacosta I, Graupner C, SanRomán J, Sarriá C, Ronderos R, Fernández C, et al. Risk of embolization after institution of antibiotic therapy for infective endocarditis. Journal of the American College of Cardiology. 2002 May;39(9):1489-1495

[33] Dickerman SA, Abrutyn E, Barsic B, Bouza E, Cecchi E, Moreno A, et al. The relationship between the initiation of antimicrobial therapy and the incidence of stroke in infective endocarditis: An analysis from the ICE prospective cohort study (ICE-PCS). American Heart Journal. 2007 Dec;**154**(6):1086-1094

[34] Mügge A, Daniel WG, Frank G, Lichtlen PR. Echocardiography in infective endocarditis: Reassessment of prognostic implications of vegetation size determined by the transthoracic and the transesophageal approach. Journal of the American College of Cardiology. 1989 Sep;**14**(3):631-638

[35] Frantz PT, Murray GF, Wilcox BR. Surgical management of left ventricular-aortic discontinuity complicating bacterial endocarditis. The Annals of Thoracic Surgery. 1980 Jan;**29**(1):1-7

[36] Utley JR, Mills J, Hutchinson JC, Edmunds LH, Sanderson RG, Roe BB. Valve replacement for bacterial and fungal endocarditis. A comparative study. Circulation. 1973 Jul;**48**(1 Suppl): III42-III47

[37] Kirklin, Kouchoukos N, Blackstone EH. Infective endocarditis. In: Cardiac Surgery. 4th ed. Philadelphia: Elsevier, Saunders; 2013. p. 682

[38] Pektok E, Sierra J, Cikirikcioglu M, Müller H, Myers PO, Kalangos A. Midterm results of valve repair with a biodegradable Annuloplasty ring for acute endocarditis. The Annals of Thoracic Surgery. 2010 Apr;**89**(4):1180-1185

[39] Thomas D, Desruennes M, Jault F, Isnard R, Gandjbakhch I. Cardiac and extracardiac abscesses in bacterial endocarditis. Archives des Maladies du Coeur et des Vaisseaux. 1993 Dec;**86**(12 Suppl):1825-1835

[40] Loire R. Cardiac lesions in bacterial endocarditis: From findings of pathology to possibilities and limits of surgery. Archives des Maladies du Coeur et des Vaisseaux. 1993 Dec;**86** (12 Suppl):1811-1818

[41] Hogevik H, Alestig K. Fungal endocarditis–a report on seven cases and a brief review. Infection. 1996 Feb;**24**(1):17-21

[42] Muehrcke DD, Lytle BW, Cosgrove DM. Surgical and long-term antifungal therapy for fungal prosthetic valve endocarditis. The Annals of Thoracic Surgery. 1995 Sep;**60**(3): 538-543

[43] Nasser RM, Melgar GR, Longworth DL, Gordon SM. Incidence and risk of developing fungal prosthetic valve endocarditis after nosocomial candidemia. The American Journal of Medicine. 1997 Jul;**103**(1):25-32

[44] Gammie JS, O'Brien SM, Griffith BP, Peterson ED. Surgical treatment of mitral valve endocarditis in North America. The Annals of Thoracic Surgery. 2005 Dec;**80**(6):2199-2204

[45] Livesey SA. Mitral valve reconstruction in the presence of infection. Heart. 2005 Oct 10; **92**(3):289-290

[46] Yamaguchi H, Eishi K, Yamachika S, Hisata Y, Tanigawa K, Izumi K, et al. Mitral valve repair in patients with infective endocarditis. Circulation Journal. 2006;**70**(2):179-183

[47] Feringa HHH, Shaw LJ, Poldermans D, Hoeks S, van der Wall EE, Dion RAE, et al. Mitral valve repair and replacement in endocarditis: A systematic review of literature. The Annals of Thoracic Surgery. 2007 Feb;**83**(2):564–570

[48] Feringa H, Bax J, Klein P, Klautz R, Braun J, Vanderwall E, et al. Outcome after mitral valve repair for acute and healed infective endocarditis. European Journal of Cardio-Thoracic Surgery. 2006 Mar;**29**(3):367-373

[49] Mihaljevic T, Paul S, Leacche M, Rawn JD, Aranki S, O'Gara PT, et al. Tailored surgical therapy for acute native mitral valve endocarditis. The Journal of Heart Valve Disease. 2004 Mar;**13**(2):210-216

[50] Doukas G. Mitral valve repair for active culture positive infective endocarditis. Heart. 2005 Oct 10;**92**(3):361-363

[51] Ruttmann E, Legit C, Poelzl G, Mueller S, Chevtchik O, Cottogni M, et al. Mitral valve repair provides improved outcome over replacement in active infective endocarditis. The Journal of Thoracic and Cardiovascular Surgery. 2005 Sep;**130**(3):765-771

[52] Bauernschmitt R, Jakob HG, Vahl C-F, Lange R, Hagl S. Operation for infective endocarditis: Results after implantation of mechanical valves. The Annals of Thoracic Surgery. 1998 Feb;**65**(2):359-364

[53] David TE, Bos J, Christakis GT, Brofman PR, Wong D, Feindel CM. Heart valve operations in patients with active infective endocarditis. The Annals of Thoracic Surgery. 1990 May;**49**(5):701-705 discussion 712–3

[54] d'Udekem Y, David TE, Feindel CM, Armstrong S, Sun Z. Long-term results of surgery for active infective endocarditis. European Journal of Cardio-Thoracic Surg Official Journal of European Association of Cardio-Thoracic Surgery. 1997 Jan;**11**(1):46-52

[55] Jault F, Gandjbakhch I, Rama A, Nectoux M, Bors V, Vaissier E, et al. Active native valve endocarditis: Determinants of operative death and late mortality. The Annals of Thoracic Surgery. 1997 Jun;**63**(6):1737-1741

[56] Larbalestier RI, Kinchla NM, Aranki SF, Couper GS, Collins JJ, Cohn LH. Acute bacterial endocarditis. Optimizing surgical results. Circulation. 1992 Nov;**86**(5 Suppl):II68-II74

[57] Middlemost S, Wisenbaugh T, Meyerowitz C, Teeger S, Essop R, Skoularigis J, et al. A case for early surgery in native left-sided endocarditis complicated by heart failure: Results in 203 patients. Journal of the American College of Cardiology. 1991 Sep;**18**(3):663-667

[58] Richardson JV, Karp RB, Kirklin JW, Dismukes WE. Treatment of infective endocarditis: A 10-year comparative analysis. Circulation. 1978 Oct 1;**58**(4):589-597

[59] Aranki SF, Adams DH, Rizzo RJ, Couper GS, Sullivan TE, Collins JJ, et al. Determinants of early mortality and late survival in mitral valve endocarditis. Circulation. 1995 Nov 1; **92**(9 Suppl):II143-II149

[60] Ting W, Silverman N, Levitsky S. Valve replacement in patients with endocarditis and cerebral septic emboli. The Annals of Thoracic Surgery. 1991 Jan;**51**(1):18-21 discussion 22

[61] Tleyjeh IM, Ghomrawi HMK, Steckelberg JM, Montori VM, Hoskin TL, Enders F, et al. Conclusion about the association between valve surgery and mortality in an infective endocarditis cohort changed after adjusting for survivor bias. Journal of Clinical Epidemiology. 2010 Feb;**63**(2):130-135

[62] Vikram HR, Buenconsejo J, Hasbun R, Quagliarello VJ. Impact of valve surgery on 6-month mortality in adults with complicated, left-sided native valve endocarditis: A propensity analysis. Journal of the American Medical Association. 2003 Dec;**290**(24, 24):3207

[63] Liang F, Song B, Liu R, Yang L, Tang H, Li Y. Optimal timing for early surgery in infective endocarditis: A meta-analysis. Interactive Cardiovascular and Thoracic Surgery. 2016 Mar; **22**(3):336-345

2

Ocular Manifestations of Endocarditis

Cheima Wathek and Riadh Rannen

Abstract

Endocarditis is an inflammation of the inside lining of the heart chambers and heart valves. Ocular manifestations are nonspecific and could reveal the disease, justifying routine ocular examination. *Staphylococcus aureus* is the most incriminated in ocular complications. Endophthalmitis, retinal arterial occlusion, Roth dots, or vitreal and retinal infiltrations could be seen with endocarditis. Ocular prognosis in endophthalmitis and retinal arterial occlusion is poor. Ocular involvement was independently associated with death in infective endocarditis.

Keywords: endocarditis, eye, endophthalmitis, retinal arterial occlusion

1. Introduction

Ocular manifestations of endocarditis are nonspecific, caused by septic embolism and in rare cases by aseptic embolism. Ocular manifestations could reveal this disease. Routine ophthalmic examination should be considered for patients with infective endocarditis.

2. Epidemiology

There are no data presenting the epidemiology of ocular manifestations of endocarditis. However, many case reports reveal that ocular manifestations are common and could be the first manifestation of the disease. Roth dots are the most commonly seen in endocarditis. Other findings are described in case reports and include focal retinitis, embolic retinopathy, subretinal abscesses, choroidal septic metastasis, choroiditis, endophthalmitis, papillitis, and optic neuritis [1].

3. Physiopathology

Infective endocarditis, especially when associated with prosthetic cardiac valves, carries a very high complication rate. Among the most dreaded complications are perivalvular abscesses, intracardiac fistulae, acute heart failure (typically from acute aortic insufficiency—a very poorly tolerated physiologic condition), complete heart block, septic emboli, and pseudoaneurysms. In fact, embolic events occur in as many as 50% of all patients with infectious endocarditis. Specific organs and/or systems involved, from most to least common, include (A) central nervous system, 65%; (B) spleen, 20%; (C) hepatic, 14%; (D) renal, 14%; (E) musculoskeletal, 11%; and (F) mesenteric, 3% [1, 2].

4. Microbiology

Streptococcus is seen in over 58% of cases of infectious endocarditis. The most common germs seen in endophthalmitis and chorioretinitis are *Staphylococcus aureus, Staphylococcus epidermidis*, and *Streptococcus viridians*. *S. aureus* can lead to ocular complications in over 56% [3, 4]. Fungal endocarditis affects intravenous drug users and severe immunodeficiency patients (onco-hematology) [5]. *Candida* is the most common seen in fungal endocarditis.

5. Ocular clinical findings

5.1. Roth dots

A Roth dot is a cluster of superficial retinal hemorrhages ovally shaped, with pale center (**Figure 1**). It is commonly seen near the optic disk.

In endocarditis, this cluster represents red blood cells which surround inflammatory cells that have collected in the area in response to a septic embolism from valvular vegetations [1].

5.2. Retinal arterial occlusion

Retinal arterial occlusion occurs as a complication of septic or aseptic embolism. Clinical manifestations depend on the localization of occlusion. We distinguish the following.

5.2.1. Central retinal arterial occlusion

Patient, if conscious, presents sudden, complete, and painless loss of vision in one eye. Fundoscopy shows pale edema of the retina, particularly in the posterior pole where the nerve fiber and ganglion cell layers are thickest. The orange reflex of the foveola with intact choroidal vasculature contrasts with the surrounding opaque neural retina, producing the cherry red spot. Central retinal arterial occlusion (CRAO) has a poor prognosis. If not treated in the first hour, it can lead to permanent loss of vision and other ocular complications [6].

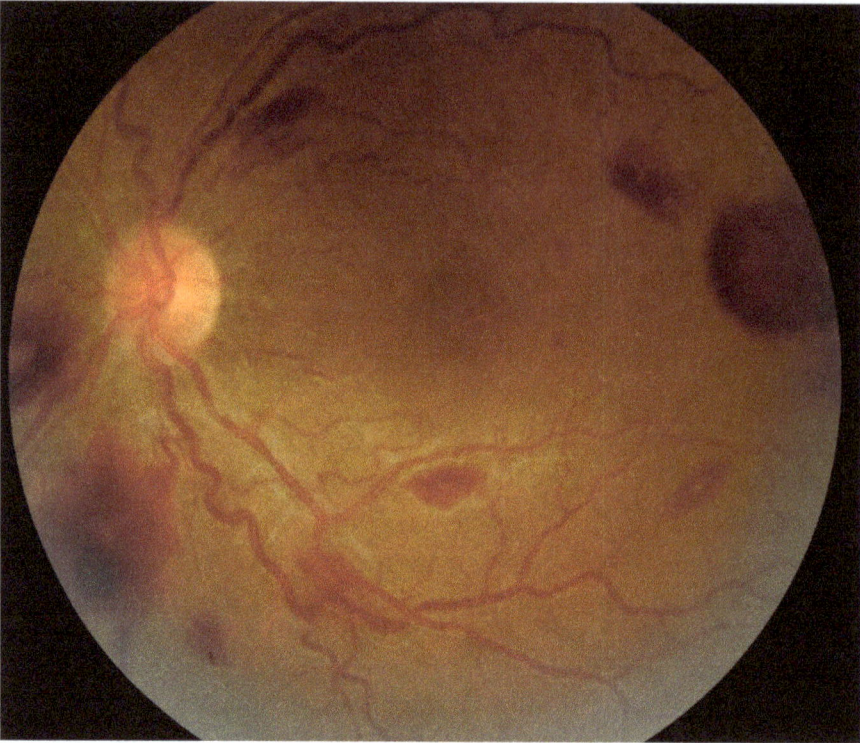

Figure 1. Fundoscopy of the left eye showing multiple Roth dots.

5.2.2. Branch retinal arterial occlusion

Branch retinal arterial occlusion (BRAO) may be clinically asymptomatic. If symptomatic, patient may report a loss of vision or visual field amputation. Fundoscopy shows a pale edema due to infarction of the inner retina in the distribution of the affected vessel. With time, the occluded vessel recanalizes, perfusion returns, and the edema resolves; however, a permanent field defect remains.

5.2.3. Ophthalmic arterial occlusion

This event is responsible for an interruption of both retinal and posterior ciliary circulations. The visual prognosis, in this entity, is usually worse. If conscious, patient presents pain, sudden and complete loss of vision. Ophthalmic examination revealed no light perception, ophthal-moplegia (**Figure 2**), and nonreactive mydriasis. Fundoscopy showed remarkable edema of the entire retina, resulting from inner and outer retinal ischemia and whitened retinal vessels (**Figure 3**). The cherry-red spot is not noted in this case because of choroidal compromise and probable retinal pigment epithelial or choroidal opacification, or both, in about 40% of eyes. Fluorescein angiography revealed impairment of retinal vascular and choroidal flows (**Figure 4**). A cherry-red spot may be initially absent, but then appear over a several-day period as choroid perfusion improves [7].

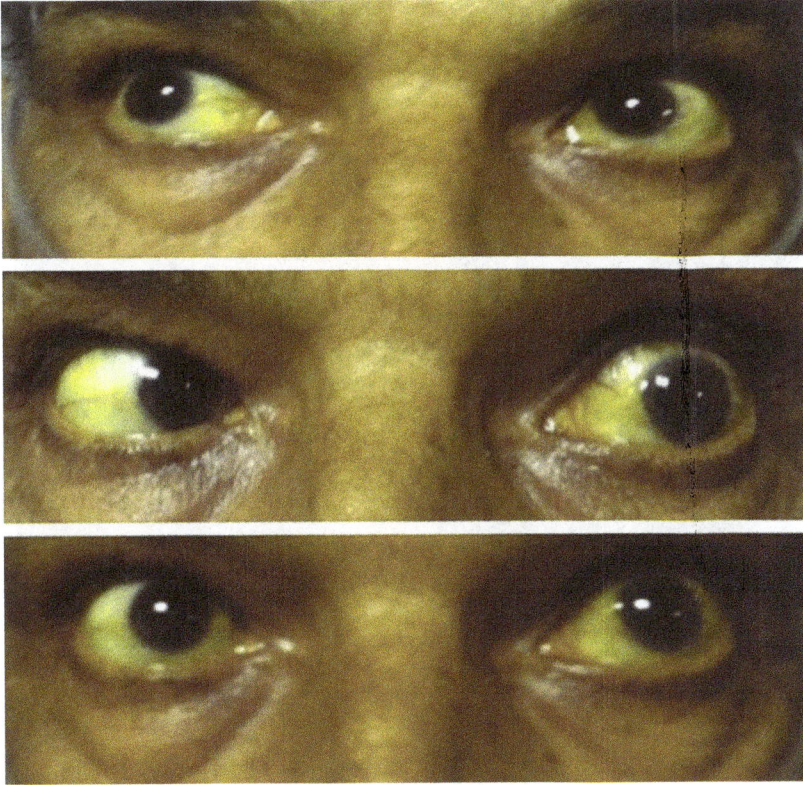

Figure 2. Ophthalmoplegia of the left eye.

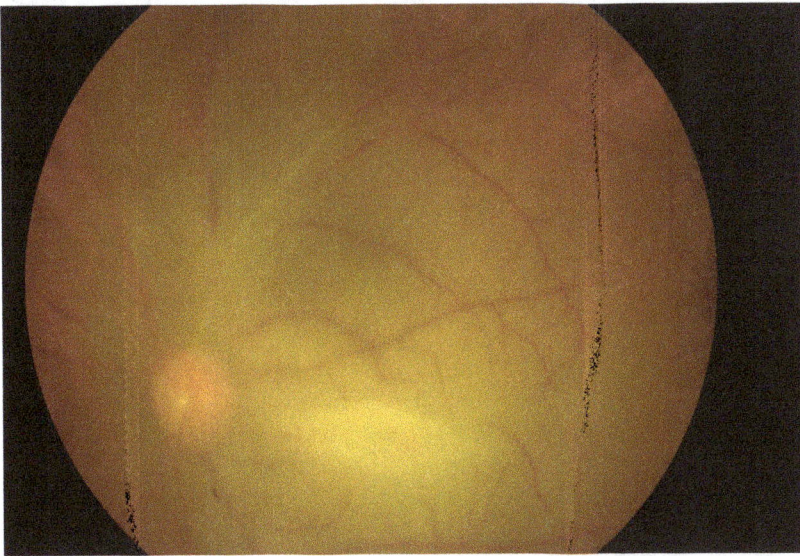

Figure 3. Fundus photograph showing edema of the entire left retina and whitened retinal vessels without cherry-red spot.

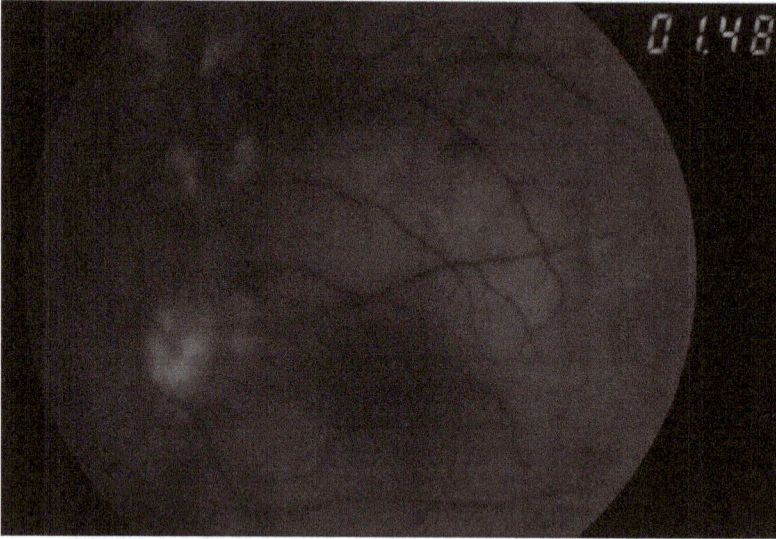

Figure 4. Fluorescein angiography showing late onset of choroidal perfusion and nonopacification of both retinal artery and vein.

5.3. Retinal and vitreal infiltration

Septic embolism can lead to posterior uveitis (retinitis, chorioretinitis, choroiditis, and vitreal infiltration). In most cases, posterior uveitis is misdiagnosed and is complicated by endophthalmitis (**Figure 5**).

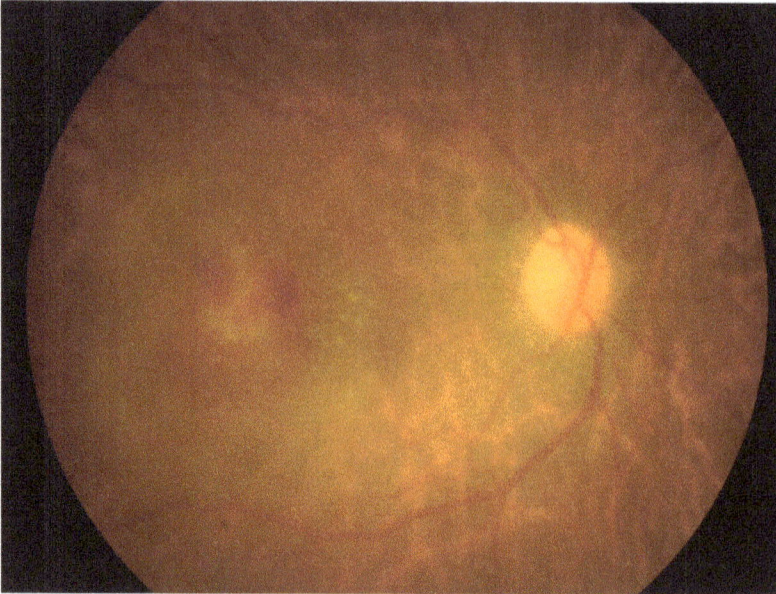

Figure 5. Fundoscopy showing retinal and vitreous infiltrations in bacterial endocarditis.

5.4. Endophthalmitis

Endophthalmitis is a condition when all the internal structures of the eye are invaded with replicating microorganisms and associated with an important inflammatory response.

Endogenous bacterial endophthalmitis is a rare pathology that affects individuals of any age and represents 2–15% of all cases. Endocarditis is the second more frequent cause of endogenous endophthalmitis after meningitis.

The rate of endophthalmitis can raise 50% with endocarditis to *S. aureus*. The right eye is generally more affected than the left eye.

The onset of the signs and symptoms depends on the pathogenic virulence. Typically, patient presents pain, chemosis, proptosis, hypopyon, and corneal melting.

Blood culture findings are positive in more than 90% of infective endocarditis cases. The most common etiological germ is *Streptococcus* 45.7% and the valvular was affected in 27.2% of the episodes. Systemic therapy may be sufficient when the vitreous cavity is not greatly involved. In the other cases, antibiotic intravitreal injections and vitrectomy are necessary [5, 8–11].

5.5. Choroidal neovascularization

Subretinal neovascularization secondary to choroidal septic metastasis was reported in two cases. Neovascularization occurs in choroidal scars with variable delay (10 months and 5 years) [12].

6. Prognosis

Ocular prognosis depends on the ocular manifestation. Functional prognosis of retinal arterial occlusion and endophthalmitis is bad in most cases. Ocular involvement was independently associated with death in infective endocarditis.

Author details

Cheima Wathek* and Riadh Rannen

*Address all correspondence to: wcheima@yahoo.fr

Military Hospital of Tunis, Ophthalmology Department, Faculty of Medicine of Tunis, Tunis El Manar University, Tunis, Tunisia

References

[1] Klig JE. Ophthalmologic complications of systemic disease. Emerg Med Clin N Am 2008;26:217–31.

[2] Gergaud JM, Breux JP, Grollier G, Roblot P, Becq-Giraudon B. Current aspects of infectious endocarditis: apropos of 53 cases. Ann Med Interne 1994;145(3): 163–7.

[3] Mainardi L. Bactériologie. Masson 2ème Edition 2011:117–18.

[4] Jung J, Lee J, Yu SN, Kim YK, Lee JY, Sung H et al. Incidence and risk factors of ocular infection caused by *Staphylococcus aureus* bacteremia. Antimicrob Agents Chemother 2016;60(4):2012–7.

[5] Silva-Vergara ML, de Camargo ZP, Silva PF, Abdalla MR, Sgarbieri RN, et al. Case report: disseminated *Sporothrix brasiliensis* infection with endocardial and ocular involvement in an HIV-infected patient. Am J Trop Med Hyg 2012;86(3):477–80.

[6] Liliana M, Pitta ML, Peresa M, Ferreirab V, Pugab MC, Severinoa D, da Silva GF. Retinal artery embolization complicating Libman-Sacks endocarditis in a systemic lupus erythematosus patient. Rev Port Cardiol 2013;32(4):345–7.

[7] Wathek C, Kharrat O, Maalej A, Nafaa MF, Rannen R, Gabsi S. Ophthalmic artery occlusion as a complication of infectious endocarditis. J Fr Ophthalmol 2014;37(10):e161–3.

[8] Zayit-Soudry S, Neudorfer M, Barak A, et al. Endogenous *Phialemonium curvatum* endophthalmitis. Am J Ophthalmol 2005;140(4):755–7.

[9] Arcieri ES, Jorge EF, de Abrea Ferreira L, et al. Bilateral endogenous endophthalmitis associated with infective endocarditis: case report. Braz J Infect Dis 2001;5(6):356–9.

[10] Shmuely H, Kremer I, Sagie A, et al. Candida tropicalis multifocal endophthalmitis as the only initial manifestation of pacemaker endocarditis. Am J Ophthalmol 1997;123(4): 559–60.

[11] Verweij PE, Rademakers AJ, Koopmans PP, et al. Endophthalmitis as presenting symptoms of group G streptococcal endocarditis. Infection 1994;22(1):56–7.

[12] Munier F, Othenin-Girard P. Subretinal neovascularization secondary to choroidal septic metastasis from acute bacterial endocarditis. Retina 1992;12:108–12.

3

Surgical Treatment for Tricuspid Valve Infective Endocarditis

Takashi Murashita

Abstract

Isolated tricuspid valve infective endocarditis is relatively rare. However, the frequency of tricuspid valve infective endocarditis in the United States is rapidly increasing, mainly due to the epidemic of intravenous drug use. A medical treatment is the first choice for this disease; however, surgical intervention is required when the patients suffer from heart failure, large vegetation, or persistent bacteremia despite appropriate medical treatment. Several techniques for tricuspid valve reconstruction have been proposed, and their outcomes have been reported to be good. However, in the cases of severe valve destruction, tricuspid valve replacement is required. Post-surgical management of drug-induced infective endocarditis is challenging due to its poor compliance to medication and high rate of reinfection. There is an ethical controversy as to surgical indication for reinfection induced by relapse of drug use. In addition, because reoperation for tricuspid valve carries high risk, there is also a controversy regarding valve choice in drug users.

Keywords: tricuspid valve infective endocarditis, intravenous drug use, surgical outcomes

1. Introduction

Infective endocarditis carries high mortality and mortality. Murdoch et al. studied 2781 adults with definite infective endocarditis admitted to 58 hospitals in 25 countries [1]. They reported that surgical treatment was performed in 48%, and in-hospital mortality was 18%. Nevertheless, surgery during the current endocarditis episode was associated with decreased risk of in-hospital death (odds ratio, 0.56; 95% confidence interval, 0.44-0.69).

Tricuspid valve infective endocarditis was relatively rare and accounted for 5 to 10% of all infective endocarditis [2]. In the study of Murdoch et al. which was reported in 2009 [1], tricuspid valve infective endocarditis was found in 12% of the entire cohort. However, the frequency of tricuspid valve infective endocarditis is rapidly increasing along with the epidemic of intravenous drug use. Seratnahaei et al. reported that the incidence of tricuspid valve infective endocarditis was 6% between 1999 and 2000, and it markedly increased to 36% between 2009 and 2010 [3]. Also reported history of intravenous drug use increased from 15 to 40%.

2. Surgery for tricuspid valve infective endocarditis

2.1. Epidemiology

The key predisposing factors for tricuspid valve infective endocarditis include intravenous drug use, cardiac implantable electronic devices, long-term central venous access catheters, and congenital heart disease [4].

In the study of Murdoch et al. [1], current intravenous drug use was found in 16% of the cohort of North America, chronic intravenous access accounted was found in 25%, implantable cardiac devices accounted was found in 12%, and congenital heart disease accounted was found in 25%.

Moss et al. reported that 41% of injection drug users with bacteremia had the evidence of endocarditis [5].

Athan et al. performed a prospective cohort study which described a 6.4% incidence of cardiac device-related infective endocarditis among 2760 patients [6]. There was coexisting valve involvement in 37.3% patients and predominantly tricuspid valve infection (24.3%). Concomitant valve infection was associated with higher mortality than no valve infection (odds ratio, 3.31; 95% confidence interval, 1.71–6.39).

2.2. Indications for surgery

The most recent guidelines from the American Heart Association stated that the surgical intervention is reasonable for patients with certain complications with class IIa recommendations, and they also stated that it is reasonable to avoid surgery when possible in patients who are intravenous drug users [7]. The 2015 European Society of Cardiology guidelines for the management of infective endocarditis stated that surgery should be considered in the following situations with class IIa recommendations: [1] right heart failure secondary to severe tricuspid regurgitation with poor response to diuretic therapy, [2] infective endocarditis caused by organisms that are difficult to eradicate (e.g. persistent fungi) or bacteremia for at least 7 days despite adequate antimicrobial therapy, and [3] tricuspid valve vegetations >20 mm that persist after recurrent pulmonary emboli with or without concomitant right heart failure [8].

Hecht et al. followed the clinical course of 121 patients with right-sided infective endocarditis caused by intravenous drug use, and reported that vegetations greater than 20 mm were associated with increased mortality [9].

Kiefer et al. performed a prospective, multicenter study enrolling over 4000 patients with infective endocarditis and known heart failure status [10]. In-hospital mortality was lower in the patients undergoing valvular surgery compared with medical therapy alone (20.6 vs. 44.8%, p < 0.001), and 1-year mortality was also lower in patients undergoing surgery compared with medical therapy alone (29.1 vs. 58.4%, p < 0.001).

2.3. Timing of surgery

The early surgical intervention for left-sided infective endocarditis has been well suggested [7, 11, 12]; however, the surgical indications for right-sided infective endocarditis are not well defined.

Akinosoglou et al. suggested that the timing of surgical management depends on the following factors: [1] cause of endocarditis (e.g. urgent in pacemaker and prosthetic infective endocarditis), [2] causative infective factors (e.g. fungal and *Staphylococcus aureus*), [3] coexistent left-sided infection, [4] response to antibiotic therapy, [5] toxicity of medical treatment, and [6] complications of disease (e.g. abscess and increased vegetation size) [13].

Early surgery should be considered if the causative organism is *Staphylococcus aureus*, which often results in large vegetations, massive valve destruction, and embolic manifestations [14]. Remadi et al. reported that early surgery was associated with reduced mortality in *Staphylococcus aureus* infective endocarditis [15].

Taghavi et al. compared the outcomes between surgical management and medical treatment for tricuspid valve endocarditis [16]. They found that patients treated surgically had clear blood cultures sooner, defervesced earlier, and demonstrated a complete resolution of vegetations. They concluded that the early surgery is warranted for patients with tricuspid valve endocarditis when they are bacteremia and/or systemically infected despite optimal medical treatment.

In contrast, Gaca et al. reviewed the surgical outcomes for isolated tricuspid valve endocarditis using the Society of Thoracic Surgeons Database, and reported that patients in the healed tricuspid valve endocarditis had lower complications rates, shorter overall length of stay, and a trend toward lower operative mortality compared with active endocarditis [17].

2.4. Tricuspid valve reconstruction

Akinosoglou et al. suggested that, in intravenous drug users who run a high risk of complications, vegetectomy and valve repair, avoiding artificial materials should be considered as that can improve late survival rate [13].

Successful surgical intervention requires radical debridement of infected tissue first [4]. In case of leaflet perforation or small defects localized to one or two leaflets can be repaired by either direct closure or patch plasty using an autologous pericardial patch [18] (**Figure 1**).

In case of limited infection on the posterior leaflet, bicuspid valve formation of the tricuspid valve can be performed by excising the posterior leaflet and mobilizing the anterior and septal leaflets [18] (**Figure 2**). Ghanta et al. reported good mid-term outcomes of suture bicuspidization of the tricuspid valve [19].

Artificial chordae using expanded polytetrafluoroethylene sutures can be applied after the resection of infected chordae [20].

Tricuspid annuloplasty is performed either with prosthetic rings or with non-prosthetic suture annuloplasty such as Kay's or De Vega's annuloplasty [13]. Although suture annuloplasty has an advantage of avoiding prosthetic materials in the setting of infection, several studies

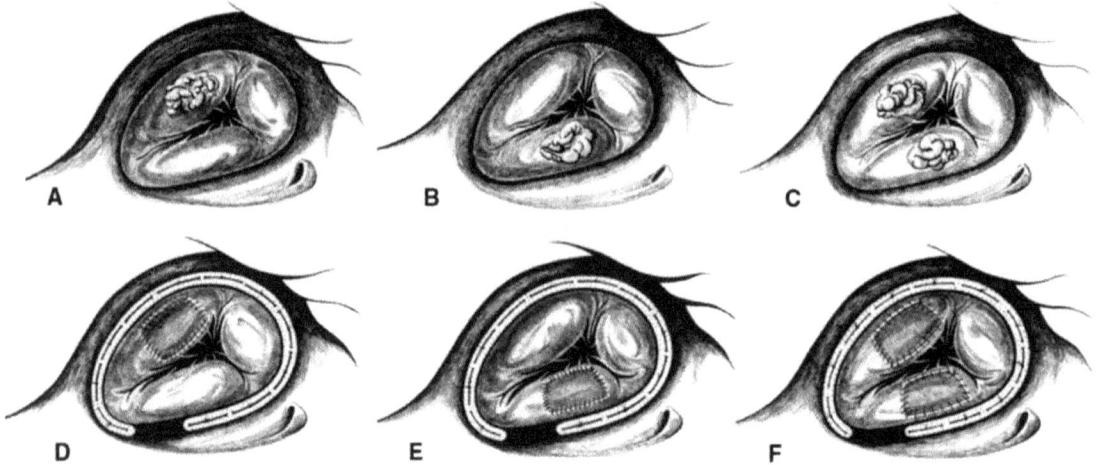

Figure 1. Endocarditic lesion on the anterior leaflet (A), the posterior leaflet (B), or on both (C), anterior and septal leaflet (D–F) after the excision of the endocarditic lesion, patch plasty, and stabilization of the valve with a tricuspid annuloplasty ring.

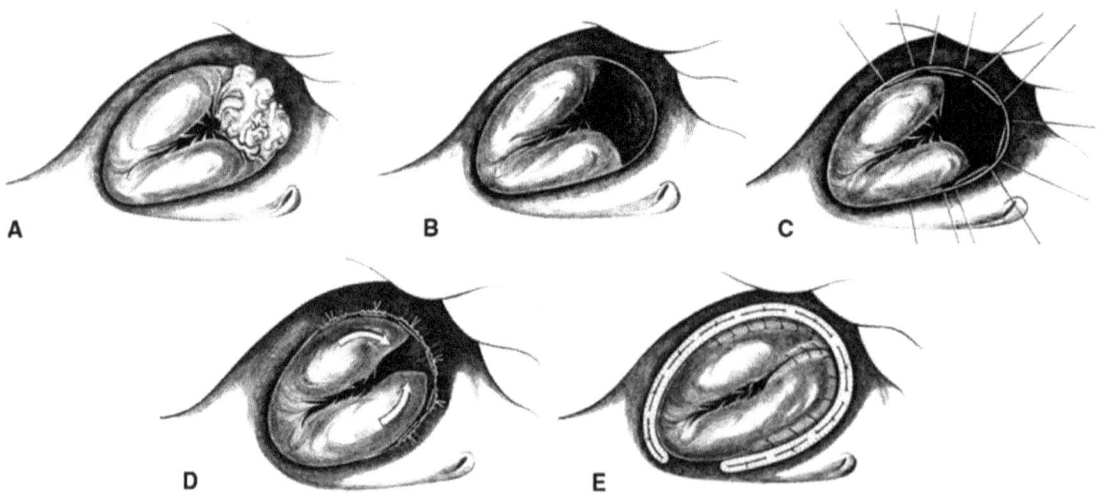

Figure 2. (A) Endocarditic lesion on the posterior leaflet. (B) Excision of the posterior leaflet. (C) Partial mobilization of the anterior and septal leaflet and preparation of plication sutures. (D) Bicuspid leaflet formation of the valve. (E) Stabilization of the valve with a tricuspid annuloplasty ring.

showed that the ring annuloplasty is superior to suture annuloplasty in terms of recurrent tricuspid regurgitation or reoperation [21–24].

2.5. Tricuspid valve replacement

In case of severe valve destruction, valve replacement is performed using either a mechanical valve or tissue valve.

Cho et al. compared surgical outcomes of mechanical tricuspid valve replacement (n = 59) and tissue tricuspid valve replacement (n = 45), and found that there was no difference in long-term valve-related complications such as thromboembolic or bleeding events [25].

Hwang et al. also reported that there was no difference in long-term survival, cardiac death rates, and thromboembolic and bleeding complication rates between mechanical and tissue tricuspid valve replacements [26].

Liu et al. performed a meta-analysis to review the results of mechanical and bioprosthetic valves in the tricuspid valve position [27]. They did not find difference in survival, reoperation, or prosthetic valve failure between two valve types.

2.6. Surgical outcomes for tricuspid valve infective endocarditis

The surgical outcomes for tricuspid valve infective endocarditis are listed in **Table 1**. Overall good surgical outcomes were reported, and the durability of tricuspid valve reconstruction was good.

Study	Year	Number of pts	Surgical technique	Mortality (%)	Recurrence of regurgitation	Recurrence of infection
Musci et al. [28]	2007	51	31 reconstructions, 17 tissue TVR, 3 mechanical TVR	11.3% for reconstruction, 12.5% for TVR	—	2 patients had reoperation due to reinfection after the tricuspid reconstruction.
Gottardi et al. [18]	2007	22	18 reconstructions, 3 tissue TVR, 1 mechanical TVR	0	3 patients had grade 1–2 TR	2 patients had recurrent endocarditis, which were treated conservatively.
Baraki et al. [29]	2013	33	15 reconstructions,14 tissue TVR, 4 mechanical TVR	9	2 patients had grade > 2 TR	3 patients underwent reoperation for recurrent endocarditis
Gaca et al. [17]	2013	910	354 reconstructions, 66 valvectomies, 490 TVR	7.6% for reconstruction, 12.1% for valvectomy, 6.3% for TVR	—	—

TVR, tricuspid valve replacement; TR, tricuspid regurgitation.

Table 1. Surgical outcomes for tricuspid valve endocarditis.

Musci et al. reported a 20-year single institution surgical experience for right-sided infective endocarditis [28]. They performed 31 tricuspid valve reconstructions and 20 valve replacements. The 30-day, 1-, 5-, 10- and 20-year survival rate after the operation was 96.2, 88.4, 73.5, 70.4 and 70.4%, respectively, for isolated right-sided infective endocarditis. The survival rate was significantly better than the patients with combined right- and left-sided infective endocarditis. Survival was not different between valve reconstruction and replacement.

Gottardi et al. performed 18 tricuspid valve repair and 4 tricuspid valve replacements for active infective endocarditis, and there was no mortality [18]. During the follow-up, three patients presented with grade 1–2 tricuspid valve regurgitation after the valve reconstruction.

Baraki et al. reviewed 33 tricuspid valve surgeries for endocarditis, which included 14 tissue valve replacements, 4 mechanical valve replacements, and 15 tricuspid valve repairs [29]. Thirty-day mortality was 9%, and advanced age, EuroSCORE, and *Staphylococcus aureus* were associated with a less long-term survival rate. Residual tricuspid valve regurgitation grade ≥2 was found in two patients.

2.7. Intravenous drug user

Intravenous drug abuse is increasing dramatically in the United States [30]. Of many medical complications caused by drug use, infective endocarditis is one of the most challenging issues given the significant risk of acute mortality as well as late recidivism, reinfection, and poor social situations.

The infection caused by the drug use can be found both on right- and left-sided heart or even on both sides. Even though the prognosis of right-sided infective endocarditis is better than left-sided, surgery may be required in at least 25% of patients [31].

The surgical outcomes for drug-induced endocarditis are summarized in **Table 2**. Overall, the short-term and long-term survival was not different between drug users and non-drug users; however, the rates of late reinfection and reoperation are higher in drug users.

The choice of valve prosthesis for intravenous drug users is controversial [32]. Rabkin et al. reported that the median survival of intravenous drug users was only 3 years, and therefore tissue valves are justified even for young patients [33]. Kaiser et al. used tissue valves more frequently in drug users than non-drug users (75 vs. 52%), even though drug users were younger [34].

In the meantime, several previous studies showed that the postoperative survival rate of drug users is similar to non-drug users [34–37]. That may imply that intravenous drug users receiving tissue valves will live long enough to require a reoperation for valve degeneration. Given the fact that the redo surgery for tricuspid valve carries high risk [38], the use of mechanical valve may be justified for selected patients who can be compliant with anticoagulation. Mechanical tricuspid valves have a risk of thrombosis with an incidence of ≤3.3% of patient-years [39].

2.8. Reinfection after surgery

Patients with intravenous drug use are high risk of reinfection. The surgical outcomes for redo tricuspid valve surgery have been reported to be poor.

Study	Year	Number of pts	Hospital	Findings
Shrestha et al. [35]	2015	536; 41 (8%) were drug users	Cleveland clinic	Short-term mortality was not different between drug users and non-drug users; however, a hazard of death or reoperation between 3 and 6 months after the operation was 10 times higher in drug users compared with non-users.
Kim et al. [36]	2016	436; 78 (17.9%) were drug users	Massachusetts General Hospital and Brigham and Women's Hospital	Operative mortality was lower among drug users; however, overall mortality was not different. Drug users had higher risk of valve-related complications principally because of higher rates of reinfection.
Rabkin et al. [33]	2012	197; 64 (32.5%) were drug users	University of Washington Medical Center	Survival was lower in drug users than non-drug users (at 30 days, 1 year, 5 years, and 10 years; 91.2 vs. 93.6%, 77.5 vs. 83.0%, 46.7 vs. 71.1%, and 41.1 vs. 52.0%, respectively, p = 0.027). Intravenous drug use was an independent risk factor for diminished survival (p = 0.03). 8 of 64 (12.5%) of drug users experienced recurrent infective endocarditis.
Kaiser et al. [34]	2007	346; 62 (17.9%) were drug users	Washington University	Long-term survival and perioperative complications were not different between drug users and non-drug users; however, reoperation for recurrent infection was higher in drug users (17 vs. 5%, p = 0.03).
Carozza et al. [37]	2006	39 drug-induced infective endocarditis and 85 non-drug-induced infective endocarditis	Second University of Naples	Although hospital and long-term survival did not significantly differ between two groups, the rate of recurrence of infection was higher in drug users.

Table 2. Surgical outcomes for drug-induced infective endocarditis.

Jeganathan et al. reviewed 68 patients who had previous history of tricuspid valve surgery and underwent reoperations on the tricuspid valve, and in-hospital mortality was 13.2% [38]. They also reported high incidence of postoperative bleeding, low cardiac output syndrome, stroke, and renal failure.

Musci et al. reported that 6 out of 79 patients underwent reoperation due to reinfection after the correction of right-sided active infective endocarditis, and only 1 of them (16.7%) survived the reoperation [28].

The prognosis of prosthetic valve infection without surgical intervention is dismal. Ivert et al. reported that 64% of the patients with prosthetic valve endocarditis died, and most deaths occurred within 3 months of the first evidence of infection [40]. Nevertheless, the surgical treatment for prosthetic valve endocarditis is also challenging [41].

Luciani et al. performed multicentre study for surgical outcomes for prosthetic valve endocarditis [42]. Among 209 patients who underwent surgery for prosthetic valve endocarditis, the in-hospital mortality was high (21.5%). Grubitzsch et al. reviewed 149 patients who underwent redo surgery for prosthetic valve endocarditis [43]. The operative mortality was 12.8%.

In the setting of high risk of surgical treatment for reinfection, a dilemma exists regarding the surgical indication for patients who are non-compliant to medical treatment, and develop reinfection due to relapsing of drug use [44]. There is a controversy as how many chances surgeons should give to non-compliant patients.

Hull et al. proposed that the patients who have a history of intravenous drug use should be encouraged to sign a contract agreeing to undergo drug rehabilitation and make a good faith effort to abstain from substance abuse in the future [45].

3. Conclusions

The incidence of tricuspid valve infective endocarditis is increasing along with the epidemic of intravenous drug use. Surgical treatment would be necessary when the patients suffer from heart failure, large vegetation, and persistent bacteremia despite appropriate antibiotic therapy. Tricuspid valve reconstruction is desirable as artificial material can be avoided; however, in cases of severe valve destruction, tricuspid valve replacement is warranted. Management of patients with intravenous drug users is challenging due to late recidivism, reinfection, and poor social situations. The operation for reinfection carries high risk. There is an ethical controversy regarding the surgical indication for reinfection induced by relapse of drug use. Surgeons can play a role by bringing the problem of epidemic of drug use to public consciousness.

Author details

Takashi Murashita

Address all correspondence to: tmurashita@gmail.com

Heart and Vascular Institute, West Virginia University, Morgantown, WV, USA

References

[1] Murdoch DR, Corey GR, Hoen B, Miró JM, Fowler VG Jr, Bayer AS, Karchmer AW, Olaison L, Pappas PA, Moreillon P, Chambers ST, Chu VH, Falcó V, Holland DJ, Jones P, Klein JL, Raymond NJ, Read KM, Tripodi MF, Utili R, Wang A, Woods CW, Cabell CH. International collaboration on endocarditis-prospective cohort study (ICE-PCS) investigators. Clinical presentation, etiology, and outcome of infective endocarditis in the 21st century: The international collaboration on endocarditis-prospective cohort study. Archives of Internal Medicine. 2009;**169**:463-473. DOI: 10.1001/archinternmed.2008.603

[2] Chan P, Ogilby JD, Segal B. Tricuspid valve endocarditis. American Heart Journal. 1989;**117**:1140-1146

[3] Seratnahaei A, Leung SW, Charnigo RJ, Cummings MS, Sorrell VL, Smith MD. The changing 'face' of endocarditis in Kentucky: An increase in tricuspid cases. American Journal of Medicine. 2014;**127, 04**:786.e1, 009-786.e6. DOI: 10.1016/j.amjmed.2014

[4] Yong MS, Coffey S, Prendergast BD, Marasco SF, Zimmet AD, McGiffin DC, Saxena P. Surgical management of tricuspid valve endocarditis in the current era: A review. International Journal of Cardiology. 2016;**202**:44-48. DOI: 10.1016/j.ijcard.2015.08.211

[5] Moss R, Munt B. Injection drug use and right sided endocarditis. Heart. 2003;**89**:577-581

[6] Athan E, Chu VH, Tattevin P, Selton-Suty C, Jones P, Naber C, Miró JM, Ninot S, Fernández-Hidalgo N, Durante-Mangoni E, Spelman D, Hoen B, Lejko-Zupanc T, Cecchi E, Thuny F, Hannan MM, Pappas P, Henry M, Fowler VG Jr, Crowley AL, Wang A. ICE-PCS investigators. Clinical characteristics and outcome of infective endocarditis involving implantable cardiac devices. JAMA. 2012;**307**:1727-1735. DOI: 10.1001/jama.2012.497

[7] Baddour LM, Wilson WR, Bayer AS, Fowler VG Jr, Tleyjeh IM, Rybak MJ, Barsic B, Lockhart PB, Gewitz MH, Levison ME, Bolger AF, Steckelberg JM, Baltimore RS, Fink AM, O'Gara P, Taubert KA. American Heart Association Committee on rheumatic fever, endocarditis, and Kawasaki disease of the council on cardiovascular disease in the young, council on clinical cardiology, council on cardiovascular surgery and anesthesia, and stroke council. Infective endocarditis in adults: Diagnosis, antimicrobial therapy, and Management of Complications: A scientific statement for healthcare professionals from the American Heart Association. Circulation. 2015;**132**:1435-1486. DOI: 10.1161/CIR. 0000000000000296

[8] Habib G, Lancellotti P, Antunes MJ, Bongiorni MG, Casalta JP, Del Zotti F, Dulgheru R, El Khoury G, Erba PA, Iung B, Miro JM, Mulder BJ, Plonska-Gosciniak E, Price S, Roos-Hesselink J, Snygg-Martin U, Thuny F, Tornos Mas P, Vilacosta I, Zamorano JL. ESC guidelines for the management of infective endocarditis: The task force for the management of infective endocarditis of the European Society of Cardiology (ESC). Endorsed by: European Association for Cardio-Thoracic Surgery (EACTS), the European Association of Nuclear Medicine (EANM). European Heart Journal. 2015;**36**:3075-3128. DOI: 10.1093/eurhe artj/ehv319

[9] Hecht SR, Berger M. Right-sided endocarditis in intravenous drug users. Prognostic features in 102 episodes. Annals of Internal Medicine. 1992;**117**:560-566

[10] Kiefer T, Park L, Tribouilloy C, Cortes C, Casillo R, Chu V, Delahaye F, Durante-Mangoni E, Edathodu J, Falces C, Logar M, Miró JM, Naber C, Tripodi MF, Murdoch DR, Moreillon P, Utili R, Wang A. Association between valvular surgery and mortality among patients with infective endocarditis complicated by heart failure. JAMA. 2011;**306**:2239-2247. DOI: 10.1001/jama.2011.1701

[11] Ghoreishi M, Foster N, Pasrija C, Shah A, Watkins AC, Evans CF, Maghami S, Quinn R, Wehman B, Taylor BS, Dawood MY, Griffith BP, Gammie JS. Early operation in patients with mitral valve infective endocarditis and acute stroke is safe. The Annals of Thoracic Surgery. 2018;**105**:69-75. DOI: 10.1016/j.athoracsur.2017.06.069

[12] Kang DH, Kim YJ, Kim SH, Sun BJ, Kim DH, Yun SC, Song JM, Choo SJ, Chung CH, Song JK, Lee JW, Sohn DW. Early surgery versus conventional treatment for infective endocarditis. The New England Journal of Medicine. 2012;**366**:2466-2473. DOI: 10.1056/NEJMoa1112843

[13] Akinosoglou K, Apostolakis E, Koutsogiannis N, Leivaditis V, Gogos CA. Right-sided infective endocarditis: Surgical management. European Journal of Cardio-Thoracic Surgery. 2012;**42**:470-479. DOI: 10.1093/ejcts/ezs084

[14] Lowes JA, Hamer J, Williams G, Houang E, Tabaqchali S, Shaw EJ, Hill IM, Rees GM. 10 years of infective endocarditis at St. Bartholomew's hospital: Analysis of clinical features and treatment in relation to prognosis and mortality. Lancet. 1980;**1**:133-136

[15] Remadi JP, Habib G, Nadji G, Brahim A, Thuny F, Casalta JP, Peltier M, Tribouilloy C. Predictors of death and impact of surgery in *Staphylococcus aureus* infective endocarditis. The Annals of Thoracic Surgery. 2007;**83**:1295-1302

[16] Taghavi S, Clark R, Jayarajan SN, Gaughan J, Brann SH, Mangi AA. Surgical management of tricuspid valve endocarditis in systemically infected patients. The Journal of Heart Valve Disease. 2013;**22**:578-583

[17] Gaca JG, Sheng S, Daneshmand M, Rankin JS, Williams ML, O'Brien SM, Gammie JS. Current outcomes for tricuspid valve infective endocarditis surgery in North America. The Annals of Thoracic Surgery. 2013;**96**:1374-1381. DOI: 10.1016/j.athoracsur.2013.05.046

[18] Gottardi R, Bialy J, Devyatko E, Tschernich H, Czerny M, Wolner E, Seitelberger R. Midterm follow-up of tricuspid valve reconstruction due to active infective endocarditis. The Annals of Thoracic Surgery. 2007;**84**:1943-1948

[19] Ghanta RK, Chen R, Narayanasamy N, McGurk S, Lipsitz S, Chen F, Cohn LH. Suture bicuspidization of the tricuspid valve versus ring annuloplasty for repair of functional tricuspid regurgitation: Midterm results of 237 consecutive patients. The Journal of Thoracic and Cardiovascular Surgery. 2007;**133**:117-126

[20] Morokuma H, Minato N, Kamohara K, Minematsu N. Three surgical cases of isolated tricuspid valve infective endocarditis. Annals of Thoracic and Cardiovascular Surgery. 2010;**16**:134-138

[21] Matsuyama K, Matsumoto M, Sugita T, Nishizawa J, Tokuda Y, Matsuo T, Ueda Y. De Vega annuloplasty and Carpentier-Edwards ring annuloplasty for secondary tricuspid regurgitation. The Journal of Heart Valve Disease. 2001;**10**:520-524

[22] McCarthy PM, Bhudia SK, Rajeswaran J, Hoercher KJ, Lytle BW, Cosgrove DM, Blackstone EH. Tricuspid valve repair: Durability and risk factors for failure. The Journal of Thoracic and Cardiovascular Surgery. 2004;**127**:674-685

[23] Murashita T, Okada Y, Kanemitsu H, Fukunaga N, Konishi Y, Nakamura K, Koyama T. Long-term outcomes of tricuspid annuloplasty for functional tricuspid regurgitation associated with degenerative mitral regurgitation: Suture annuloplasty versus ring annuloplasty using a flexible band. Annals of Thoracic and Cardiovascular Surgery. 2014;**20**:1026-1033. DOI: 10.5761/atcs.oa.13-00292

[24] Hata H, Fujita T, Miura S, Shimahara Y, Kume Y, Matsumoto Y, Yamashita K, Kobayashi J. Long-term outcomes of suture vs. ring tricuspid annuloplasty for functional tricuspid regurgitation. Circulation Journal. 2017;81:1432-1438. DOI: 10.1253/circj.CJ-17-0108

[25] Cho WC, Park CB, Kim JB, Jung SH, Chung CH, Choo SJ, Lee JW. Mechanical valve replacement versus bioprosthetic valve replacement in the tricuspid valve position. Journal of Cardiac Surgery. 2013;28:212-217. DOI: 10.1111/jocs.12093

[26] Hwang HY, Kim KH, Kim KB, Ahn H. Propensity score matching analysis of mechanical versus bioprosthetic tricuspid valve replacements. The Annals of Thoracic Surgery. 2014;97:1294-1299. DOI: 10.1016/j.athoracsur.2013.12.033

[27] Liu P, Qiao WH, Sun FQ, Ruan XL, Al Shirbini M, Hu D, Chen S, Dong NG. Should a mechanical or biological prosthesis be used for a tricuspid valve replacement? A meta-analysis. Journal of Cardiac Surgery. 2016;31:294-302. DOI: 10.1111/jocs.12730

[28] Musci M, Siniawski H, Pasic M, Grauhan O, Weng Y, Meyer R, Yankah CA, Hetzer R. Surgical treatment of right-sided active infective endocarditis with or without involvement of the left heart: 20-year single center experience. European Journal of Cardio-Thoracic Surgery. 2007;32:118-125

[29] Baraki H, Saito S, Al Ahmad A, Fleischer B, Schmitto J, Haverich A, Kutschka I. Surgical treatment for isolated tricuspid valve endocarditis- long-term follow-up at a single institution. Circulation Journal. 2013;77:2032-2037

[30] Ferraris VA, Sekela ME. Missing the forest for the trees: The world around us and surgical treatment of endocarditis. The Journal of Thoracic and Cardiovascular Surgery. 2016;152:677-680. DOI: 10.1016/j.jtcvs.2016.05.014

[31] Gould FK, Denning DW, Elliott TS, Foweraker J, Perry JD, Prendergast BD, Sandoe JA, Spry MJ, Watkin RW. Working Party of the British Society for Antimicrobial Chemotherapy. Guidelines for the diagnosis and antibiotic treatment of endocarditis in adults: A report of the Working Party of the British Society for Antimicrobial Chemotherapy. The Journal of Antimicrobial Chemotherapy. 2012;67:269-289. DOI: 10.1093/jac/dkr450

[32] Carozza A, Della Corte A, Ursomando F, Cotrufo M. The choice of valve prosthesis for infective endocarditis in intravenous drug users: Between evidence and preference. The Annals of Thoracic Surgery. 2008;85:1141. DOI: 10.1016/j.athoracsur.2007.04.090

[33] Rabkin DG, Mokadam NA, Miller DW, Goetz RR, Verrier ED, Aldea GS. Long-term outcome for the surgical treatment of infective endocarditis with a focus on intravenous drug users. The Annals of Thoracic Surgery. 2012;93:51-57. DOI: 10.1016/j.athoracsur.2011.08.016

[34] Kaiser SP, Melby SJ, Zierer A, Schuessler RB, Moon MR, Moazami N, Pasque MK, Huddleston C, Damiano RJ Jr, Lawton JS. Long-term outcomes in valve replacement surgery for infective endocarditis. The Annals of Thoracic Surgery. 2007;83:30-35

[35] Shrestha NK, Jue J, Hussain ST, Jerry JM, Pettersson GB, Menon V, Navia JL, Nowacki AS, Gordon SM. Injection drug use and outcomes after surgical intervention for infective endocarditis. The Annals of Thoracic Surgery. 2015;100:875-882. DOI: 10.1016/j.athoracsur.2015.03.019

[36] Kim JB, Ejiofor JI, Yammine M, Ando M, Camuso JM, Youngster I, Nelson SB, Kim AY, Melnitchouk SI, Rawn JD, MacGillivray TE, Cohn LH, Byrne JG, Sundt TM 3rd. Surgical outcomes of infective endocarditis among intravenous drug users. The Journal of Thoracic and Cardiovascular Surgery. 2016;**152**:832-841. DOI: 10.1016/j.jtcvs.2016.02.072

[37] Carozza A, De Santo LS, Romano G, Della Corte A, Ursomando F, Scardone M, Caianiello G, Cotrufo M. Infective endocarditis in intravenous drug abusers: Patterns of presentation and long-term outcomes of surgical treatment. The Journal of Heart Valve Disease. 2006;**15**:125-131

[38] Jeganathan R, Armstrong S, Al-Alao B, David T. The risk and outcomes of reoperative tricuspid valve surgery. The Annals of Thoracic Surgery. 2013;**95**:119-124. DOI: 10.1016/j.athoracsur.2012.08.058

[39] Kunadian B, Vijayalakshmi K, Balasubramanian S, Dunning J. Should the tricuspid valve be replaced with a mechanical or biological valve? Interactive Cardiovascular and Thoracic Surgery. 2007;**6**:551-557

[40] Ivert TS, Dismukes WE, Cobbs CG, Blackstone EH, Kirklin JW, Bergdahl LA. Prosthetic valve endocarditis. Circulation. 1984;**69**:223-232

[41] Mahesh B, Angelini G, Caputo M, Jin XY, Bryan A. Prosthetic valve endocarditis. The Annals of Thoracic Surgery. 2005;**80**:1151-1158

[42] Luciani N, Mossuto E, Ricci D, Luciani M, Russo M, Salsano A, Pozzoli A, Pierri MD, D'Onofrio A, Chiariello GA, Glieca F, Canziani A, Rinaldi M, Nardi P, Milazzo V, Trecarichi EM, Santini F, De Bonis M, Torracca L, Bizzotto E, Tumbarello M. Prosthetic valve endocarditis: Predictors of early outcome of surgical therapy. A multicentric study. European Journal of Cardio-Thoracic Surgery. 2017;**52**:768-774. DOI: 10.1093/ejcts/ezx169

[43] Grubitzsch H, Schaefer A, Melzer C, Wernecke KD, Gabbieri D, Konertz W. Outcome after surgery for prosthetic valve endocarditis and the impact of preoperative treatment. The Journal of Thoracic and Cardiovascular Surgery. 2014;**148**:2052-2059. DOI: 10.1016/j.jtcvs.2014.05.025

[44] DiMaio JM, Salerno TA, Bernstein R, Araujo K, Ricci M, Sade RM. Ethical obligation of surgeons to noncompliant patients: Can a surgeon refuse to operate on an intravenous drug-abusing patient with recurrent aortic valve prosthesis infection? The Annals of Thoracic Surgery. 2009;**88**:1-8. DOI: 10.1016/j.athoracsur.2009.03.088

[45] Hull SC, Jadbabaie F. When is enough enough? The dilemma of valve replacement in a recidivist intravenous drug user. The Annals of Thoracic Surgery. 2014;**97**:1486-1487. DOI: 10.1016/j.athoracsur.2014.02.010

4

The Ethics in Repeat Heart Valve Replacement Surgery

Julie M. Aultman, Emanuela Peshel,
Cyril Harfouche and Michael S. Firstenberg

Abstract

The treatment of patients with intravenous drug use (IVDU) has evolved to include a wide range of medications, psychiatric rehabilitation, and surgical interventions, especially for life-threatening complications such as infective endocarditis (IE). These interventions remain at the discretion of physicians, particularly surgeons, whose treatment decisions are influenced by several medical factors, unfortunately not without bias. The stigma associated with substance use disorder is prevalent, which leads to significant biases, even in the healthcare system. This bias is heightened when IVDU patients require repeat valve replacement surgeries for IE due to continued drug use. Patients who receive a valve replacement and continue to use illicit drugs intravenously often return to their medical providers, months to a few years later, with a reinfection of their bioprosthetic valve; such patients require additional surgeries which are at the center of many ethical discussions due to high mortality rates, for many complex medical and social reasons, associated with continuous chemical dependency after surgical interventions. This chapter examines the ethics of repeat heart valve replacement surgery for patients who are struggling with addiction. Considerations of justice, the fiduciary therapeutic relationship, and guiding ethical principles justify medically beneficial repeat heart valve replacement surgeries for IVDU patient populations.

Keywords: replacement valve surgery, ethics, justice, addiction, intravenous drug use

1. Introduction

The treatment of patients with intravenous drug use (IVDU) has evolved to include a wide range of medications, psychiatric rehabilitation, and surgical interventions, especially for life-threatening complications such as infective endocarditis (IE). These interventions, how-ever, remain at the discretion of surgeons, and the healthcare team, whose treatment deci-sions are influenced by several medical factors, unfortunately not without bias. The stigma associated with substance use disorder is prevalent, especially toward IVDU, which leads to significant biases, even in the healthcare system [1]. This bias is heightened when IVDU patients require multiple or repeat valve replacement surgeries for IE due to continued drug use, which can be quite costly for healthcare institutions.

We explore various barriers when considering repeat heart valve surgeries, especially the implicit bias that can negatively influence the duty of physicians and their decision to provide comprehensive patient care. Patients who receive a valve replacement and continue to use illicit drugs intravenously, often return to their medical providers months to years later with a re-infection of their prosthetic valve; many of these patients have several medical comor-bidities and require extensive care. The topic of multiple or repeat heart valve surgeries are the center of many ethical discussions due to the high mortality rates associated with both the inherent mortality from ongoing drug abuse and the risks of often complex and technically challenging high-risk re-operative cardiac surgery.

This chapter examines the ethics of repeat heart valve replacement surgery for patients who are struggling with addiction, and the important factors that ought to guide health care pro-fessionals in making future treatment decisions. Considerations of justice, the fiduciary thera-peutic relationship, and guiding ethical principles justify medically beneficial repeat heart valve replacement surgeries for IVDU patient populations. We will present and analyze two cases, which were presented to a hospital ethics committee, and provide justification for a narrative-based ethical approach to identify those factors for when patients ought to receive multiple heart valves and the conditions for pursuing this surgical intervention despite chem-ical dependency challenges.

To better examine the ethical and social issues significant to discussions about heart valve replacement surgery among IVDU populations, particularly those seeking repeat surgeries due to chemical dependency relapse, it is important to understand the current climate in the United States with respect to IVDU and IE, as well as the need for comprehensive surgical and mental health care for patients who are committed to their recovery.

2. A brief examination of the literature

There is an increasing body of literature prompted by the rapid increase of prescription and non-prescription opioid drugs in the United States that emerged in the 1990s and is at epi-demic levels today. In 2016, 64,000 Americans died from drug overdoses, which was a 21% increase from the year before [2]. Some states are struggling more than others to combat this leading cause of death among Americans under age 50 [2]. Unfortunately, there is more discussion about public health and law enforcement interventions, rather than focusing on individualized medical care in persons who are in critical need of comprehensive therapy, which includes high-risk surgeries, detoxification programs, and extensive mental health care for chemical dependency among other related mental health disorders. Helping the addict is discussed less frequently as an important step to fight this epidemic [3], which is relevant to our ethical and social examination as to why we need to re-think the standards of medical care and treat patients holistically by incorporating mental health care into every aspect of their overall care. This is especially pertinent to the treatment of IE secondary to IVDU.

2.1. Relationship of intravenous drug use and infective endocarditis

With the rise of the opioid epidemic in the past few years, high-risk valve replacement surgeries have become a growing medical, financial, and ethical burden. Historically, IVDU represented a small percentage of patients with IE. In one study, the proportion increased from 14.8% in 2002–2004 to 26% in 2012–2014 during which time, heroin use doubled [4, 5]. Today, approximately 11% of IVDU are at risk for developing IE [6], which is characterized by infection of the inner lining of the heart, leading to the growth of vegetation on heart valves that disrupt the ability to pump blood. Overall, IE is an extremely morbid disease: in-hospital mortality rates range from 11 to 26% with an estimated 5-year mortality of up to 50% [7]. Complications include heart failure, valve insufficiency, embolic strokes, and intra-cerebral hemorrhage. IE secondary to IVDU is most commonly caused by bacteremia from *Staphylococcus aureus* and *Enterococcus faecalis* that are abundantly found on the skin and gastrointestinal tract, or by particulates in illicit drugs that cause micro-damage to tissues as they circulate [8, 9] following injection. Treatment is often sufficient using high-dose antibiotics, but 60 to 70% of severe cases require surgical intervention [4].

Studies have shown that patients with IE secondary to IVDU are younger than patients with no IVDU and more likely to be young Caucasian males, with some regional variability among populations [4]. The average age of patients who suffer from IE secondary to IVDU is 30 years old, and 90% of them are heroin addicts [7, 8]. Approximately 75% of individuals admitted to treatment for heroin abuse or dependency reported using injection as the primary method of drug use [10].

Despite IVDU representing a significantly younger patient population with less cardiovascular and comorbid risk factors, long-term outcomes are compromised by reinfection [4] and continued drug abuse. A patient who receives a valve replacement yet continues to use intravenous drugs is likely to re-infect their bioprosthetic or homograft valves, requiring additional valve replacement surgeries. However, such treatment opportunities may not be offered to this patient population due to high mortality rates. For example, studies have found that patients who resume IVDU after their initial valve replacement have high mortality compared to patients who abstain from drug use after their surgery [11]. A patient who resumes IVDU may get an extra 1–5 years of life out of their new valve rather than the 10–15 years of life that a new valve (mechanical or biological) can give without IVDU. Such decision-making must also be done in the setting of the overall poor and limited (but somewhat incompletely defined) life-expectancy of the habitual use of IV drugs.

2.2. Factors contributing to stigma and the refusal of care

In general, many surgical professionals identify repeat valve replacement surgery as non-beneficial for patients with IVDU, and thus, refuse or are reluctant to offer this procedure or refer patients to other surgeons who are willing to treat this patient population. Even when the valve replacement surgery may provide some benefit and give a few more years of quality life for patients, surgical professionals and the healthcare team may feel as though the financial burdens to patients and healthcare institutions is a reasonable justification for not replacing infected valves. This is especially true given the high relapse rates for IVDU and readmission with active IVDU. In addition, because the IVDU patient population contributes to increased unemployment and reliance on publicly funded insurance [12], some health care professionals may feel as though they have a duty to the community by not prolonging the lives of patients with IE secondary to IVDU, and thus adding additional financial burdens for communities and an already resource-limited health system.

Smyth et al. (2010) conducted a prospective study of patients who were dependent on opioids and admitted to a residential chemical dependency service for treatment. The authors found that 91% of 109 patients interviewed had relapsed; 59% relapsed just within one week of discharge [13]. Those who had earlier relapse were characteristic of our patient population; patients are younger in age, have a history of IVDU, did not complete the recommended length of time in the addiction program, and did not enter in or commit to aftercare programs. The authors also found that delayed relapse occurred among those who completed their entire program, as well as those individuals who were in a relationship with an opiate user, which was an unexpected finding and deserves further research [13].

Furthermore, given the significant rise of IVDU with the opiate epidemic in the United States, further research on relapse is needed, including the multitude of factors that contribute to relapse. Without addressing the factors that contribute to relapse, the rate will continue to rise, perpetuate stigma, fuel healthcare professionals' reluctance to provide multiple heart valve replacement surgeries, among other medical interventions. A study in China examined heroin addiction relapse and the effects of detoxification medications (methadone) combined with psychological counseling and social support measures, which were found to be essential to on-going recovery and reduction of relapse rates along with patient compliance [14]. Additional studies have found that patients who recur to IVDU after the initial valve replacement procedure have very high mortality compared to patients who undergo rehabilitation [15].

From a medical perspective, the relationship between IE and substance use disorder is no different than nephropathy and diabetes, coronary artery disease and smoking, or the countless other chronic medical problems that are worsened by "life-style" choices. However, the negative connotations and stigma associated with IVDU lead to patients being treated differently in the health care system and among physicians, who deny life-saving care and devalue their patients as persons in need of advocacy and support to combat their addictions.

2.3. Gaps in the literature

Unfortunately, little research has been done on the value of extensive psychiatric and behavioral health interventions prior to, during, and following surgical treatment and the overall clinical, psychosocial, and legal outcomes (e.g., improved medical compliance, reduced recidivism in drug use and criminal acts). One study found that only 7.8% of patients treated for IE were discharged with plans to receive medication-assisted treatment during the 10-year period of the study. In that same study, 25% of patients were readmitted with active IVDU [16]. Aggressive treatment for IE, including antibiotics and valve transplants, is neither effective nor advantageous without targeting the underlying addictive behaviors that contribute to poor health outcomes and mortality.

Addiction treatment, particularly for opioid users, is limited by factors that are beyond the control of physicians and drug users who may be willing to seek recovery. A study published by Jones *et al.* in 2015 reported that nationally, 96% of states (48 out of 50) had lower opioid treatment program capacity rates than their corresponding opioid abuse or dependence rates. The study also reported that 38 states had over 75% of their opioid treatment programs operating at an 80% capacity or more [17]. These numbers are indicative of a severe national shortage in treatment options, which could in part explain the ongoing struggle in IVDU achieving or maintaining their recovery.

Furthermore, little theoretical work has been done to identify the complex ethical issues surrounding this IVDU patient population who qualify for valve replacement surgery but who may be denied this life-sustaining intervention due to a number of factors including, but not limited to, financial cost, perceived poor quality of life, suspected non-compliance in post-surgical care and addiction treatment, and social worth. This chapter aims to start closing these gaps and to provide guidance to surgeons and healthcare teams when confronted with difficult medical, social, and ethical dilemmas.

Thus, through the presentation of two cases of IE secondary to IVDU, we will identify the medical, social, and ethical issues, recommendations for whether we should provide repeat valve replacements, and how we ought to treat patients who are struggling with mental health issues, including, but not limited to chemical dependency. Our case analyses will also identify the limits of justice and the duty of health care professionals in providing repeat heart valve surgeries.

3. Case presentation

The following two case presentations are based on actual patients with identifying information removed so as to protect their identities. These cases were presented to an ethics committee for an initial recommendation; however, the analysis and discussion presented here extends beyond committee consultation or even those guiding ethical principles that contribute to decision-making and resolution. These cases reveal a need for a narrative ethical approach to best understand individual patients and their medical, psychosocial, and value-based needs from diagnosis through recovery. The cases presented in this chapter are montages of health care team members' stories about their interactions with patients through medical evidence, patient interviewing, and clinical observation. However, there is an equal need for the medical team and the patient to co-author or construct a joint narrative of illness and medical care [18, 19]. These cases, however, do represent the multiple voices of the multidisciplinary medical team about the patient in a brief, accessible case presentation. The features of these cases serve as valuable starting points for understanding the complexity of medical decision-making, unifying repeat heart valve replacement, post-operative care, and mental health treatment, and the need for ongoing recognition of the patient's story.

3.1. Case 1: a unified care model

A 24-year-old homeless, female patient is brought into the emergency department by a family member and presents for sepsis related to IVDA. The patient has a 10-year history of drug use with previous endocarditis, requiring cardiac surgery and debridement of an infected tricuspid valve approximately 14 months prior to the current admission. She has a history of untreated depression. The patient is admitted for complaints of joint pain, swelling, and general malaise. She reports injecting heroin and crack cocaine in her extremities (feet, arms, and hands) daily. The patient was drug-free for a short period of time with the assistance of residential treatment and hospitalization at a nursing facility where she received IV antibiotics for the endocarditis. However, the patient missed a dose of Suboxone (buprenorphine and naloxone) due to lack of transportation, did not seek support from health care professionals, and was unsuccessfully attempting to stop her persistent drug use on her own. Her continued drug use and failure of medical management have resulted in the need for pre-operative cardiac surgery for large vegetation in the tricuspid valve. The patient is willing to pursue addiction treatment following surgery and post-operative care and has had a history of taking Suboxone as an effort to stay clean and sober. An ethics consult is called to provide a recommendation on whether it is ethically permissible to re-operate in this patient with infective endocarditis from persistent IVDU. The ethics committee further weighed in on recommendations for achieving a unified care model in which the immediate medical needs namely, heart valve replacement, antibiotic therapy, and acute peri-operative pain management. Critical in the discussion was also providing a pathway that includes comprehensive mental health care for the patient's depression and addiction.

3.2. Case 2: resistance to IVDU treatment

A 29-year-old married male with a history of depression, multiple suicide attempts, poly-substance intravenous drug use (heroin and methamphetamines), and a history of endocarditis was brought to the emergency department by EMS following a suspected overdose. The patient was unresponsive until EMS delivered multiple doses of naloxone in route to the emergency department. Upon arrival, the patient was alert but had difficulty speaking. The patient's wife, who is a recovering addict, alerted EMS to her husband's overdose. Upon questioning the patient's current drug use, he admits to using methamphetamine cut with Fentanyl over the past week. The patient was drug-free for approximately 1.5 months after a prior hospital admission for septic mitral valve endocarditis due to IVDA, as well as renal failure, which was resolved following treatment. He received a bioprosthetic mitral valve and antibiotic therapy. Aside from his brief period drug-free, he has never been in treatment specifically for his chemical dependency and currently feels like he doesn't need such treatment. The patient suffers from multiple cerebral septic emboli with hemorrhagic transformation, aphasia, and distal limb emboli. He currently reports feeling feverish with body chills, headache, and joint pain; lab results show *Serratia* bacteremia, hypokalemia, transaminitis, anemia, and thrombocytopenia (I do not think we need these labs after *Serratia* bacteremia). An ethics committee is called upon to guide the treating surgeon whether this patient should receive a repeat valve replacement if he medically qualifies for this intervention. Additional ethical guidance is sought to determine what are the ethical obligations of the healthcare team when the patient does not believe he needs chemical dependency treatment and is likely to have repeated events of IE secondary to IVDU.

4. Ethics case analyses: a need for comprehensive just care and patient illness narratives

The above cases are representative of several medical, social, and ethical issues presented when patients are suffering from IE secondary to IVDU and who may require a repeat heart valve surgery and extensive mental health care for addiction and other related mental disorders (e.g., depression). In situations where patients have IE secondary to IVDU and need a new heart valve—their first surgical intervention—surgeons and others are more likely to treat the typical young patient with a probable successful surgical outcome without a need to seek ethical counsel. In our experiences, while most patients receive minimal chemical dependency treatment post-surgery, relapse (as discussed above) is likely, and a comprehensive mental health care program with monitoring, social support, and a recognition of the social determinants that contribute to the relapse are often not sufficiently addressed.

Thus, these patients return with IE and in need of a second, third, or more heart valve replacement surgeries. Surgeons and other healthcare professionals, particularly those working in community hospitals with limited financial resources, may question their duties to this patient population while considering their obligations to their medical community and society at large. Heart valve replacement surgeries, post-operative care, and addiction treatment are costly, and the financial burdens to patients, healthcare institutions, and the general community may deter surgeons from moving forward despite the patient's need. We can add the statistic about how the cost is increasing using the data from NC either here or in the paragraph with all the other statistics. Furthermore, the social stigma and biases against drug-addicted patients impact medical decisions, particularly when combined with the potential risk to health outcome measures, which can affect individual health care professional evaluations, work satisfaction, and trust among the general patient population.

The emotional impact of providing surgical care with the likelihood the patient will be back again for repeat heart valves due to IVDU can prompt moral distress, cynicism, and resentment of this patient population regardless of the moral obligations to treat when medically necessary, or beneficial. All of these considerations for repeat heart valve replacement surgeries should not be dismissed. They are essential for building a case for comprehensive just care, which is guided by core ethical principles of beneficence, non-maleficence, and justice, as well as a recognition of the individual patient's story through narrative medicine. Narrative medicine prompts healthcare professionals to absorb, interpret, and co-author the dynamic story-telling in patient care. By co-authoring the illness narratives of patients, providers are able to acquire deeper insight into each patient's understanding of their illness, their goals for recovery, and the triggers that act as obstacles to recovery. Furthermore, through these illness narratives, providers will bear witness to the individuality of medical cases and recognize that some patients really can be helped even with the likelihood of relapse and future harm, which can reduce moral distress and clinical cynicism (e.g., "why try to help if these patients will end up abusing drugs again") [20–22]. However, the illness narratives need to be sustained; patients' stories do not end once they complete their post-operative care (e.g., antibiotic therapy).

It is our general position that repeat heart valves for patients with IE secondary to IVDU ought to be given if they are medically beneficial and if the patient is willing to commit to addiction recovery and ongoing, comprehensive mental health treatment that aims to address the social triggers, existing mental health disorders, and other factors that influence the chemical dependency. This is not the responsibility of the surgeon alone, but a medical team that has access to hospital and community resources, appropriate skills, knowledge to address the whole patient and their medical and psychosocial needs, and the ability to combat social stigma by treating the patient as a person with a very specific narrative. When repeat heart valves are not medically necessary or ethically beneficial, may cause undue suffering, and/ or the patient is unwilling to commit to a comprehensive treatment program after thorough guidance by the health care team, then it is ethically justifiable to refuse surgery. However, each case is unique, and there may arise unique considerations that have not yet been previously addressed or ethically analyzed. Thus, it is essential that a narrative ethical approach that calls attention to the nuances of the case, i.e., the elements of the patient's story, is automatically part of the medical assessment and a sustainable chronic care plan.

4.1. Case I analysis: establishing standards of care

In this first case, there are a number of social factors that are contributing to the patient's current medical state. First, this is a young, homeless patient who does not have the means to acquire sustainable basic human needs. Regardless of whether her drug use led to the homelessness or vice versa, she is surviving in an unhealthy, unsupportive, and harmful environment, which is an obstacle to addiction recovery and overall health. When living in a residential treatment facility, she was able to have security, shelter, food, warmth, and community support, in addition to, medical treatment, all of which are essential for a recovering addict who, unfortunately, did not have these resources prior to her first valve surgery. However, these resources are limited; they are only available for the duration of her medical treatment for the endocarditis, and not for the ongoing recovery for her addiction. Her lack of essential resources, social instability, and homelessness are likely to have played a role in her subsequent relapse while on Suboxone; this demonstrates the necessity for holistic and comprehensive care in order to fully rehabilitate a patient with a chronic condition. Furthermore, this patient has a history of untreated depression—another significant factor that could have led to her current medical state.

The use of IV drugs to combat feelings of depression and despair are not uncommon among untreated patients. Reasons for why she did not seek medical attention for her depression are unknown, but given the difficulties of navigating the health care system, federal insurance programs, and community programs that can aid a patient in accessing mental health care, it is not surprising that her depression went untreated. A person already addicted to IV drugs may have even more difficulty accessing mental health care due to the cognitive effects of the drugs, the stigma of drug use, and the lack of social support in seeking help. This patient tried to stop her drug use, but could not stop without the necessary social support and addiction therapy. Because she was previously successful at recovery, is a good surgical candidate for a medically indicated tricuspid valve replacement, and has a strong commitment to seeking post-operative care and addiction treatment, the surgical intervention should be granted. An ethics committee convened with this case and further recommended that it is critical for a team-based approach to be utilized for patients with IVDU who are seeking valve replacements.

A range of medical specialists and addiction experts, along with the surgical team, are essential for developing and implementing a treatment plan. It is also recommended that these patients sign a behavioral agreement in addition to the standard surgical consent form that details the patient's level of understanding about the risks and benefits of the surgery, addiction interventions, and any other medical and psychosocial care that promotes a good clinical outcome. Clinical outcomes are often determined by the success of the surgeries and post-operative care. However, we need to begin to look more critically at the long-term success of recovery, factors contributing to relapse, and how a team-based approach can aid the patient in quickly getting back into recovery. Recovery is a life-long process and a good clinical outcome may take years to fully measure and understand despite the more immediate surgical successes.

In the end, this patient did receive re-operative tricuspid and aortic tissue valve replacement. However, the behavioral contract, a non-legally binding contract, was not used. This contract prompts the patient to understand the need to get comprehensive treatment beyond a valve replacement, as well as empower the patient to take charge of her life, and maintain physical and mental health through ongoing counseling, therapy, and pharmaceutical interventions to treat her depression and addiction. The value of the contract is that it is a way to understand the patient's illness narrative and her commitment to recovery; although not used for this particular patient, it is a useful tool that can be beneficial for other patients. Of course, basic human needs (home, food, social support) are also needed, yet securing these resources for patients can be a challenge without having social work, nursing, and community support. There are limitations to what a surgeon can do beyond immediate surgical care, so it is critical for a wider health care community to recognize their ethical obligations to this patient population.

4.2. Case 2 analysis: a deeper understanding of medical need

In regard to the second case, this young male patient is struggling with mental health issues—particularly untreated depression and addiction—and is married to a recovering addict, who either can be a positive or negative influence in his recovery depending on their willingness to work together toward mutual recovery. Without mental health treatment, his depression, suicidal ideations, and addiction will continue. One of the primary problems with this case is the patient's reluctance (which might be confounded by potential neurologic dysfunction due to his embolic strokes) to mental health treatment, feeling as though he does not need it despite the magnitude of health complications arising from his pervasive drug use. Specifically, the IVDU has led to multiple hospitalizations, a mitral valve replacement, and multiple, serious co-morbidities that have left him with ongoing physical pain and cognitive impairment. Prior to testing for valve functionality, this patient, too, was presented to an ethics committee, which prompted discussion regarding whether valve re-operation would be beneficial to this patient with serious comorbidities that may increase his surgical risk and lead to a poorer quality of life.

Similar to the first case, discussions surrounding addiction stigma, the need for social support, a need for the patient's commitment to seek addiction treatment, and a team-based approach to patient care were presented. However, unlike the first case, this particular patient is suffering from a number of medical issues that each need to be taken into consideration in the evaluation for a replacement valve, as well as an acknowledgment of the patient's lack of commitment to comprehensive mental health treatment. The ethical guidance sought is grounded in the principles of beneficence and non-maleficence, as well as a narrative-based justice approach that details the specifics of the patient's medical history, social support, quality of life, and his preferences and commitment to recovery. The goals of the medical team, from an ethical perspective, are to very carefully look at his medical condition, and whether he even has a chance for survival and future quality of life with a second valve replacement surgery. Second, it is critical for the medical team to revisit the topic of comprehensive mental health care, including treatment for depression and chemical dependency. Objective consideration must also be given if there are overwhelming evidence of medical/surgical futility — but this concept can be extremely difficult to determine in young patients.

The need for aggressive inpatient chemical dependency treatment is essential to this patient's recovery. However, unlike the first case in which valve replacement surgery and addiction treatment are simultaneously discussed as a holistic approach to patient care, for this patient, the addiction treatment becomes an interesting topic of discussion due to the gravity of his medical condition and his resistance to treatment. That is, the first case had less medical ambiguities in terms of the surgical candidacy for valve replacement combined with a clear indication of the patient's commitment to recovery. Thus, due to the immediate and justifiable medical need, the decision to move forward with surgery came simultaneously with a team-based plan and patient contract for recovery. Here, the patient's condition warrants an initial discussion about whether replacement valve surgery would be non-beneficial treatment. Causing further harm either during surgery or postoperatively should be avoided so as to ensure the best quality of life while living with a terminal condition. Furthermore, if the replacement valve surgery would be deemed beneficial, there remains the issue of the patient's lack of commitment to recovery. If there is persistent resistance to mental health care, ethically it would be unjust to proceed with a surgical intervention.

Following the ethics consult, the patient's valves with small vegetation were functioning, and his bacteremia was responding well to antibiotic therapy. The surgical team determined that after he completed extended care, he then should seek aggressive inpatient chemical dependency treatment to limit the risk of relapse and recurrence. However, the medical team may be at an impasse given the patient's current resistance and lack of commitment to addiction recovery.

While it is recommended the medical team should have ongoing dialog with the patient to understand his reluctance at undergoing mental health treatment, and continuing to identify providers, care facilities, etc., that could aid in his recovery, additional steps may be needed before proceeding with any future medical interventions (e.g., valve replacement). If medical therapy alone fails e.g. progression of disease, worsening valve functioning, or recurrent emboli that lead to further complications, treatment options will need to be re-evaluated. Depending on his medical state, the patient may not be a future candidate for a replacement valve, and thus other medical resources and personnel, such as palliative care, may be required for the care of this patient.

In our first case, it is recommended the patient sign a behavioral contract to strengthen her existing commitment toward recovery, which further illustrates she does not have to go through recovery alone, i.e., the medical team will not give up on her if she maintains her commitment. In this second case, however, a behavioral contract may not be enough, since such non-legally binding contracts are symbolic gestures of the medical team's medical/social/legal relationship to a patient the shared responsibilities of both parties. When a patient is not willing to share responsibilities in the relationship and is resistant to addressing serious mental health disorders, the first step is to understand why.

4.3. Addressing the ethical and social problems of repeat valve replacements and the limits of justice

Valve replacements in IVDU must be administered regardless of the negative connotations associated with addiction or illicit drug use, with the patient's health, surgical success, and access to comprehensive addiction treatment being the goals of treatment. Both conscious and unconscious biases can affect clinical judgments that lead to unjust decision-making and disrespectful treatment of patients.

Similar to the health disparities we see in organ transplantation cases, where racial and ethnic biases have affected the length of time on a transplant waiting list, or lifestyle behaviors (e.g., alcohol addiction) have affected judgments about probability of success for organ replacement surgeries, medical judgments are not immune to bias when determinations about medical outcomes are being made. That is, it is all too easy for a surgeon to determine that her patient does not qualify for a valve replacement because of the high surgical risk, which may be based on the patient's untreated addiction, probability of relapse, and co-morbidities due to the effects of IVDU (e.g. the inherent risks of recurrent overdoses), rather than on the patient's survivability on the surgical table and success of the valve replacement itself. A surgeon may also exhibit conscious biases toward her patient when considering the continued burden of having to provide ongoing treatment, which increases the financial and personnel cost to the medical institution. Thus, such attitudes and feelings lead to a biased clinical judgment, but may also be generated out of concern for professional evaluation and outcomes-based, performance measures.

The first step in reducing the need for repeat valve replacement and improving patient health outcomes and survivability is to understand the patient's own unique story that prompted the IVDU, their goals for treatment, and their overall understanding of their own responsibilities toward successful, comprehensive treatment. By motivating them with a behavioral contract that speaks to the healthcare team's responsibility to the patient's care and the patient's own commitment, this may be a positive step.

Second, patients will not have a chance for successful recovery if they are not provided with needed resources and appropriate guidance to motivate them to seek long-term treatment. Such treatment should involve methods ranging from psychotherapy to pharmaceutical interventions.

Unfortunately, most current care is focused on the infective pathology; in IE patients only the acute problem is addressed, but no effort seems to be placed on preventing readmissions or improving the patient's quality of life. Addressing the lack of care and support IVDU patients are receiving, rather than trying to limit patient access to replacement procedures provides the just treatment these patients deserve, in addition to reducing the financial burden on healthcare systems and society. Health care providers often fail to identify addiction as the significant comorbidity that it is, and do not treat it as aggressively and appropriately using drugs that specifically target opioid use disorders; this results in under-treatment of addiction [16]. Such a limited care approach needs to change.

Third, surgeons and the healthcare team also require the support of ethics teams when complex social and ethical questions arise with patients. Personal biases lead to social stigmatization of patients with IVDU, influence medical decisions, lead to provider burnout, moral distress, and cynicism among health care providers. Having ongoing team-based discussions about these negative experiences, attitudes, and emotions is one step in the right direction, Recognizing the ethical and social issues that penetrate the medical problems can also help navigate and resolve dilemmas and elicit a deeper understanding of the individual patient and their illness narrative. It is important for healthcare providers to engage in self-care, and to have the opportunity to address issues before they devolve into negative emotions and attitudes that can be harmful to self and other.

Finally, it is critical for the health care team to know when additional treatment is futile. There are limits to justice. However, such limits to therapies must be based upon objective evidence supported by the medical literature rather than poorly grounded assumptions, biases, and outdated, or erroneous knowledge or datasets.

5. Conclusions

Unless physicians treat the chronic and acute illnesses in patients with IE due to IVDU, their ethical duties toward their patients remain unfulfilled, and they fail to provide just care. This issue becomes more precarious when considering patients who require additional valve replacements due to continued IVDU.

The American Medical Association's *Code of Medical Ethics* states that is the physician's ethical obligation "to place patients' welfare above their own self-interest and above obligations to other groups and to advocate for their patients' welfare" [23]. It is the duty of physicians to promote the health of their patients through comprehensive, beneficial treatment based on evidence-based medicine, and to respect them as persons with dignity, uninfluenced by social stigma and clinical bias. For patients with IE secondary to IVDU, it is important to treat both the psychiatric, social and infectious etiologies: the substance use disorder, homelessness, and food insecurity, as well as the IE, along with any additional comorbidities that are present. Although every patient with IE secondary to IVDU differs in the severity of presentation and comorbid conditions, patients with a positive prognosis should have the opportunity to achieve health and life with medical assistance.

Unfortunately, it is not unusual for patients with recurrent IE secondary to IVDU to experience social stigmatization and bias at the hands of the healthcare system and to be denied the comprehensive care that is needed in such cases. While some patients are justifiably denied due to a significant medical risk over benefit, patients are also denied simply because they are perceived as non-compliant, or because their potentially risky surgical treatments may negatively affect the health reviews and ratings of the surgeons performing the valve replacements. It is not ethically just to penalize viable surgical candidates when their addiction has neither been addressed nor treated. Citing high rates of treatment failure and non-compliance is not a valid excuse when the substance use disorder has not been treated as aggressively as the IE, especially when taking into considerations the lack of resources available for these patients to seek and maintain recovery.

Conflict of interest

The authors have no conflict of interest.

Author details

Julie M. Aultman[1]*, Emanuela Peshel[1], Cyril Harfouche[1] and Michael S. Firstenberg[1,2]

*Address all correspondence to: jmaultma@neomed.edu

1 Northeast Ohio Medical University, Rootstown, Ohio, United States

2 The Medical Center of Aurora, Aurora, CO, United States

References

[1] Cami J, Farre M. Drug addiction. The New England Journal of Medicine. 2003;**349**:975-986

[2] Katz J. Drug Deaths In America Are Rising Faster Than Ever. New York: New York Times; June 5, 2017. https://www.nytimes.com/interactive/2017/06/05/upshot/opioid-epidemic-drug-overdose-deaths-are-rising-faster-than-ever.html?_r=0

[3] McGinty EE, Kennedy-Hendricks A, Baller J, Niederdeppe J, Gollust S, Barry CL. Criminal activity or treatable health condition? News media framing of Opioid analgesic abuse in the United States, 1998-2012. Psychiatric Services. 2016;**67**(4):405-411

[4] Kim JB, Ejiofor JI, Yammine M, et al. Surgical outcomes of infective endocarditis among intravenous drug users. The Journal of Thoracic and Cardiovascular Surgery. 2016 Sep; **152**(3):832-841

[5] Huynh TN, Kleerup EC, Wiley JF, et al. The frequency and cost of treatment perceived to be futile in critical care Terrance. JAMA Internal Medicine. 2013;**173**(20):1887-1894

[6] Phillips KT, Stein MD. Risk practices associated with bacterial infections among injection drug users in Denver, Colorado. The American Journal of Drug and Alcohol Abuse. 2010;**36**:92-97

[7] Wurcel AG, Anderson JE, Chui KKH, et al. Increasing infectious Endocarditis admissions among young people who inject drugs. Open Forum Infectious Diseases. 2016;**3**(3): ofw157. DOI: 10.1093/ofid/ofw157

[8] Kaiser SP, Melby SJ, Zierer A, et al. Long-term outcomes in valve replacement surgery for infective endocarditis. The Annals of Thoracic Surgery. 2007;**83**:30-35

[9] Mathew JMD, Addait TMD, Anand AMD, et al. Clinical features, site of involvement, bacteriologic findings, and outcome of infective Endocarditis in intravenous drug users. Archives of Internal Medicine. 1995;**155**(15):1641-1648

[10] Westling K, Aufwerber E, Ekdahl C, et al. Swedish guidelines for diagnosis and treatment of infective endocarditis. Scandinavian Journal of Infectious Diseases. 2007;**39**:929

[11] Arbulu A, Asfaw I. Management of Infective Endocarditis: Seventeen Years' experience. The Annals of Thoracic Surgery. 1987;**43**:144-149

[12] O'Toole TP, Pollini R, Gray P, et al. Suboptimal addiction interventions for patients hospitalized with injection drug use-associated infective Endocarditis. Journal of Substance Abuse Treatment. 2007 Jul;**33**(1):51-59

[13] Smyth BP, Barry J, Keenan E, Ducray K. Lapse and relapse following inpatient treatment of opiate dependence. Irish Medical Journal. 2010 Jun;**103**(6):176-179

[14] Rong C, Jiang HF, Zhang RW, Zhang LJ, Zhang JC, Zhang J, Feng XS. Factors associated with relapse among heroin addicts: Evidence from a two-year community based follow up study in China. International Journal of Environmental Research and Public Health. 28 January 2016;**13**(2):177

[15] Riddick FA. The code of medical ethics of the American Medical Association. Ochsner J. Spring. 2003;**5**(2):6-10

[16] Substance Abuse and Mental Health Services Administration. Center for Behavioral Health Statistics and Quality Treatment Episode Data Set (TEDS): 2000-2010. National Admissions to Substance Abuse Treatment Services. DASIS Series S-61, HHS Publication No. (SMA) 12-4701. Rockville, MD: Substance Abuse and Mental Health Services Administration; 2012

[17] Jones CM, Campopiano M, Baldwin G, McCance-Katz E. National and state treatment need and capacity for Opioid agonist medication-assisted treatment. American Journal of Public Health. August 1, 2015;**105**(8):e55-e63

[18] Brody H. My story is broken; can you help me fix it? Medical ethics and the joint construction of narrative. Literature and Medicine. 1994;**13**:79-92

[19] Jones AH. Narrative in medical ethics. BMJ [British Medical Journal]. 1999;**318**(7178): 253-256

[20] Anyanwu AC. The vagaries of patient selection in cardiovascular surgery. The Journal of thoracic and cardiovascular surgery. 2016 Sep 1;**152**(3):842-846

[21] Peters MJ. Head to head: Should smokers be refused surgery? BMJ [British Medical Journal]. 2007 Jan 6;**334**(7583):20

[22] Heath J, Braun MA, Brindle M. Smokers' rights to coronary artery bypass graft surgery. JONA'S Healthcare Law, Ethics and Regulation. 2002 Jun 1;**4**(2):32-35

[23] Riddick FA. The code of medical ethics of the American Medical Association. The Ochsner Journal. 2003;**5**(2):6-10

5

Prosthetic Valve Endocarditis

Ahmed Fayaz, Medhat Reda Nashy,
Sarah Eapen and Michael S. Firstenberg

Abstract

The management of infections of the cardiac structures—specifically native heart valves—remains a difficult clinical challenge. Patients often present with a systemic infection that is made worse by embolic complications, such as strokes, along with pathophysiologic sequelae of acute valvular dysfunction. The timing of interventions has a significant impact on short- and long-term outcomes. The challenges and management decisions are even more complex when the infection involves a prosthetic valve—as risks of reoperative cardiac surgery can be substantial. The goal of this chapter is to discuss the history of prosthetic valve endocarditis, review the current literature on the management of specific valvular involvement (i.e., aortic and/or mitral), and illustrate the challenging problems and outcomes that drive clinical decision making. While many of the indications for surgery are similar to those associated with native valve infections, there is increased risk with reoperative surgery, often difficulties in clearing infection due to prosthetic material being in place. Unfortunately, antibiotics alone are not always effective, and frequent communications between the cardiac surgeon and infectious disease physicians are often necessary to find the "sweet spot" to perform the surgery.

Keywords: endocarditis, valve disease, aortic valve, mitral valve, cardiac surgery, prosthetic heart valves, infections

1. Introduction

Prosthetic valve endocarditis (PVE) is a rare, but serious complication of cardiac valve replacement surgery. As the prevalence of prosthetic valves increases, the incidence of PVE also rises. PVE constitutes approximately 20% of all cases of endocarditis, now greater than previous estimates of 1–5% [1]. The incidence of PVE is estimated at 0.3–1% per patient-year, with a cumulative risk of 3% at 5 years and 5% at 10 years [1, 2]. The incidence of PVE in the aortic position is significantly higher than in the mitral position [3]. In comparison, the mitral valve is more commonly affected than the aortic valve in native valve endocarditis [4]. Patients undergoing simultaneous aortic and mitral valve replacement have an even greater risk of PVE than with a single valve replacement [5, 6].

2. Historical note

In 1885, Osler observed an association between perioperative bacteremia and endocarditis [7]. In 1935, Okell and Elliott noted that 11% of patients with poor oral hygiene had positive blood cultures for *Streptococcus viridans*, and that 60% of patients had bacteremia associated with dental extraction [8]. Not long after, initial reports of valve replacements by Starr and Harken, the first reports of PVE appeared in the literature [9, 10]. Before the routine use of prophylactic antibiotics, Geraci and Stein reported incidences of early PVE of 10 and 12%, respectively [11, 12]. The use of routine prophylactic antibiotics was noted to reduce the incidence of early PVE to 0.2% [11]. From the outset, the surgical management of PVE has been a formidable challenge. In the 1960s and 1970s, surgery for PVE was associated with an extremely high mortality rate. Discouraged by early operative experience, cardiac surgeons avoided intervention in cases of PVE despite recognition that antibiotic therapy alone was ineffective and often fatal. Surgery for PVE was reserved for high risk cases, and the surgical outcomes were predictably poor. Hence, a vicious cycle developed in which surgery was avoided for fear of poor surgical outcomes, and poor surgical outcomes achieved in high risk cases reinforced this fear.

In 1972, Ross successfully performed an aortic root replacement for PVE using an aortic homograft [13]. His report stressed surgical principles still true today: complete surgical debridement of all infected tissue, the use of homograft for reconstruction, and the minimal use of foreign material in the infected area [13]. In 1977, Olinger and Maloney reported replacement of an infected aortic prosthesis and external felt buttressing for correction of aortoventricular discontinuity [14]. In 1980, Frantz reported successful repair of an aortoventricular discontinuity from endocarditis and abscess formation by aortic root replacement using a synthetic valved conduit [15]. In 1981, Reitz successfully applied this technique to the treatment of prosthetic aortic valve endocarditis [16]. In 1982, Symbas combined aortic valve replacement with patch repair of a periannular abscess cavity [17]. In 1987, David and Feindel described techniques to reconstruct the mitral annulus with pericardium after debridement for PVE [18].

Surgical treatment of PVE remains a significant challenge, but outcomes improved in the 1990s. Factors that contributed to improved outcomes included:

1. widespread use of transthoracic and trans-esophageal echocardiography in making an early, accurate diagnosis,

2. an appreciation that, like surgical infections elsewhere, surgery for PVE requires radical debridement of infected and devitalized tissue,

3. improvements in myocardial protection, including routine use of retrograde cardioplegia, permitted longer and safer cardiac operations, and

4. cryopreserved homograft availability. Combined with resistance to reinfection, homografts provided flexibility in cardiac reconstruction after debridement. Currently, homograft aortic root replacement is considered the procedure of choice in the treatment of complex aortic PVE.

3. Risk

The risk of PVE to the patient is lifelong. However, as assessed by hazard function analysis, the risk of infection is greatest during the first 3 weeks after valve implantation [19]. Most deaths occur within 3 months of PVE development [18]. By clinical convention, PVE is classified as early or late [20]. Early PVE is acquired perioperatively and accounts for approximately one-third of all cases [20, 21]. Although traditionally defined as occurring within 60 days of initial valve replacement, the contemporary literature variably defines early PVE as occurring within 2, 6, or 12 months of initial valve replacement [20–22]. Late PVE results from infection unrelated to the initial valve operation and accounts for the remaining two-thirds [20]. The prognosis for early PVE is significantly worse than that of late PVE and often requires surgical intervention [20].

The distinction between early and late PVE provides insight into the acquisition of infection, expected clinical course, and appropriate management. Early PVE arises from the contamination of the valve during the perioperative period of valve implantation [20]. However, a patient with a prosthetic valve placed more than 12 months prior remains at risk for PVE commonly related to a healthcare-associated infection [20]. In a prospective, multicenter study of 171 patients with prosthetic heart valves by Fang et al., 43% developed endocarditis [23]. At the time, bacteremia was discovered, 33% had prosthetic valve endocarditis. These cases were described as having endocarditis at the outset. In comparison, 11% developed endocarditis at a mean of 45 days after the bacteremia was discovered. These cases were described as having new endocarditis. All cases of new endocarditis were health care associated with 33% developing bacteremia from intravascular devices [23].

Patients with central venous catheters are at particular risk for bacteremia. In the United States, approximately 80,000 central venous catheter-related cases of bacteremia are reported annually [24]. Urinary catheters are another source of bacteremia [25]. Catheter-associated bacteriuria develops at a rate of 8% per day in the first week of catheterization [25]. After the tenth day of catheterization, over 50% of patients are bacteriuric. Bacteremia develops in 0.4–4% of patients with catheter-associated bacteriuria [25]. Bacteremia per se does not invariably cause PVE. In a 10-year review of 890 patients by Parker et al., 3.6% undergoing cardiac valve replacement developed bacteremia in the early postoperative period. Only 6% of bacteremic patients developed PVE, though uniformly fatal [26]. Other authors have suggested that the risk of PVE may be significantly higher in cases of bacteremia; Murray reported an infective endocarditis rate of up to 25% in cases of *Staphylococcus aureus* bacteremia [27].

Although PVE secondary to candidemia is rare, accounting for 5–10% of all cases, it carries a high mortality rate [28]. In a retrospective study of 44 cases of nosocomial fungemia in patients with prosthetic heart valves by Nasser et al., 9% developed fungal endocarditis at a mean of 232 days after documented candidemia [29]. Hence, patients with candidemia must be treated aggressively in the acute setting and be provided close long-term follow-up.

Implantation of a prosthetic valve in the setting of native valve contamination without known active infection may increase the risk of PVE. For this reason, many surgeons routinely culture excised valve leaflets to ensure that the new valve is not contaminated at the time of implantation. In a study of 222 patients by Campbell et al., 14.4% who underwent elective valve replacement had positive valve cultures [30]. Coagulase-negative *Staphylococcus* was the most common bacterial isolate [30]. None of these patients had clinical evidence of infection. Only 3% of patients with positive valve cultures developed PVE. Most positive native valve cultures were thought to be false positives. Campbell concluded that positive cultures did not predict PVE and recommended against routinely obtaining native valve cultures [30].

Nonetheless, the potential morbidity and mortality of PVE may justify the practice of culturing excised valve tissue and treating patients with positive cultures. Intraoperative contamination at the time of valve implantation may occur from a variety of sources. Cardiac surgical procedures are complex and entail numerous intravascular monitoring devices as well as the circuit of the cardiopulmonary bypass machine. This complexity may contribute to the incidence of positive intraoperative blood cultures. In 1969, Ankeney and Parker reported positive intraoperative blood cultures in 19% of patients undergoing open cardiac surgery [31]. In a 1974 study of 66 patients undergoing open cardiac surgery, Kluge et al. reported a 71% incidence of positive intraoperative cultures from at least one site and a 20% incidence from two or more sites [32]. Several decades later, the issue remains unresolved.

In a 2004 study of 64 patients who underwent cardiovascular surgery, Shindo et al. reported positive intraoperative blood cultures in 16% of patients who underwent cardiopulmonary bypass [33]. Intraoperative blood salvage is routinely used in cardiac surgical procedures to avoid homologous blood transfusion. Autotransfusion is associated with lower risk of hypersensitivity reactions and infections compared to transfusion of homologous blood [33]. However, intraoperative blood salvage is associated with a high incidence of positive cultures. Shindo et al. reported positive blood cultures in 67% of cases using intraoperative blood salvage, excluding cardiopulmonary bypass [33]. In a 1992 study of 31 patients, Bland et al. reported positive cultures in 97% of cases using intraoperative blood salvage [34]. In a 1999 study of 10 patients by Reents et al., 90% of cases using a cell-saving device had bacterial contamination [35].

Hemodialysis has also been associated with endocarditis, particularly with the increasing prevalence of dialysis dependence. In a study of 329 patients with endocarditis by Cabell et al., 20.4% were hemodialysis dependent [36]. Hemodialysis was independently associated with the development of *Staphylococcus aureus* endocarditis. The frequency of hemodialysis dependence also significantly increased during the 7-year study period, from 6.7 to 21% [36]. There was a corresponding significant increase in *Staphylococcus aureus* endocarditis during the study period, from 10 to 68.4% [36]. The prognosis of endocarditis in hemodialysis patients is poor, with in-hospital death rates of 25–45% and 1-year death rates of 46–75% [37].

Healthcare-associated infections are a significant source of PVE, accounting for 10–34% of all cases [38]. The majority of cases of healthcare-associated PVE develop more than 72 h following hospital admission [38]. The source of healthcare-associated PVE is frequently an intravascular device, such as a pacemaker or implantable cardioverter defibrillator. PVE is classified as healthcare-associated if it occurs within 1 year of device insertion [38].

4. Type of prosthesis

The incidence of PVE in mechanical and bioprosthetic valves is comparable [39]. Patients with mechanical prostheses have a higher risk of PVE in the first 3 months following valve replacement than those with bioprostheses [19]. The reason for higher risk of PVE in the early postoperative period with mechanical prostheses is unclear. Allografts lack prosthetic material and have a very low incidence of PVE in the early postoperative period. This suggests that mechanical prostheses have a tendency to develop early PVE, attributed to surface contamination at the time of surgery [19].

PVE in mechanical and bioprosthetic valves differs in anatomic involvement [40]. Infection of mechanical valves involves the junction between the sewing ring and annulus. This leads to the development of perivalvular abscesses, valve dehiscence, pseudoaneurysms, and fistulas. In comparison, infection of bioprosthetic valves is localized to the leaflets, leading to vegetations, cusp rupture, and perforation [40]. Endocarditis after mitral valve repair is rare. In a study of 30 patients, Gillinov et al. reported only 3% of cases of failed mitral valve repair as being caused by endocarditis [41]. In a study of 1275 mitral valve repairs over a 9-year period, Karavas et al. reported a 0.7% incidence of mitral valve endocarditis requiring surgical intervention [42]. The reason for this low incidence is likely related to less prosthetic material for potential infection with mitral valve repair than replacement.

4.1. Aortic valve prosthetic valve endocarditis

Aortic PVE is associated with substantial early morbidity and mortality. Regardless of the type of infected valve, mechanical or bioprosthetic, extensive tissue destruction may complicate aortic PVE. In a 20-year study of surgical treatment of aortic PVE by Perrotta et al., perivalvular abscess was reported in 83% of patients [43]. Comparably, Sabik et al. reported a 78% abscess rate in 103 patients with aortic PVE [44]. Abscess formation may be complicated by pseudoaneurysm and fistulisation [40]. Complete aortoventricular discontinuity has been reported in 40% of patients with aortic PVE [44]. Medical therapy alone has been associated with mortality rates as high as 70%, improved to 4–20% with surgical intervention. Significant risk factors for mortality include older age, higher preoperative creatinine, shorter interval from initial valve operation to reoperation for PVE, and fistula development. Mortality results from sepsis and multiple organ failure [44].

Aortic PVE is characterized by varying degrees of annular involvement. Extension of infection into the annular and periannular structures is a major determinant of both early and late surgical outcomes. The extent of valvular destruction relates to the virulence of the infecting organism and the duration of infection [45]. The inflammatory process of aortic PVE begins at the prosthetic sewing ring and extends through the aortic annulus, commonly in the region of aortomitral continuity [46]. The spectrum of periannular infection ranges from simple localized abscess to larger subannular aneurysm, with or without perforation into adjacent cardiac chambers. Progressive periannular infection may disrupt aortoventricular continuity or the aortomitral trigone, leading to intracardiac fistulae [44].

The goals of surgical intervention for aortic PVE include [44]:

1. complete debridement of infected and nonviable tissue,

2. repair of associated cardiac defects,

3. reconstruction of the aortic root, and

4. placement of a competent valve.

Reconstruction is complicated by severe destruction of the aortic root seen in PVE, characterized by development of abscesses, fistulas, aortoventricular discontinuity, and ventricular septal defects [47]. Achievement of the goals of surgical intervention for aortic PVE may require radical cardiac debridement. Failure to adhere to these principles poses significant risk for recurrent infection and valve dehiscence.

Following complete debridement, appropriate surgical reconstruction is guided by specific circumstances. In the majority of cases, an aortic root replacement is indicated [48]. A tension-free repair, excluding attenuated areas from high pressures, is essential [48]. If necessary, transmural sutures may be used to secure the conduit to the interventricular crest. Surgical principles dictate minimal use of synthetic material in the infected area. Aortic homograft is considered the replacement valve-conduit of choice in the treatment of aortic PVE [49]. Homograft vascular tissue is significantly more resistant to infection than prosthetic material. Aortic root replacement with homograft minimizes prosthetic material in the area of infection, thereby reducing risk of recurrent infection. The incidence of reinfection is low, ranging from 0 to 6.8% [49].

The use of allograft provides greater flexibility in the reconstruction of debrided areas [50]. Implantation may exclude abscess cavities from circulation by sewing the proximal anastomosis of the allograft to the inferior border of the abscess cavity [50]. Use of an aortic homograft with its attached mitral leaflet is particularly valuable in this regard [51].

The Ross operation, using pulmonary allograft, has been proposed as an alternative surgical option for the treatment of complex aortic PVE [51]. An initial study in 1994 by Joyce et al. of pulmonary allograft replacement reported success in six patients between 10 and 32 years of age with aortic valve endocarditis, with no mortality or reinfection [52]. In 2002, a retrospective study of 343 patients who underwent the Ross procedure by Takkenberg et al. reported low operative mortality, but limited durability due to progressive dilation of the autograft root causing severe aortic valve regurgitation [53]. The Ross procedure is typically performed in critically ill patients and is used very selectively in PVE.

Morbidity and mortality associated with allograft aortic root replacement in the setting of PVE with involvement of the periannular region is significant [54]. A retrospective study of 32 patients with complicated aortic PVE who underwent allograft aortic root replacement by Dossche et al. reported annular abscess in 81%, aortomitral discontinuity in 43%, and aortoventricular discontinuity in 34%. There was a 9.4% operative mortality rate in this study, attributed to multiple organ failure and low cardiac output. The reported 5-year survival rate was 97.3%, and 5-year freedom from recurrent endocarditis was 96.5% [54]. As described, Sabik et al. reported similar rates of periannular abscess and aortoventricular discontinuity at 78 and 40%, respectively [44]. Reconstruction with cryopreserved allograft was associated with an in-hospital mortality rate of 3.9% in this study. Long-term survival rates at 1, 2, 5, and 10 years were 90, 86, 73, and 56%, respectively. Only 3.9% of patients required reoperation for recurrent PVE; 95% were free of recurrent PVE at 2 years [44].

Despite the advantages provided by allografts in the treatment of aortic PVE, their availability is limited. This has led to the use of mechanical valve-conduits for aortic root reconstruction with excellent results in the treatment of aortic PVE. Hagl et al. reported favorable results in a retrospective study of 28 patients who underwent aortic root replacement for PVE using prosthetic material rather than homograft [55]. Reported in-hospital mortality was 11%, and the incidence of recurrent endocarditis requiring reoperation was only 4% [55].

A study of 127 patients by Avierinos et al. compared the treatment of aortic endocarditis with aortic homograft in 43% and with conventional prosthesis in 57% [56]. In-hospital mortality was comparable between homograft and prosthesis at 11 and 8%, respectively. Prosthetic valve endocarditis was the only variable independently associated with in-hospital mortality. This mortality rate was not influenced by the type of valvular substitute, even in cases of annular abscess. There was no significant difference in endocarditis recurrence, prosthesis dysfunction, or cardiovascular mortality between aortic homograft and prosthesis at 10 years [56].

Aortic root replacement with stentless porcine xenografts has been developed as a surgical alternative in aortic PVE [57]. The stentless valve provides flexibility in reconstruction of the debrided myocardium. However, it places prosthetic material in the infected area, risking infection of the prosthetic valve-conduit. A study of 132 patients who underwent aortic root replacement with stentless porcine xenografts by LeMaire et al. reported a 7.6% mortality rate. There was a 6.8% incidence of late valve-related complications, including prosthetic endocarditis and annular pseudoaneurysm [57]. Reconstruction with cryopreserved allograft remains the preferred surgical strategy.

In addition to the difficulty associated with extensive resection of the prosthetic valve-conduit and surrounding tissue, two particular challenges must be overcome to replace the infected valve-conduit. The first challenge is reimplantation of the coronary artery ostia into the allograft. Scarring from the initial procedure may make it difficult to effectively mobilize the left and right main coronary ostia for anastomosis to the allograft without undue tension. Raanani et al. described surgical reconstruction of the left main coronary artery using an autologous pericardial or saphenous vein patch [58]. The second challenge is achieving adequate resection and debridement of the distal graft-to-aorta anastomosis, which may require deep hypothermia and circulatory arrest. Furthermore, an allograft may not have sufficient length to reach the distal aortic anastomosis. Sabik et al. described the use of a second allograft to bridge the distance between the first allograft and the aorta [44].

High operative mortality rates have been reported for the replacement of infected valve-conduits, attributed to the degree of surgical difficulty. In a study of 11 patients with infected ascending aortic grafts who underwent composite valve graft placement by LeMaire and Coselli in 2007, a 30-day mortality rate of 46% was reported [59]. In comparison, a study of 12 patients who underwent composite replacement of the aortic valve and ascending aorta for infective endocarditis by Ralph-Edwards et al. reported an operative survival rate of 91.7% [60]. In this series, extensive debridement was performed, often requiring resection of the infected portion of the left ventricular outflow tract with circumferential reconstruction using bovine pericardium. It was often necessary to extend the length of the coronary arteries with saphenous vein or expanded polytetrafluoroethylene grafts to facilitate reimplantation as well [60]. As described, in a study of 23 patients who underwent ascending aorta and aortic valve replacement with the prosthetic material for acute PVE, Hagl et al. reported an 11% in-hospital mortality rate and a 4% incidence of recurrent endocarditis requiring reoperation at 4 months [55].

4.2. Mitral prosthetic valve endocarditis

Endocarditis is rare after mitral valve repair. The rate of freedom from endocarditis at 10 years following mitral valve repair is estimated at 95–99% [61]. Although native valve endocarditis can often be managed medically, PVE typically requires early operation. In a study of 22 patients with endocarditis after mitral valve repair by Gillinov et al., 68.1% underwent repeat mitral valve operations. Mitral valve replacement was required in 73.3%, and rerepair was performed in 26.7%. Following reoperation, 30-day, 1-year, and 5-year rates of freedom from reoperation were 65, 41, and 26%, respectively [61]. The principles of surgical management include the removal of all infected and devitalized tissue as well as the removal of the annuloplasty ring. If rerepair is not possible, replacement is necessary. Destruction of the mitral annular region is less common than periaortic annular destruction. Surgical debridement and resection of abscess formation in the posterior mitral annulus or in the region of aortomitral continuity is a significant surgical challenge, associated with a high operative mortality.

The mitral annulus may be reconstructed with autologous pericardium after debridement, as described by David and Feindel [62]. If the posterior mitral annular region requires reconstruction, this may be done with pericardium as well [15]. If necessary, the new mitral prosthesis may be translocated onto either the atrial or ventricular side of the annulus. If technically feasible, ventricular translocation may prevent exposure of the attenuated area to high pressure [15]. Aortomitral discontinuity is uncommon and particularly difficult to reconstruct. This trigonal region may be reconstructed using a modification of the technique described by Rastan et al. [63].

5. Operations with recent stroke

Neurologic sequelae occur in 25–70% of cases of infective endocarditis and portend increased mortality [64]. The mechanisms of neurologic injury include ischemic infarction secondary to embolization, hemorrhagic transformation of ischemic infarction, pyogenic arteritis, and rupture of intracranial mycotic aneurysm [65]. Systemic embolization occurs in 12.9% of patients with left-sided endocarditis after initiation of antibiotic therapy [66]. Of those with embolic events, 52% affect the central nervous system, and 65% occur within 2 weeks of initiation of antibiotic therapy [66]. Risk factors for embolization include vegetation size and mobility [66, 67]. There is no significant difference in incidence of embolization between native and prosthetic valve endocarditis. The risk of embolization is higher in mitral endocarditis than in aortic endocarditis [66].

The most common neurologic complication is ischemic stroke [65]. From a surgical perspective, the primary concern is hemorrhagic transformation of an ischemic infarct as a consequence of anticoagulation required during cardiopulmonary bypass [65]. Asymptomatic cerebral infarctions may occur in 30–40% of patients with endocarditis [64]. For this reason, it may be advisable to exclude an ischemic stroke with preoperative computed tomography. Clinically, silent or small infarcts should not delay cardiac surgery, since the risk of progression is low [64]. However, with the evidence of larger infarcts or intracerebral hemorrhage, surgical intervention should be delayed up to 4 weeks due to the associated risk of a significant neurologic event during cardiopulmonary bypass [64]. In such patients, the need for valve replacement should be balanced with high perioperative neurologic risk.

6. Indications for surgery

While there are a variety of resources available to assist in the decision making regarding interventions for prosthetic valve endocarditis, the key principles of therapy have been advocated by both American [68, 69] and European societies [70].

1. *Indications for surgery.*[1]

- Valve dysfunction resulting in symptoms of heart failure (Class I).

- Left-sided infectious endocarditis caused by S. aureus, fungal, or other highly resistant microorganisms (Class I).

- Relapsing infection (Class IIa).

- Recurrent emboli and persistent vegetations despite appropriate antibiotic therapy (Class IIa).

---

[1]Adapted from The American Association of Thoracic Surgeons consensus statement on the management of infectious endocarditis [68].

2. *Timing of surgery.*

- Once an indication for surgery is established, the patient should be operated on within days (Class I). Earlier surgery (emergency or within 48 hours) is reasonable for patients with large, mobile vegetations (Class IIa).

- Patients should be on appropriate antibiotic therapy at the time of surgery (Class I). Once a patient is on an appropriate antibiotic regimen, further delay of surgery is unlikely to be beneficial (Class IIa).

3. *Neurologic complications and surgery for PVE.*

- An operative delay of 3 weeks or more is reasonable among patients with recent intra-cranial hemorrhage (Class IIa).

- Patients with PVE and neurologic symptoms should undergo brain imaging (Class I); it is reasonable to screen patients with left-sided IE for possible stroke or intracranial bleeding prior to operation (Class IIa).

4. *Technical considerations.*

- Aortic PVE. If the root and the annulus are preserved after radical debridement in prosthetic aortic valve IE, implantation of a new prosthetic valve (tissue or mechanical) is reasonable (Class IIa). If there is annular destruction and invasion outside the aortic root, then the root reconstruction and use of an allograft or a biologic tissue root are preferable to a prosthetic valved conduit (Class IIa).

- Mitral PVE. When there are annular destruction and invasion, the annulus is reconstructed and the new prosthetic valve anchored to the ventricular muscle or to the reconstruction patch in a way to prevent leakage and pseudoaneurysm development (Class IIa).

- Among patients on dialysis, normal indications for surgery are reasonable, but additional comorbidities must be factored into assessments of risks and outcomes (Class IIa). Shorter durability of bioprostheses and allografts may be considered in the choice of valve prostheses used (Class IIa).

7. Conclusions

Without a doubt, the incidence of native valve endocarditis is growing-the reasons for this are multifactorial and, in general, reflect a greater access to advanced cardiac surgical therapies. Sicker patients, older patients, and more patients are undergoing valve replacement surgery for an ever-expanding list of indications. Increased used of vascular access, be it for chronic electrical system therapies (i.e., pacemakers and defibrillators), medical therapies (i.e., chemotherapy, dialysis), or as an extension of intravenous substance abuse, all have contributed to a growing incidence of both native and prosthetic valve infections. Regardless, any prosthetic valve replacement leads to a life-time risk that these patients for the development of prosthetic valve infections-either as a result of their initial operation, their ongoing (and potentially worsening) comorbidities, or simply as a function of patients living longer and with a cumulative annual risk. The development of prosthetic valve endocarditis is often, and appropriately so, viewed as a catastrophic event due to its association with devastating complications (i.e., strokes), substantial risk for operative morbidity and/or mortality, and baseline comorbidities and functional status at the time of presentation. More than most other medical and surgical therapies, a timely engagement by a multidisciplinary team is crucial to the establishment of a short- and long-term treatment plan. Clearly, much like native valve endocarditis, patients with prosthetic valve infections have shown benefit from early and aggressive surgical therapies-once established indications for surgery have been met or it has been demonstrated that optimized medical therapies have failed. Such therapies, despite substantial perioperative risks, must be focused on with aggressive debridement and elimination of all prosthetic and infected material. While prolonged courses of antibiotics and nonoperative management may have a role in select patients with limited disease burden, or for those in whom surgical reintervention is deemed to be a prohibitive, it must be recognized that the risk of treatment failure in such patients often results in worse complications or premature death. In conclusion, the medical and specific surgical decisions when dealing with a prosthetic valve infection must be individualized to provide the patient with the best opportunity for a cure.

Conflict of interest

None of the authors of this chapter have any disclosures or conflicts of interest to report in the context of the material presented.

Author details

Ahmed Fayaz[1]*, Medhat Reda Nashy[1], Sarah Eapen[2] and Michael S. Firstenberg[3,4]

*Address all correspondence to: drfayaz@gmail.com

1 King Fahd Hospital of University, Khobar, Saudi Arabia

2 Summa Akron City Hospital, Akron, Ohio, United States

3 The Medical Center of Aurora, Aurora, Colorado, United States

4 Northeast Ohio Medical Universities, Rootstown, Ohio, United States

References

[1] Wang A, Athan E, Pappas MS, et al. Contemporary clinical profile and outcome of prosthetic valve endocarditis. JAMA. 2007;**297**:1354-1361

[2] Rutledge R, Kim BJ, Applebaum RE. Actuarial analysis of the risk of prosthetic valve endocarditis in 1,598 patients with mechanical and bioprosthetic valves. Archives of Surgery. 1985;**120**:469

[3] Arvay A, Lengyel M. Incidence and risk factors of prosthetic valve endocarditis. European Journal of Cardio-Thoracic Surgery. 1988;**2**:340-346

[4] McDonald JR. Acute infective endocarditis. Infectious Disease Clinics of North America. 2009;**23**:643-664

[5] Calderwood SB, Swinski LA, Waternaux CM, Karchmer AW, Buckley MJ. Risk factors for the development of prosthetic valve endocarditis. Circulation. 1985;**72**:31-37

[6] Grover FL, Cohen DJ, Oprian C, Henderson WG, Sethi G, Hammermeister KE. Determinants of the occurrence of and survival from prosthetic valve endocarditis: Experience of the veterans affairs cooperative study on valvular heart disease. The Journal of Thoracic and Cardiovascular Surgery. 1994;**108**:207-214

[7] Osler W. The Gulstonian lectures on malignant endocarditis: Lecture II. British Medical Journal. 1885;**1**:522-526

[8] Okell CC, Elliot SD. Bacteraemia and oral sepsis with special reference to the aetiology of subacute endocarditis. Lancet. 1935;**2**:869-872

[9] Starr A, Edwards ML. Mitral replacement: Clinical experience with a ball-valve prosthesis. Annals of Surgery. 1961;**154**:726-740

[10] Harken DE, Taylor WJ, Lefemine AA, et al. Aortic valve replacement with a caged ball valve. The American Journal of Cardiology. 1962;**9**:292-299

[11] Wilson WR, Jaumin PM, Danielson GK, Giuliani ER, Washington JA II, Geraci JE. Prosthetic valve endocarditis. Annals of Internal Medicine. 1975;**82**:751-756

[12] Stein PD, Harken DE, Dexter L. The nature and prevention of prosthetic valve endocarditis. American Heart Journal. 1966;**71**:393-407

[13] Lau JKH, Robles A, Cherian A, Ross DN. Surgical treatment of prosthetic endocarditis: Aortic root replacement using a homograft. The Journal of Thoracic and Cardiovascular Surgery. 1984;**97**:712-716

[14] Olinger GN, Maloney JV. Repair of left ventricular-aortic discontinuity complicating endocarditis from an aortic valve prosthesis. The Annals of Thoracic Surgery. 1977;**23**:576-577

[15] Frantz PT, Murray GF, Wilcox BR. Surgical management of left ventricular-aortic discontinuity complicating bacterial endocarditis. The Annals of Thoracic Surgery. 1980;**29**:1-7

[16] Reitz BA, Stinson EB, Watson DC, Baumgartner WA, Jamieson SW. Translocation of the aortic valve for prosthetic valve endocarditis. The Journal of Thoracic and Cardiovascular Surgery. 1981;**81**:212-218

[17] Symbas PN, Vlasis SE, Zacharopoulos L, Lutz JF. Acute endocarditis: Surgical treatment of aortic regurgitation and aortico-left ventricular discontinuity. The Journal of Thoracic and Cardiovascular Surgery. 1982;**84**:291-296

[18] David TE, Feindel CM, Armstrong S, Sun Z. Reconstruction of the mitral annulus. A ten-year experience. The Journal of Thoracic and Cardiovascular Surgery. 1995;**10**:1323-1332

[19] Ivert TSA, Dismukes WE, Cobbs CG, Blackstone EH, Kirklin JW, Bergdahl LAL. Prosthetic valve endocarditis. Circulation. 1984;**69**:223-232

[20] Gnann JW, Dismukes WE. Prosthetic valve endocarditis: An overview. Herz. 1983;**8**: 320-331

[21] Tornos P. Management of prosthetic valve endocarditis: A clinical challenge. Heart. 2003;**89**:245-246

[22] Nonaka M, Kusuhara T, An K, et al. Comparison between early and late prosthetic valve endocarditis: Clinical characteristics and outcomes. The Journal of Heart Valve Disease. 2013;**22**:567-574

[23] Fang G, Keys TF, Gentry LO, et al. Prosthetic valve endocarditis resulting from noso-comial bacteremia: A prospective, multicenter study. Annals of Internal Medicine. 1993;**119**:560-567

[24] Mermel LA. Prevention of intravascular catheter-related infections. Annals of Internal Medicine. 2000;**132**:391-402

[25] Conway LJ, Liu J, Harris AD, Larson EL. Risk factors for bacteremia in patients with urinary catheter-associated bacteriuria. American Journal of Critical Care. 2016;**26**:43-52

[26] Parker FB, Greiner-Hayes C, Tomar RH, Markowitz AH, Bove EL, Marvasti MA. Bacte-remia following prosthetic valve replacement. Annals of Surgery. 1983;**197**:147-151

[27] Murray RJ. *Staphylococcus aureus* infective endocarditis: Diagnosis and management guidelines. Internal Medicine Journal. 2005;**35**:S25-S44

[28] Nguyen MH, Nguyen ML, Yu VL, McMahon D, Keys TF, Amidi M. Candida prosthetic valve endocarditis: Prospective study of six cases and review of the literature. Clinical Infectious Diseases. 1996;**22**:262-267

[29] Nasser RM, Melgar GR, Longworth DL, Gordon SM. Incidence and risk of develop-ing fungal prosthetic valve endocarditis after nosocomial candidemia. The American Journal of Medicine. 1997;**103**:23-32

[30] Campbell WN, Tsai W, Mispireta LA. Evaluation of the practice of routine culturing of native valves during valve replacement surgery. The Annals of Thoracic Surgery. 2000;**69**:548-550

[31] Ankeney JL, Parker RF. *Staphylococcal endocarditis* following open heart surgery related to positive intraoperative blood cultures. In: Brewer LA III, editor. Prosthetic Heart Valves. Springfield, IL: Charles C Thomas; 1969. pp. 719-730

[32] Kluge RM, Calia FM, McLaughlin JA, et al. Sources of contamination in open heart surgery. JAMA. 1974;**230**:1415-1418

[33] Shindo S, Matsumoto H, Kubota K, Kojima A, Matsumoto M. Temporary bacteremia due to intraoperative blood salvage during cardiovascular surgery. American Journal of Surgery. 2004;**188**:237-239

[34] Bland MA, Villarino ME, Arduino MJ, et al. Bacteriologic and endotoxin analysis of salvaged blood used in autologous transfusions during cardiac surgery. The Journal of Thoracic and Cardiovascular Surgery. 1992;**103**:582-588

[35] Reents W, Babin-Ebell J, Misoph MR, Schwarzkopf A, Elert O. Influence of different autotransfusion devices on the quality of salvaged blood. The Annals of Thoracic Surgery. 1999;**68**:58-62

[36] Cabell CH, Jollis JG, Peterson GE, et al. Changing patient characteristics and the effect on mortality in endocarditis. Archives of Internal Medicine. 2002;**162**:90-94

[37] Hoen B. Infective endocarditis: A frequent disease in dialysis patients. Nephrology, Dialysis, Transplantation. 2004;**19**:1360-1362

[38] Francischetto O, Silva LA, Senna KM, et al. Healthcare-associated infective endocarditis: A case series in a referral hospital from 2006 to 2011. Arquivos Brasileiros de Cardiologia. 2014;**103**:292-298

[39] Sidhu P, O'Kane H, Ali N, et al. Mechanical or bioprosthetic valves in the elderly: A 20-year comparison. The Annals of Thoracic Surgery. 2001;**71**:S257-S260

[40] Habib G, Badano L, Tribouilloy C, et al. Recommendations for the practice of echocardiography in infective endocarditis. European Journal of Echocardiography. 2010;**11**:202-219

[41] Gillinov AM, Cosgrove DM, Blackstone EH, et al. Durability of mitral valve repair for degenerative disease. The Journal of Thoracic and Cardiovascular Surgery. 1998;**116**: 734-743

[42] Karavas AN, Filsoufi F, Mihaljevic T, Aranki SF, Cohn LH, Byrne JG. Risk factors and management of endocarditis after mitral valve repair. The Journal of Heart Valve Disease. 2002;**11**:660-664

[43] Perrotta S, Jeppsson A, Frojd V, Svensson G. Surgical treatment of aortic prosthetic valve endocarditis: A 20-year single-center experience. The Annals of Thoracic Surgery. 2016;**101**:1426-1433

[44] Sabik JF, Lytle BW, Blackstone EH, Marullo AGM, Pettersson GB, Cosgrove DM. Aortic root replacement with cryopreserved allograft for prosthetic valve endocarditis. The Annals of Thoracic Surgery. 2002;**74**:650-659

[45] Martinez G, Valchanov K. Infective endocarditis. Continuing Education in Anaesthesia, Critical Care & Pain. 2012;**12**:134-139

[46] Akay MH, Danch MA, Cohn WE, Frazier OH. Reconstruction of the fibrous trigone. Texas Heart Institute Journal. 2009;**36**:475-476

[47] Kang N, Wan S, Ng CSH, Underwood MJ. Periannular extension of infective endocardi-tis. Annals of Thoracic and Cardiovascular Surgery. 2009;**15**:74-81

[48] Mahesh B, Angelini G, Caputo M, Jin XY, Bryan A. Prosthetic valve endocarditis. The Annals of Thoracic Surgery. 2005;**80**:1151-1158

[49] Perrotta S, Zubrytska Y. Valve selection in aortic valve endocarditis. Polish Journal of Thoracic and Cardiovascular Surgery. 2016;**13**:203-209

[50] Kirklin JK, Kirklin JW, Pacifico AD. Aortic valve endocarditis with aortic root abscess cavity: Surgical treatment with aortic valve homograft. The Annals of Thoracic Surgery. 1988;**45**:674-677

[51] Lopes S, Calvinho P, Oliveira F, Antunes M. Allograft aortic root replacement in complex prosthetic endocarditis. European Journal of Cardio-Thoracic Surgery. 2007;**32**:125-132

[52] Joyce F, Tingleff J, Aagaard J, Pettersson G. The Ross operation in the treatment of native and prosthetic aortic valve endocarditis. The Journal of Heart Valve Disease. 1994;**3**:371-376

[53] Takkenberg JJM, Dossche KME, Hazekamp MG, et al. Report of the Dutch experience with the Ross procedure in 323 patients. European Journal of Cardio-Thoracic Surgery. 2002;**22**:70-77

[54] Dossche KM, Defauw JJ, Ernst SM, et al. Allograft aortic root replacement in prosthetic aortic valve endocarditis: A review of 32 patients. The Annals of Thoracic Surgery. 1997;**63**:1644-1649

[55] Hagl C, Gall JD, Lansman SL. Replacing the ascending aorta and aortic valve for acute prosthetic valve endocarditis: Is using prosthetic material contraindicated? The Annals of Thoracic Surgery. 2002;**74**:S1781-S1785

[56] Avierinos JF, Thuny F, Chalvignac V, et al. Surgical treatment of active aortic endocar-ditis: Homografts are not the cornerstone of outcome. The Annals of Thoracic Surgery. 2007;**84**:1935-1942

[57] LeMaire SA, Green SY, Sharma K, et al. Aortic root replacement with stentless porcine xenografts: Early and late outcomes in 132 patients. The Annals of Thoracic Surgery. 2009;**87**:503-513

[58] Raanani E, Kogan A, Shapira Y, Sagie A, Kornowski R, Vidne BA. Surgical reconstruc-tion of the left main coronary artery: Fresh autologous pericardium or saphenous vein patch. The Annals of Thoracic Surgery. 2004;**78**:1610-1613

[59] LeMaire SA, Coselli JS. Options for managing infected ascending aortic grafts. The Journal of Thoracic and Cardiovascular Surgery. 2007;**134**:839-843

[60] Ralph-Edwards A, David TE, Bos J. Infective endocarditis in patients who had replace-ment of the aortic root. The Annals of Thoracic Surgery. 1994;**58**:429-433

[61] Gillinov AM, Faber CN, Sabik JF, et al. Endocarditis after mitral valve repair. The Annals of Thoracic Surgery. 2002;**73**:1813-1816

[62] David TE, Feindel CM, Ropchan GV. Reconstruction of the left ventricle with autologous pericardium. The Journal of Thoracic and Cardiovascular Surgery. 1987;**94**:710-714

[63] Rastan D. Aortic and aortic-mitral annular enlargement. The Journal of Thoracic and Cardiovascular Surgery. 1996;**109**:818-819

[64] Morris NA, Matiello M, Lyons JL, Samuels MA. Neurologic complications in infective endocarditis: Identification, management, and impact on cardiac surgery. The Neurohospitalist. 2014;**4**:213-222

[65] Masuda J, Yutani C, Waki R, Ogata J, Kuriyama Y, Yamaguchi T. Histopathological analysis of the mechanisms of intracranial hemorrhage complicating infective endocarditis. Stroke. 1992;**23**:843-850

[66] Vilacosta I, Graupner C, San Román JA, et al. Risk of embolization after institution of antibiotic therapy for infective endocarditis. Journal of the American College of Cardiology. 2002;**39**:1489-1495

[67] Deprèle C, Berthelot P, Lemetayer F, et al. Risk factors for systemic emboli in infective endocarditis. Clinical Microbiology and Infection. 2004;**10**:46-53

[68] Pettersson GB, Coselli JS, Hussain ST, Griffin B, Blackstone EH, Gordon SM, LeMaire SA, Woc-Colburn LE. 2016 The American Association for Thoracic Surgery (AATS) consensus guidelines: surgical treatment of infective endocarditis: Executive summary. The Journal of Thoracic and Cardiovascular Surgery. 2017;**153**(6):1241-1258

[69] Baddour LM, Wilson WR, Bayer AS, Fowler VG, Tleyjeh IM, Rybak MJ, Barsic B, Lockhart PB, Gewitz MH, Levison ME, Bolger AF. Infective endocarditis in adults: Diagnosis, antimicrobial therapy, and management of complications: A scientific statement for healthcare professionals from the American Heart Association. Circulation. 2015;**132**(15):1435-1486

[70] Habib G, Lancellotti P, Antunes MJ, Bongiorni MG, Casalta JP, Del Zotti F, Dulgheru R, El Khoury G, Erba PA, Iung B, Miro JM. 2015 ESC guidelines for the management of infective endocarditis: the task force for the management of infective endocarditis of the European Society of Cardiology (ESC) endorsed by: European Association for Cardio-Thoracic Surgery (EACTS), the European Association of Nuclear Medicine (EANM). European Heart Journal. 2015;**36**(44):3075-3128

6

Antibiotic Prophylactic Regimens for Infective Endocarditis in Patients Undergoing Dental Procedures

Miguel Castro, Javier Álvarez, Javier F. Feijoo,
Marcio Diniz, Lucía García-Caballero, Pedro Diz and
Jacobo Limeres

Abstract

Up to date causal relationship has been demonstrated between dental manipulations and the onset of infective endocarditis (IE). However, since 1955, numerous expert committees have proposed antibiotic prophylaxis (AP) to prevent bacteraemia of oral origin. Controversy regarding the efficacy of AP prior to the dental procedures has intensified in recent years because of the lack of conclusive evidence on its efficacy for the prevention of IE and on its cost-effectiveness, as well as the possibility of allergic reactions and the emergence of antibiotic resistance. Accordingly, AP is now maintained exclusively for patients at highest risk and who require the manipulation of the gingival or periapical regions of the teeth or perforation of the oral mucosa. In the context of a restrictive policy, the National Institute for Health and Clinical Excellence (NICE) of the United Kingdom published a new guideline in 2008 stating that "AP against IE is not recommended for persons undergoing dental procedures", regardless of risk status and of the nature of the procedure to be performed. The NICE guideline has generated further controversy, and expert committees in other countries continue to publish prophylactic regimens for the prevention of IE secondary to dental procedures. In this chapter, we discuss the principal guidelines currently applicable in Europe, the USA and Australia, and we draw particular attention to the need for randomised clinical trials.

Keywords: infective endocarditis, bacteraemia, dental procedures, dentistry, antibiotic prophylaxis

1. Historical perspectives

In 1955, the American Heart Association (AHA) was the first medical society to establish the need for a prophylactic antibiotic regimen to prevent infective endocarditis (IE) in at-risk patients undergoing various surgical procedures, including tooth extractions and other dental manipulations that affect the gum.

In the pre-antibiotic era, reports based on clinical observations described cases of IE of streptococcal aetiology in which there was a history of professional dental manipulation. This suggested the possibility that "transient bacteraemia during dental procedures may lead to subacute endocarditis in subjects with abnormal heart valves" [1].

The 1955 AHA Committee on the Prevention of Rheumatic Fever and Bacterial Endocarditis concluded that patients undergoing dental procedures must be protected by high concentrations of antibiotic present in the blood at the time of the procedure. Penicillin administered parenterally was preferred, although oral penicillin V was introduced as second choice. In cases of sensitivity to penicillin, other antibiotics such erythromycin or tetracycline were recommended [2].

Since that time, the scientific community has universally accepted the need for antibiotic prophylaxis in patients susceptible to developing IE. Experimental models developed in the 1970s provided evidence of the efficacy of prophylaxis in animals and demonstrated the ability of antibiotics to prevent *Streptococcus sanguinis* endocarditis [3]. However, the different antibiotic regimens to prevent IE in dental patients were developed based on empirical criteria.

In 1982, the British Society for Antimicrobial Chemotherapy included amoxicillin in the prophylactic antibiotic regimen against IE [4]. Amoxicillin has a broad antibacterial spectrum and a more favourable pharmacokinetic profile than penicillin V for oral administration; this has made it the drug of choice in all current guidelines on the use of antibiotics to prevent IE.

The main inclusion criteria for the prophylactic regimens established by the first committees were the rheumatic heart disease and congenital malformations, but fundamental changes have been introduced since that time regarding "patients considered to be at risk of IE". The campaigns for the prevention of rheumatic fever, the increase in the prevalence of intravenous drug abuse and the growth in cardiovascular interventions have transformed the microbiological patterns of IE, with a relative decrease in the incidence of streptococcal endocarditis and a significant increase in endocarditis due to staphylococci and other less common organisms.

These changes make it difficult to draw reliable epidemiological conclusions on the efficacy of antibiotics for the prevention of IE. In general, the majority of studies indicate that, despite the universal implantation of antibiotic prophylaxis prior to the dental treatment, no global reduction in the prevalence of IE has been achieved [5].

This has been one of the main arguments put forward by the British health authorities to revoke the indications for antibiotic prophylaxis in patients undergoing dental, digestive tract or genitourinary interventions. A few years ago, the National Institute for Health and Clinical

Excellence (NICE) in the United Kingdom published a proposal that surprised the scientific community by considering that "antibiotic prophylaxis for IE was not recommended for persons undergoing dental treatment". This recommendation was even applicable to "high-risk patients, independently of the type of dental procedure they were to undergo" [6].

This scepticism of the British health authorities to the prophylactic efficacy of antibiotics in IE is not shared by other scientific societies, which continue to include antibiotic cover for dental procedures in patients at risk of developing IE.

Epidemiological observations and statistical analyses made after the cessation of prophylaxis in the United Kingdom suggest the need for antibiotic cover in patients at maximum risk of IE of poor prognosis. In this setting, current guidelines maintain the need for prevention for patients considered to be at high risk of developing IE, such as individuals with prosthetic heart valves, the presence of certain congenital cardiopathies and patients who have had a previous episode of IE.

2. Impact of the nice recommendations

In the controversial document published in 2008, NICE brought about the complete cessation of antibiotic prophylaxis for all patients at risk of IE undergoing dental interventions [6]. The main premises on which the British experts based this decision was the quantifiable risk of antibiotic administration to the individual patient, the potential appearance of unnecessary antimicrobial resistance and the economic analysis of the cost-effectiveness of prophylaxis.

The recommendation was based on the limited available evidence on antibiotic prophylaxis as an effective method to reduce the incidence of IE when given before an interventional procedure. Furthermore, the existence of transient bacteraemia during activities of daily living, such as toothbrushing or chewing, diminishes the significance of dental procedures as a cause of IE, making antibiotic prophylaxis virtually ineffective for preventing the disease.

Consequently, NICE did not recommend antibiotic prophylaxis against IE in persons undergoing dental procedures or digestive, respiratory or genitourinary tract interventions, except for manipulations at an infected non-dental site.

The expert committees across the rest of the world, including the AHA and the European Society of Cardiology (ESC), have continued to recommend antibiotic prophylaxis in high-risk individuals, and these protocols are followed by most cardiologists and cardiac surgeons.

The first studies on the epidemiological repercussions of the implementation of the NICE guideline showed a substantial reduction in the prescription of antibiotics in its area of influence and the data gathered showed no significant changes in the general upward trend in cases of IE [7].

In 2013, a case of IE was reported in which aetiological analysis suggested a very strong association with a previous dental intervention performed without antibiotic cover. The affected patient had a metallic aortic valve and developed a fatal episode of *S. sanguinis* endocarditis 10 days after undergoing a dental procedure without antibiotic prophylaxis, following the NICE recommendations. The dental history of the patient showed that he had received antibiotic prophylaxis during dental sessions over the previous 10 years with no adverse outcomes [8].

The most recent epidemiological studies have identified a significant increase in the incidence of IE after implementation of the NICE guideline. A retrospective study was performed in England to investigate the effect of antibiotic prophylaxis versus no prophylaxis on the incidence of IE [9]. The data collected and the subsequent analysis suggested that after March 2008—the year of publication of the NICE guideline—the number of cases of IE increased significantly above the expected historical trend.

According to some experts, these data are mainly observational and do not prove that the lower level of antibiotic prophylaxis was the cause of the increase in IE. However, no other satisfactory explanation for this increase in the incidence of IE has yet been put forward [10].

Despite this, NICE has reviewed all evidence relating to the effectiveness of IE prophylaxis as a precaution but, at present, they have found no need to change any of the existing 2008 guideline. They have, however, made an additional research recommendations on antibiotic prophylaxis against IE as summarised in **Table 1**.

Field of research	Importance
1. National register of infective endocarditis	To provide a cohort of patients able to generate sufficient evidence from well-conducted national studies
2. Cardiac conditions and infective endocarditis	To use a population-based cohort study design to allow direct comparison between acquired heart valve disease and structural congenital heart disease to estimate relative and absolute IE risk
3. Interventional procedures and infective endocarditis	To determine the frequency and intensity of bacteraemia caused by non-oral daily activities
4. Antibiotic prophylaxis against infective endocarditis	A randomised controlled trial with long-term follow-up comparing antibiotic prophylaxis with no antibiotic prophylaxis in adults and children with underlying structural heart defects undergoing interventional procedures

Note: https://nice.org.uk/guidance/CG64/chapter/Recommendations-for-research#4-antibiotic-prophylaxis-against-infective-endocarditis

Table 1. NICE recommendations for research. Antimicrobial prophylaxis against infective endocarditis in adults and children undergoing interventional procedures (updated in 2015).

3. Current antibiotic protocols

Antibiotic prophylaxis protocols against IE have undergone relevant changes in recent years. There is no doubt that the categorical 2008 NICE recommendations and their implementation in their area of influence constitute an event with significant epidemiological repercussions that will serve to evaluate the efficacy of antibiotic prophylaxis for the prevention of IE. The scientific societies responsible for this question continue detailed follow-up in order to incorporate their conclusions as relevant data arise.

Among the different prophylaxis guidelines proposed by expert committees around the world, those that represent their corresponding geographical areas stand out for their scientific relevance. In the USA, the AHA has been pioneer in the introduction of antibiotic prophylaxis against IE; its most recent guideline was published in 2007 [11]. In Australia, the Infective Endocarditis Prophylaxis Expert Group (AIEPEG) published a guideline in 2008 that has been supported by the principal health associations in its area of influence [12]. In Europe, the ESC published the 2015 review of its protocols in the European Heart Journal, stating the official position of that scientific society on this subject [13]. These three guidelines coincide on two major points:

• All propose amoxicillin as the antibiotic of choice.

• All propose clindamycin as the alternative antibiotic of choice to amoxicillin.

3.1. Amoxicillin as the antibiotic of choice for prophylaxis

The standard regimens of the three guidelines mentioned above recommend the oral administration of 2 g of amoxicillin between 30 and 60 min before a dental procedure in adults. In the case of children, the recommended dose is 50 mg/kg body weight. When oral administration is not possible, amoxicillin can be administered intramuscularly or intravenously at the same dose.

Amoxicillin was introduced into the IE prophylaxis protocols in 1982 [4] and since that time it has become the drug of choice in the prophylactic guidelines internationally. From a pharmacological point of view, amoxicillin has optimal characteristics due to its rapid absorption after administration by mouth, achieving maximum plasma concentrations within 1–2 h after ingestion, and therapeutic levels are maintained for a minimum of 6 h. Amoxicillin is highly active against streptococci and also covers anaerobes and gram-negative bacteria. It is thus effective against the majority of microorganisms present in bacteraemia of oral origin. However, it is considered that between 5 and 35% of the microorganisms detected in blood cultures from patients undergoing dental treatment can be resistant to the antibiotic. This finding, together with the increased prevalence of IE caused by penicillin-resistant staphylococci and other unusual microorganisms, could justify the introduction of antibiotics other than amoxicillin into standard prophylaxis protocols in the future in order to improve the antimicrobial spectrum in certain circumstances.

3.2. Alternative drugs to amoxicillin

The three guidelines incorporate cephalosporins for parenteral administration as an alternative to amoxicillin. The cephalosporins are also recommended in patients with penicillin allergy, though this proposal is accompanied by a warning that the use of cephalosporins is contraindicated in individuals with a history of anaphylaxis.

About 10% of patients attending dental consultations are allergic to penicillin and its derivatives, although a large majority of these reported allergic reactions are no more than minor side-effects or late hypersensitivity reactions presenting as pruritus or rash, but not IgE-mediated. Urticaria (hives) is IgE-mediated; it only accounts for 10% of all exanthematous drug reactions, but may be interpreted as a clinical sign of immediate hypersensitivity that could progress to an episode of acute (fulminant) anaphylaxis.

The main antigenic determinant of the anaphylactic reaction to penicillins is the β-lactam ring, a part of the molecule that is essential for its bactericidal activity and that also forms part of the chemical structure of the cephalosporins and clavulanates (clavulanic acid), among others. Drug-related anaphylaxis is a life-threatening medical emergency and, as a result, the administration of β-lactam drugs is contraindicated in patients who give a history of penicillin allergy until such time as allergy testing establishes the true risk of anaphylaxis in each individual case [14].

The three main guidelines coincide on the oral or intravenous administration of 600 mg of clindamycin as the antibiotic of choice in patients allergic to penicillins (**Table 2**). Clindamycin has intrinsic in vitro activity against streptococci, staphylococci and anaerobes, it rarely causes allergic reactions and it has a low incidence of side-effects, making it an ideal alternative antibiotic based on its antimicrobial spectrum and biosafety. However, some authors have demonstrated that it is ineffective in preventing bacteraemia following dental procedures [15].

Australia (AIEPEG)	Europe (ESC)	USA (AHA)
Clindamycin	Clindamycin	Clindamycin
Lincomycin		Azithromycin
Vancomycin		Clarithromycin
Teicoplanin		

Abbreviations: AIEPEG, Australian Infective Endocarditis Prophylaxis Expert Group; ESC, European Society of Cardiology; AHA, American Heart Association.

Table 2. Alternative antibiotics for prophylaxis against infective endocarditis in patients allergic to penicillins and their derivatives.

The 2007 AHA guideline describes in great detail specific situations that could require changes to the application of the prophylactic regimens in clinical practice. For example, intramuscular injections should be avoided in patients receiving anticoagulants. In patients attending the dental clinic whilst on treatment with penicillins for other causes, it is preferable to delay dental therapy for at least 10 days; it is accepted that viridans group streptococci in the oral cavity of patients on long-term antibiotic therapy could be relatively resistant to penicillin or amoxicillin, and the cessation of antibiotic therapy allows the usual oral flora to be re-established. When the dental intervention cannot be postponed, the health professional should select a different class of antibiotic rather than increase the dose of the current antibiotic; options include clindamycin, azithromycin and clarithromycin, though only for patients with the highest-risk cardiac conditions [11].

Azithromycin and clarithromycin are macrolides with similar activity to erythromycin on the oral streptococci, but they show better gastrointestinal tolerance and a more favourable pharmacokinetic profile. Erythromycin is unstable under acidic gastric conditions, shows poor absorption and has a limited spectrum of activity. Azithromycin, on the other hand, causes fewer gastrointestinal side-effects, rapidly reaches high tissue concentrations and displays a better antibacterial spectrum, making it a good candidate for IE prophylaxis [16].

The Australian guideline includes a parenteral regimen of lincomycin, vancomycin or teicoplanin for patients with penicillin hypersensitivity and for those on long-term penicillin therapy or who have taken penicillin or related β-lactam antibiotics more than once in the previous month [12].

Finally, the ESC guideline is the most restrictive, recommending clindamycin as the only alternative antibiotic. In contrast to the proposal of the Australian expert committee, the European guideline states that the glycopeptides, such as vancomycin and teicoplanin, are not recommended because their efficacy has not been fully demonstrated and there is a potential for the induction of resistance [13].

4. At-risk patients

In its conclusions, the 2007 AHA guideline states that IE prophylaxis for dental procedures is a reasonable practice only for patients with underlying heart conditions associated with the highest risk of an adverse outcome [11]. New pathophysiological concepts and risk-benefit analyses justify the current tendency of the scientific community towards more limited indications for antibiotic prophylaxis in IE (**Table 3**).

1.	Bacteraemia occurs repeatedly and frequently during routine daily activities such as toothbrushing, flossing or chewing, and even more frequently in patients with poor dental health.
2.	Most case-control studies did not report an association between invasive dental procedures and the occurrence of infective endocarditis.
3.	The estimated risk of infective endocarditis following dental procedures is very low.
4.	Although antibiotic administration carries a small risk of anaphylaxis, it may become significant in the event of widespread use.
5.	Widespread use of antibiotics may result in the emergence of resistant microorganisms.
6.	Although efficacy of antibiotic prophylaxis on bacteraemia and the occurrence of infective endocarditis has been proven in animal models, the effect on bacteraemia in humans is controversial.
7.	No prospective randomised controlled trial has investigated the efficacy of antibiotic prophylaxis on the occurrence of infective endocarditis.

Table 3. Arguments for the restriction of the indication for prophylaxis against infective endocarditis [13].

Epidemiological evidence also supports this restrictive policy, as the incidence of IE and its associated mortality have not varied in recent decades despite the use of antibiotic prophylaxis. At the present time, we are seeing an increase in the number of cases of IE due to *Staphylococcus aureus* and of unknown aetiology and a fall in the incidence of cases of IE of streptococcal aetiology [17]. This has occurred despite the evident, considerable increase in the number of dental interventions and in the ratio of dentists to population in recent years.

In this context and awaiting relevant new data, NICE in the UK continues its recommendation to universally cease antibiotic prophylaxis for medical interventions, although the majority of cardiologists and cardiac surgeons consider antibiotic prophylaxis necessary for patients at highest risk of adverse outcomes from endocarditis [9].

- Isolated secundum atrial septal defect.
- Surgical repair of atrial septal defect, ventricular septal defect, or patent ductus arteriosus (without residua beyond 6 months).
- Previous coronary artery bypass graft surgery.
- Mitral valve prolapse without valvar regurgitation.
- Physiologic, functional or innocent heart murmurs.
- Previous Kawasaki disease without valvar dysfunction.
- Previous rheumatic fever without valvar dysfunction.
- Cardiac pacemakers (intravascular and epicardial) and implanted defibrillators.

Table 4. Patients in whom prophylaxis against infective endocarditis is not recommended [18].

The 1997 AHA guideline was the first to stratify cardiac conditions into high, moderate and low risk for IE [18]. AHA experts stated that the risk of suffering IE assumed by low-risk patients undergoing dental treatment could be considered negligible, no higher than in the general population, and, as a result, they recommended abolishing antibiotic prophylaxis for routine dental treatment in these patients. This 1997 recommendation was particularly helpful in clinical practice because heart murmurs, pacemakers and minor congenital defects were frequently reported by dental patients in their medical records. The establishment of a restrictive position on the part of the health authorities regarding antibiotic prophylaxis created a framework of medico-legal protection in dental practice. The 1997 AHA guideline thus provided dentists with a certain capacity to evaluate the prescription of prophylaxis in patients with a history of cardiac disease and moderate their natural tendency to prescribe universal antibiotic cover derived from a fear of missing one of the numerous indications (**Table 4**). This conceptual change was further strengthened 10 years later when the 2007 AHA committee eliminated antibiotic prophylaxis for patients considered to be in the moderate risk category in the 1997 guideline (**Table 5**), on the basis that *"previously published AHA guidelines for the prevention of IE contained ambiguities and inconsistencies and were often based on minimal published data or expert opinion, they were subject to conflicting interpretations among patients, healthcare providers, and the legal system about patient eligibility for prophylaxis and whether there was strict adherence by healthcare providers to AHA recommendations for prophylaxis"* [11].

The current result of this policy limiting the indications for antibiotic prophylaxis to the highest risk cardiac conditions is stated even more restrictively in the 2015 ESC guideline (**Table 6**). In their recommendation, the ESC excludes prophylaxis even in heart transplant recipients who develop heart valve disease; this is considered a true high-risk condition in the AHA and Australian guidelines. The Australian recommendations also include rheumatic heart disease in indigenous Australians, a population in which unusually high prevalence and mortality related to this disease have been detected [19].

- Congenital cardiac conditions

    ✓ Ductus arteriosus

    ✓ Ventricular septal defect

    ✓ Ostium primum atrial septal defect

    ✓ Coarctation of the aorta

    ✓ Bicuspid aortic valve

- Acquired valve dysfunction

    ✓ Rheumatic

    ✓ Collagen vascular disease

    ✓ Others

- Hypertrophic cardiomyopathy

- Mitral valve prolapse with valve regurgitation and/or thickened leaflets

---

Table 5. Cardiac conditions that carry a moderate risk of infective endocarditis [18].

Finally, dental surgeons show a degree of concern over the need for prophylaxis when performing dental procedures on patients with implanted cardiac devices such as pacemakers, stents and implantable defibrillators. In 2007, Lockhart et al. published an interesting literature review on this subject, revealing widely differing opinions, a situation that usually leads dentists to contact physicians for advice on management. Interestingly, most physicians, surgeons and medical specialists want their patients to receive antibiotic prophylaxis for all invasive dental procedures to prevent distant site infection of organs, tissues or prosthetic materials, and a number of them do so for medico-legal rather than scientific reasons. The majority of the literature sources agree that there is no indication for prophylaxis in patients with cardiac devices. Bacterial seeding of a graft site via a haematogenous route is an uncommon event and most of infections occurring in the first 2 months are due to *Staphylococcus* spp. and non-oral bacteria, probably as result of the manoeuvres of graft placement [20].

Based on these premises, it could be stated that patients with implantable cardiac devices may be cautiously covered with antibiotic prophylaxis exclusively during the early post-implantation period, though this is mainly for medico-legal reasons. Considering the current IE prophylaxis guidelines, there is no reason for antibiotic use during routine dental treatment in patients with implantable cardiac devices, unless individual cases present concomitant diseases that could justify such a decision.

1.	Patients with any prosthetic valve, including a transcatheter valve, or those in whom any prosthetic material was used for cardiac valve repair.
2.	Patients with a previous episode of infective endocarditis.
3.	Patients with congenital heart disease (CHD):
a.	Any type of cyanotic CHD.
b.	Any type of CHD repaired with a prosthetic material, whether placed surgically or by percutaneous techniques, up to 6 months after the procedure or lifelong if residual shunt or valvular regurgitation remains.

Table 6. Cardiac conditions associated with the highest risk of adverse outcomes of endocarditis according to the European Society of Cardiology guideline [13].

5. Risk-related dental procedures

In 1935, Okell and Elliott detected positive blood cultures in more than half of patients undergoing dental manipulations, with a particularly high prevalence among those with deficient oral health. Since that time, the relationship between bacteraemia of oral origin and dental interventions constituted proof that endocardial infection could be precipitated by oral streptococci mobilised during dental manipulation [21].

Transient bacteraemia has been widely documented as a common finding during dental procedures, associated particularly with the manipulation of teeth and periodontal tissues. Non-surgical tooth extraction is the dental procedure that most frequently provokes bacteraemia of oral origin, with a detection rate of positive blood cultures of 58–100% (**Figure 1**).

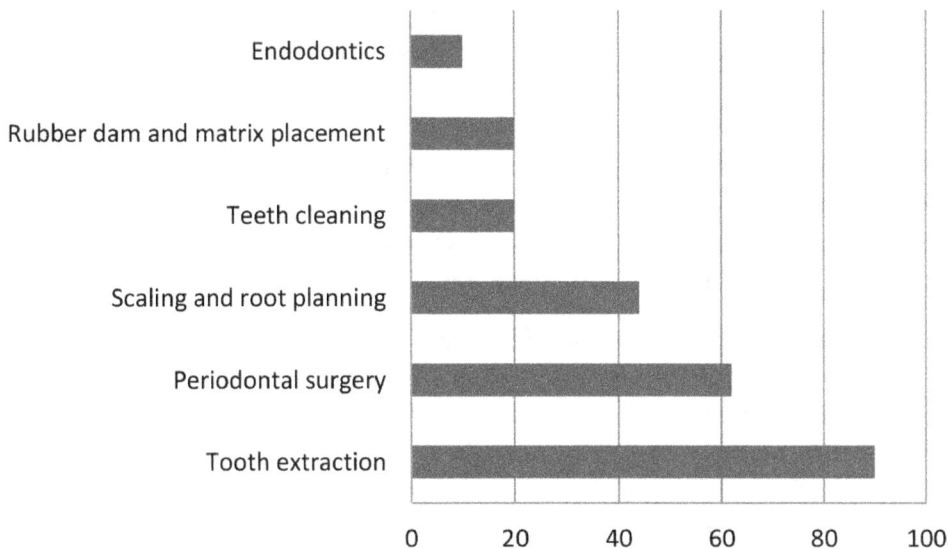

Figure 1. Prevalence of oral bacteraemia after dental procedures (inferred from [11]).

From early studies, it was generally accepted that the incidence and magnitude of bacteraemia of oral origin during dental procedures was directly proportional to the degree of inflammation and infection in the mouth. However, more recent series have found no relationship between the number of caries or the presence of periapical lesions and increased risk of post-intervention bacteraemia. Similarly, it is also accepted that the grade of gingival and periodontal health does not affect the presence or intensity of bacteraemia during interventions, and an increase in the prevalence of bacteraemia has only been demonstrated after tooth extractions in the setting of an acute infectious condition.

Studies that have investigated the bacteriological spectrum of bacteraemia of oral origin show a wide variability in their results due to the different sampling and detection techniques employed. However, *Streptococcus* spp.—the bacterial species most frequently implicated in IE of oral origin—is detected in at least 30% of cases [22]. This inoculum of streptococci that reaches the bloodstream has intrinsic pathogenic potential to colonise susceptible endocardial tissue in highest-risk patients. Structurally, streptococci have surface proteins (adhesins) that have been shown experimentally to have high affinity for the extracellular matrix, making the microorganisms capable of easily colonising vegetations and medical devices that become coated with matrix proteins after implantation. After colonisation, the bacterial biofilm acts as a propitious environment to perpetuate infection. The resulting fibrin and platelet deposition over the biofilm contributes to organise an actual bacteria-release clot which is able to create the recurrent bacteraemias that characterise IE.

A number of experimental studies have been able to reproduce these pathological events in animal models, but it remains to be seen whether oral bacteraemia secondary to dental interventions could promote identical results in humans [23].

A prospective study recently performed on patients diagnosed with IE appears to indicate that the mouth is a potential portal of entry (POE) for IE. A sample of 318 patients diagnosed with IE was examined prospectively by different specialists selected according to the natural habitat or site of colonisation of the causal diagnosed microorganism. A potential oral POE was detected by a stomatologist in 68 cases (21%), of which only 12% were considered possibly related to previous professional manipulation. Interestingly, the highest percentage of patients (88%) with oral and dental POEs was therefore made up of patients with no history of dental interventions. It was assumed that these patients presented a deficient state of oral health in the form of dental, endodontal or periodontal infection (**Table 7**).

These results agree strongly with those of Lockhart et al. [11] who presented a comparative study on the presence of bacteraemia in patients undergoing tooth extractions and toothbrushing. They found that the risk of oral bacteraemia was significantly associated with poor oral hygiene during toothbrushing. However, they did not find any association in the extraction group, even when performed without antibiotic cover. This is consistent with statements that patients at risk of IE have greater exposure to the action of oral bacteria during activities of daily living, such as toothbrushing or chewing, particularly if the individual has poor oral hygiene.

	N	%
Related to dental procedures (previous 3 months)	8	12
Tooth extraction	4	6
Scaling	1	1.5
Endodontics	1	1.5
No details	2	3
Not related to dental procedures	60	88
Dental focus of infection (decay, fracture, trauma)	9	13.3
Dental focus of infection (no further details)	22	32.1
Periodontal disease	7	10.3
Endodontal and periodontal disease	12	17.5
Radiological dental infectious focus with no clinical lesion	9	13.3
Vigorous tooth brushing with frequent bleeding	1	1.5

Table 7. Infective endocarditis patients with identified oral and dental portals of entry (n = 68) [24].

These observations highlight the importance of maintaining oral hygiene in patients at highest risk of IE, and provide an important argument that dental care could have greater repercussions than antibiotic prophylaxis on the incidence of IE of oral origin.

6. Evidence of the efficacy of antibiotic prophylaxis

Since the 1955 AHA statement, Ref. [2] antibiotic prophylaxis has been continuously recommended to clinicians for IE prevention among patients undergoing interventional medical procedures. Since that early paper, antibiotic prophylaxis for IE has been considered "good medical and dental practice" and it has been said that the "exact dosage and duration of therapy are somewhat empirical". Now, more than 50 years later, AHA experts continue to consider that the basis for the recommendations for IE prophylaxis are still not well established and that the quality of evidence is based on expert opinion, a few case-controlled studies, clinical experience and descriptive studies [11]. All these circumstances lead antibiotic prophylaxis against IE to be included in class C evidence (**Table 8**).

Level A	Data derived from multiple randomised clinical trials or meta-analyses
Level B	Data derived from a single randomised trial or non-randomised studies
Level C	Only expert consensus, case studies or standard of care

Table 8. Classification of the levels of evidence.

Despite this, intense research into this subject has been undertaken from three main perspectives:

- The prevention of bacterial endocarditis in experimental animal models.

- The efficacy of antibiotics for the prevention of bacteraemia secondary to dental procedures.

- Epidemiological studies.

6.1. The prevention of bacterial endocarditis in experimental animal models

The induction of IE in experimental animals was first achieved in 1970. The technique consisted of introducing a polyethylene catheter into the right side of the heart of the animal to induce a nonbacterial thrombotic endocarditis. Bacteria were then injected via the catheter to induce experimental bacterial endocarditis that served as a suitable model for the study of bacteriological, pathological and immunological aspects of IE [25].

Although experimental studies make it possible to investigate the efficacy of prophylactic antibiotic regimens against IE, there are difficulties associated with animal models both in their methodology and in the extrapolation of results. The plastic catheter acts as a foreign body delaying the successful treatment of established infection in animals, and the pharmacokinetics of antimicrobials in animals differ considerably from those in man [26].

The percentage of positive post-extraction blood cultures in experimental animals receiving antibiotic prophylaxis fell slightly with respect to the controls. However, it was observed that the administration of amoxicillin effectively prevented the onset of IE, allowing the researchers to suggest that the antibiotics had some protective mechanism over and above their bactericidal activity.

Animal research continues to be very useful for the preliminary evaluation of the efficacy and safety of drugs, and studies are being performed on the usefulness of other, alternative drugs to antibiotics for the prevention of IE in at-risk patients [27].

6.2. Efficacy of antibiotics in the prevention of bacteraemia secondary to dental procedures

The majority of studies show that amoxicillin is effective in the control of bacteraemia of oral origin, reducing the rate of positive blood cultures after dental interventions in a range that varies between 70 and 100%. There are a number of reports on the efficacy of alternative antibiotics to amoxicillin for the prevention of bacteraemia of oral origin. Results are heterogeneous as they are conditioned by numerous factors such as geographical situation, previous patient oral health status, blood culture sampling technique, microbiological analysis, resistance maps, etc.; however, in general, alternative antibiotics show a lower efficacy in the control of bacteraemia.

Interestingly, clindamycin constitutes the alternative antibiotic of choice to amoxicillin in the three main guidelines (AHA, ESC and AIEPEG). Although some studies have concluded that clindamycin was useful to reduce oral bacteraemia, more recently published studies have found that clindamycin prophylaxis does not produce a significant reduction in the incidence of oral bacteraemia during dental procedures [15, 28, 29]. Some authors have proposed moxifloxacin as an alternative to amoxicillin, given its efficacy in experimental endocarditis [30] and in the prevention of bacteraemia following dental procedures in humans [15]. However, endocarditis expert committees appear to be ignoring this antibiotic at the present time.

S. aureus is now the most common pathogen in IE. This circumstance could justify the use of amoxicillin in association with a β-lactamase inhibitor, such as clavulanate, to broaden the bactericidal spectrum of antibiotic prophylaxis against IE. A recent study suggests that intravenous amoxicillin/clavulanate could be effective in the prevention of oral bacteraemia, virtually eliminating post-procedure inocula [29]. This observation opens the door to further research into the efficacy of oral amoxicillin/clavulanate in the prevention of bacteraemia. In any case, given its unusual demonstrated effectiveness in the elimination of oral bacteraemia, the intravenous prophylactic regimen of amoxicillin/clavulanate could be a high-efficacy alternative for patients with cardiac risk factors and severe systemic alterations, such as immune compromise, who require curative interventional dental treatment.

6.3. Epidemiological studies

Up to 2008, epidemiological studies did not support the hypothesis for the use of prophylactic antibiotics for medical procedures as a preventive method against IE. Case-control studies indicated that most IE events occurred independently of medical interventions and of the administration of antibiotic prophylaxis. A further argument was that despite the universal application of antibiotic prophylaxis, the incidence of IE and its associated mortality had not varied over decades [5].

In 2008, cessation of the NICE recommendation for antibiotic prophylaxis introduced a new epidemiological context into the study of IE, and analysis will serve to establish reliable conclusions in its area of influence. Implementation of the NICE guideline in England provides an opportunity for retrospective studies to investigate the comparative effect of antibiotic prophylaxis versus no prophylaxis on the incidence of IE.

Initially, the data suggest a significant increase in the incidence of IE after implantation of the NICE guideline, rising above the projected historical trend. This observation could lead to the hypothesis that the increased incidence of IE could be related to medical procedures in susceptible individuals performed without appropriate antibiotic cover. With regard to the dental procedures, we should observe an increase in the incidence of IE caused by oral viridans group streptococci but, at the present time, no data are available on pathogen-specific causal microorganisms [30].

7. Detractors of antibiotic prophylaxis

In view of the lack of scientific evidence on the prophylactic efficacy of the antibiotics for the prevention of IE, the British health authorities have focused their attention on the principle problems of the indiscriminate administration of antibiotics [6]:

- Quantifiable risk to the individual patient.

- Creation of unnecessary antimicrobial resistance.

- Economic burden.

However, a recent study on the incidence and nature of adverse reactions to antibiotics prescribed for endocarditis prophylaxis in England from 2004 estimates that reported adverse drug reaction rates from amoxicillin prescribed as antibiotic prophylaxis are low, without a single fatal reaction for nearly 3 million prescriptions [31].

The emergence of antibiotic resistance is a serious public health problem, but prophylactic antibiotic regimens for IE would only have a very limited effect as evidence shows that bacteria acquire resistance to antibiotics only after the administration of several consecutive doses.

With regard to the cost to the national health systems of the systematic administration of prophylaxis, cost-efficacy analyses of antibiotic prophylaxis for at-risk patients undergoing dental treatment provided contradictory results. In some countries, such as the USA, it has been estimated that prophylaxis constitutes a considerable expense, [32] but their results cannot be extrapolated to other countries in which the administration of prophylactic antibiotics to high-risk patients only represents a very small percentage of all the antibiotics that dentists prescribe.

Research into the control of bacteraemia shows that the administration of amoxicillin significantly reduces bacteraemia of oral origin, though it does not completely eliminate the possibility that this could occur. Alternative antibiotics such as clindamycin have shown poor results in the reduction of bacteraemia after dental interventions, leading us to deduce that the efficacy of prophylactic antibiotics in the prevention of IE in high-risk patients undergoing dental manipulations is limited.

8. Future research

Studies published to date on antibiotic prophylaxis against IE have a series of limitations that hinder their extrapolation, and attention must be focused on this aspect in future research:

- Regarding participants, it has been suggested that the prevalence of post-extraction bacteraemia may be related to age [33]. Age is also a determining factor in the pharmacokinetics of the antibiotic, and the efficacy of specific prophylaxis regimens may differ between children and adults. The oral health status may also influence the prevalence of post-dental manipulation bacteraemia, although this is still a controversial issue [34].

- The mode of anaesthesia, particularly general anaesthesia, can determine the appearance of post-extraction bacteraemia and prolong its duration. Comparative studies should therefore be performed using local and general anaesthesia [35].

- The prevalence of bacteraemia secondary to dental treatment and probably the predominant bacterial species are determined by the nature of the procedure. We therefore do not know whether antibiotic prophylaxis will be equally effective for different dental procedures [22].

- It is not known whether the dose and route of administration for the majority of current antibiotic prophylaxis regimens has a bearing on antibacterial activity.

- The fact that positive post-dental-manipulation blood cultures are not detected after the administration of antibiotic prophylaxis does not guarantee that bacteraemia does not occur due to bacteria that cannot be cultured in the usual culture media and/or whose inoculum is below the threshold of the method of detection employed.

Author details

Miguel Castro, Javier Álvarez, Javier F. Feijoo, Marcio Diniz, Lucía García-Caballero, Pedro Diz* and Jacobo Limeres

*Address all correspondence to: pedro.diz@usc.es

Special Needs Unit and OMEQUI Research Group, School of Medicine and Dentistry, Santiago de Compostela University, Santiago de Compostela, Spain

References

[1] Elliot SD. Bacteraemia and oral sepsis. Proc R Soc Med 1939; 32: 747–754.

[2] American Heart Association. Prevention of rheumatic fever and bacterial endocarditis through control of streptococcal infections. Circulation 1955; 11: 317–320.

[3] Pelletier LL Jr, Durack DT, Petersdorf RG. Chemotherapy of experimental streptococcal endocarditis. IV. Further observations on prophylaxis. J Clin Invest 1975; 56: 319–330.

[4] British Society for Antimicrobial Chemotherapy. The antibiotic prophylaxis of infective endocarditis. Lancet 1982; 2: 1323–1326.

[5] Prendergast BD. The changing face of infective endocarditis. Heart 2006; 92: 879–885.

[6] National Institute for Health and Clinical Excellence. Prophylaxis against infective endocarditis. Antimicrobial prophylaxis against infective endocarditis in adults and children undergoing interventional procedures 2008. http://nice.org.uk/CG064

[7] Thornhill MH, Dayer MJ, Forde JM, et al. Impact of the NICE guideline recommending cessation of antibiotic prophylaxis for prevention of infective endocarditis: before and after study. BMJ 2011; 342: d2392.

[8] Lopez R, Flavell S, Thomas C. A not very NICE case of endocarditis. BMJ Case Rep 2013: bcr2012007918.

[9] Dayer MJ, Jones S, Prendergast B, Baddour LM, Lockhart PB, Thornhill MH. Incidence of infective endocarditis in England, 2000–2013: a secular trend, interrupted time-series analysis. Lancet 2015; 385: 1219–1228.

[10] Thornhill MH, Dayer M, Lockhart PB, et al. Guidelines on prophylaxis to prevent infective endocarditis. Br Dent J 2016; 220: 51–56.

[11] Wilson W, Taubert KA, Gewitz M, et al. Prevention of infective endocarditis. Guidelines from the American Heart Association. J Am Dent Assoc 2007; 138: 739–745, 747–760.

[12] Moulds RF, Jeyasingham MS. Infective Endocarditis Prophylaxis Expert Group, Therapeutic Guidelines Limited. Antibiotic prophylaxis against infective endocarditis: time to rethink. Med J Aust 2008; 189: 301–302.

[13] Habib G, Lancellotti P, Antunes MJ, et al. 2015 ESC Guidelines for the management of infective endocarditis: the task force for the management of infective endocarditis of the European Society of Cardiology (ESC). Endorsed by: European Association for Cardio-Thoracic Surgery (EACTS), the European Association of Nuclear Medicine (EANM). Eur Heart J 2015; 36: 3075–3128.

[14] Becker DE. Drug allergies and implications for dental practice. Anesth Prog 2013 Winter; 60: 188–197.

[15] Diz Dios P, Tomás Carmona I, Limeres Posse J, Medina Henríquez J, Fernández Feijoo J, Álvarez Fernández M. Comparative efficacies of amoxicillin, clindamycin, and moxifloxacin in prevention of bacteremia following dental extractions. Antimicrob Agents Chemother 2006; 50: 2996–3002.

[16] Addy LD, Martin MV. Azithromycin and dentistry—a useful agent?. Br Dent J 2004; 197: 141–143.

[17] Vogkou CT, Vlachogiannis NI, Palaiodimos L, Kousoulis AA. The causative agents in infective endocarditis: a systematic review comprising 33,214 cases. Eur J Clin Microbiol Infect Dis 2016; 35: 1227–1245.

[18] Dajani AS, Taubert KA, Wilson W, et al. Prevention of bacterial endocarditis: recommendations by the American Heart Association. Clin Infect Dis 1997; 25: 1448–1458.

[19] Davies SB, Hofer A, Reeve C. Mortality attributable to rheumatic heart disease in the Kimberley: a data linkage approach. Intern Med J 2014; 44: 1074–1080.

[20] Lockhart PB, Loven B, Brennan MT, Fox PC. The evidence base for the efficacy of antibiotic prophylaxis in dental practice. J Am Dent Assoc 2007; 138: 458–474.

[21] Okell CC, Elliott SD. Bacteraemia and oral sepsis with special reference to subacute endocarditis. Lancet 1935; 226: 869–887.

[22] Diz Dios P, Tomás Carmona I, Limeres Posse J. ***Bateriemias producidas por inter-venciones odontológicas (chap. 13). In: Patología Periodontal y Cardiovascular. Coordinators: De Teresa E, Noguerol Rodríguez B. Editorial: Panamericana S.A., Madrid, 2011: 159–167.

[23] Veloso TR, Amiguet M, Rousson V, et al. Induction of experimental endocarditis by continuous low-grade bacteremia mimicking spontaneous bacteremia in humans. Infect Immun 2011; 79: 2006–2011.

[24] Delahaye F, M'Hammedi A, Guerpillon B, et al. Systematic search for present and potential portals of entry for infective endocarditis. J Am Coll Cardiol 2016; 67: 151–158.

[25] Garrison PK, Freedman LR. Experimental endocarditis I. *Staphylococcal endocarditis* in rabbits resulting from placement of a polyethylene catheter in the right side of the heart. Yale J Biol Med 1970; 42: 394–410.

[26] Petersdorf RG. Antimicrobial prophylaxis of bacterial endocarditis. Prudent caution or bacterial overkill? Am J Med 1978; 65: 220–223.

[27] Veloso TR, Mancini S, Giddey M, et al. Vaccination against *Staphylococcus aureus* experimental endocarditis using recombinant *Lactococcus lactis* expressing ClfA or FnbpA. Vaccine 2015; 33: 3512–3517.

[28] Maharaj B, Coovadia Y, Vayej AC. A comparative study of amoxicillin, clindamycin and chlorhexidine in the prevention of post-extraction bacteraemia. Cardiovasc J Afr 2012; 23: 491–494.

[29] Limeres Posse J, Álvarez Fernández M, Fernández Feijoo J, et al. Intravenous amoxi-cillin/clavulanate for the prevention of bacteraemia following dental procedures: a randomized clinical trial. J Antimicrob Chemother 2016; 71: 2022–2030.

[30] Sakka V, Galani L, Pefanis A, et al. Successful moxifloxacin prophylaxis against experimental streptococcal aortic valve endocarditis. J Antimicrob Chemother 2005; 56: 1160–1162.

[31] Thornhill MH, Dayer MJ, Prendergast B, Baddour LM, Jones S, Lockhart PB. Incidence and nature of adverse reactions to antibiotics used as endocarditis prophylaxis. J Antimicrob Chemother 2015; 70: 2382–2388.

[32] Lockhart PB, Blizzard J, Maslow AL, Brennan MT, Sasser H, Carew J. Drug cost implications for antibiotic prophylaxis for dental procedures. Oral Surg Oral Med Oral Pathol Oral Radiol 2013; 115: 345–353.

[33] Lockhart PB, Brennan MT, Kent ML, Norton HJ, Weinrib DA. Impact of amoxicillin prophylaxis on the incidence, nature, and duration of bacteremia in children after intubation and dental procedures. Circulation 2004; 109: 2878–2884.

[34] Lockhart PB, Brennan MT, Thornhill M, et al. Poor oral hygiene as a risk factor for infective endocarditis-related bacteremia. J Am Dent Assoc 2009; 140: 1238–1244.

[35] Barbosa M, Carmona IT, Amaral B, et al. General anesthesia increases the risk of bacteremia following dental extractions. Oral Surg Oral Med Oral Pathol Oral Radiol Endod 2010; 110: 706–712.

7

The Role of Modern-Era Echocardiography in Identification of Cardiac Risk Factors for Infective Endocarditis

John F. Sedgwick and Gregory M. Scalia

Abstract

This chapter provides an updated overview of the scientific literature on cardiac pathology predisposing to infective endocarditis and the estimated risk associated with selected lesion-specific abnormalities, in an era of changing epidemiology and advanced echocardiographic imaging. Importantly, with the evolution of modern-era echo, subtle changes in valve structure and function are now easily detectable and a proportion of cases of apparently 'normal' valves involved with IE, may in fact have subtle pre-existing pathological and/or haemodynamic abnormalities. The chapter will have a clinical focus with an aim to provide the Physician with up-to-date and practical information on cardiac risk factor identification for infective endocarditis.

Keywords: echocardiography, infective endocarditis, risk factors, valvular heart disease, congenital heart disease, degenerative valve disease, rheumatic heart disease, cardiac pathology, disease incidence, modern-era

1. Introduction

Infective endocarditis (IE) risk is strongly associated with underlying cardiac disease. This chapter will review the pathology, mechanisms and estimated risks according to lesion-specific groups. Echocardiographic predictors of IE will be discussed along with the increasingly reported occurrence of IE in 'normal valves'.

2. Predisposing cardiac disease: a changing epidemiology

Since mid-last century, the epidemiology of IE has continued to change across high-income countries (HIC), from predominantly young patients with rheumatic heart disease (RHD) to the current era of an ageing population with IE, infrequent RHD and prevalent degenerative valve disease (DVD). A history of acute rheumatic fever (ARF) in patients with IE had declined from ~38 to 22.5% in the 30 years up to 1967 [1]. By the 1980s, this had reduced to 6% [2]. According to data from the International Collaboration on Endocarditis—Prospective Cohort Study (ICE-PICS), DVD is the most common underlying pathology in IE, with significant mitral regurgitation (MR) and aortic regurgitation (AR) accounting for 43.3 and 26.3% of cases, respectively, compared with rheumatic mitral valve, present in only 3.3% cases. Prosthetic valve endocarditis (PVE) accounts for up to 22.2% of cases [3], whilst the prevalence of cardiac device-related infective endocarditis (CDRIE) has increased along with health-care associated IE (HCAIE) [4]. Endocarditis patterns in congenital heart disease (CHD) have changed due to patients surviving into adulthood with more complex disease, the availability of improved surgical techniques and implantation of prosthetic material [5, 6].

The 2015 European Society of Cardiology IE management guidelines now consider the following cardiac conditions to pose the highest risk of IE: (i) prosthetic cardiac valves and/or repairs with prosthetic material, (ii) previous IE, (iii) cyanotic CHD, and (iv) any CHD that has been repaired for up to 6 months post procedure or indefinitely if a residual defect or valve incompetence persists. Repair or intervention includes both surgical and transcatheter procedures. Antibiotic prophylaxis is recommended for these patients when exposed to procedures considered high-risk [7].

3. Estimating risk of infective endocarditis: methodological issues

There are methodological challenges with investigating risk of acquiring IE. Two major limitations are: i) low incidence of IE in the general population and ii) selection bias associated with tertiary referral hospitals. Variations in study design and methodology also contribute to the difficulties faced in drawing generalised conclusions.

4. Pathogenesis of infective endocarditis with underlying cardiac disease

The major predisposing categories of underlying cardiac pathology are DVD, CHD and RHD. Platelet-fibrin aggregates form on damaged or inflamed endothelium, resulting in nonbacterial thrombotic endocarditis (NBTE), a precursor of IE [8]. Microorganisms are able to attach to this nidus via adhesion molecules and stimulate a host inflammatory response [8].

Regurgitant valves are at higher risk of IE than stenotic valves [9]. In a large clinical-pathological study on native valve endocarditis (NVIE), 84% of valves were regurgitant [10]. Another found the majority of cases of IE presenting to surgery were for regurgitant valves compared to a control-group of non-IE cases undergoing surgery (9% of regurgitant bicuspid aortic valves (BAV), 1.2% of calcified BAVs, 1.6% of calcified trileaflet aortic valves (AV) and 7% of mitral valve prolapse (MVP)) [11]. Aortic regurgitation (AR) is a predisposing lesion in 17–36% of cases of IE, whilst mitral regurgitation (MR) accounts for 10–18% [12].

The pathogenesis of IE in structural cardiac abnormalities is characterised by the hydrody-namic theory [13]. A high velocity turbulent jet exerts a shearing effect on endothelium, at the site of a restrictive orifice (e.g. ventricular septal defect (VSD) or MR jet) and/or a distal point of contact (jet lesion). The narrowest diameter of flow is the vena contracta (VC), just distal to the restricted anatomical orifice. This is where the pressure is minimal and retrograde flow may occur, permitting platelets and bacteria to deposit [13]. The typical location of vegetation is on the upstream side of the valve, that is, the atrial aspect of the MV, tricuspid valve (TV) and ventricular aspect AV, pulmonary valve (PV) [9].

Structurally normal native right-sided valves in the absence of significant pulmonary hyperten-sion, are exposed to lower pressure flows and are far less commonly involved with IE. In children, without CHD, native right-sided IE involving normal valves is rare but may occur in association with trauma to the valve from central lines or catheters [14, 15]. Other factors are important in risk of acquiring IE and include an interplay between microorganism virulence, altered host defence mechanisms, predisposing systemic illness, and environmental and social factors [16].

5. Structurally normal native cardiac valves

Infective endocarditis does occur in some patients without pre-existing known structural abnormalities. Whether the valves were completely normal is uncertain. Early degenerative changes can be present without clinical detection [17]. Modern-era echo with high image reso-lution and careful scrutiny of valve morphology and function, has the potential to shed more light on this research question.

There is an increasing prevalence of IE involving structurally normal cardiac valves, account-ing for 26–43% of native left-sided IE cases [2, 18, 19]. Sun et al. [18] reported the commonest underlying cardiac predisposition was mitral valve prolapse (MVP) followed by normal valves (26%). Olmas et al. [20] found in an IE cohort, normal left-sided native valves in 39.8% of patients aged >65 years and in 53.8% of those aged ≤65 years, whilst DVD comprised 23.4% of the cohort. However, details regarding Doppler valve function were not available. This is important, for even normal valves may be regurgitant, exposing endothelium to shear-ing forces. Limitations include assessing valves for pre-existing pathology when already involved by infection and absence of pathological correlation to exclude subtle underlying pathology. In vitro studies have demonstrated certain microorganisms can attach to and/or be internalised by healthy valve endothelium, however in vivo, animal studies have required trauma to the endothelium to initiate IE following an inoculum of bacteria [9]. This raises the question—are the valves 'normal' or are there subtle pathological changes or haemodynamic disturbance, which predispose to IE. This was also raised by Que and Moreillon [21] and Baddour et al. [9].

To assess normal valve thickness according to age, 200 normal valves were reviewed at autopsy [22]. There was approximately double the thickness of the aortic cusps and mitral leaflets with age [22]. In a separate study, transoesophageal echo (TOE) identified normal MV thickness overall to be ≤3 mm and AV≤2 mm in those aged <60 years [23]. The prevalence of normal valves with physiological regurgitation was investigated in a retrospective echocardiographic study of 1333 patients without a history of cardiac disease or hypertension [24]. Physiological MR and TR were defined as structurally normal valves on 2-D imaging, with a regurgitant jet area occupying <20% of the left atrial (LA) area and <5 cm² within the right atrium (RA), respectively. Aortic regurgitation with jet to LVOT width ratio <25% and normal leaflets was considered physiological. Non-organic MR was detected in 1/3rd or patients aged 10–19 years and approximately 2/3rd of persons aged >30 years. Non-organic TR was identified in over 4/5th of persons across all age cohort groups (10–89 years). Non-organic AR was present in <10% of patients under 50 years, with an increase in prevalence corresponding to each decade, up to 46% of those aged 80–89 years [24].

5.1. Risk of endocarditis in normal valves with physiological regurgitation

Data is not readily available on the risk of IE in patients with left-sided non-organic regurgitation. However, one study did assess the risk of IE in structurally normal right-sided cardiac valves in adult patients with CHD and pulmonary hypertension (PHTN) [25]. Both TVs and PVs had physiological regurgitation. The presence of PHTN was responsible for increased regurgitant velocities across the valves and thought to mimic the haemodynamic forces experienced by incompetent left-sided valves. High velocity flow was defined as PR jet ≥3.2 m/s and TR≥4.7 m/s. A small subset of valves was inspected at necropsy with the majority of TVs and minority of PVs revealing mild nodular degenerative changes along leaflet closure margins. The echocardiograms were said to be normal in appearance. There were 0.61 and 7.17 cases of IE per 1000 patient-years in the normal valve group compared to the CHD control group, respectively. The risk was therefore small, but inconclusive due to insufficient patient numbers [25].

6. Degenerative valve disease

6.1. Degenerative disease of the aortic valve

The prevalence of nonrheumatic AS increases with ageing [26]. In a cohort of older patients with IE, the prevalence of acquired MR and AS was reported as 57 and 28% respectively, compared with 38 and 10% in patients <65 years [26, 27].

6.1.1. Fibro-calcific degeneration

Age-related findings often begin on the aortic valve in early or middle adulthood and include the following: (i) noduli arantii—fibroelastic proliferation on the ventricular surface of the cusps, from early adulthood, most pronounced on the noncoronary cusp, (ii) ridge-like thickening at the base of cusps where mechanical forces are highest; occurs in early adulthood in 20–40% persons, and (iii) commissural adhesion, due to fibroelastic hyperplasia, affecting 10–20% of older persons [28]. With ageing, endothelial dysfunction and hemodynamic stress lead to degenerative changes, inciting an inflammatory process, not unlike atherosclerosis. Histological changes include subendothelial thickening, lipid and protein accumulation, inflammatory cell proliferation, fibrosis and calcification within the valve fibrosa [29]. The process is accelerated over the age of 55 years, and onset in males is marginally earlier than females [28]. Initially there is no significant restriction to cusp opening and the diagnosis of aortic sclerosis is confirmed with echo.

6.1.1.1. Aortic sclerosis and echocardiography

The presence of aortic sclerosis (focal thickening, no commissural fusion, peak velocity <2.0 m/s) is associated with an increased risk of death [30]. Caution should be exercised not to over diagnose sclerosis on echo [31]. Artefactual thickening and echogenicity can appear with harmonic imaging and over-gained signals. Optimising transthoracic (TTE) image settingsand use of both harmonic and fundamental frequencies can overcome these limitations [31]. Transoesophageal imaging has higher resolution and anatomical detail is superior [31].

6.1.1.2. Aortic stenosis and risk of endocarditis

Eventually large calcified deposits occupy the body of the leaflet and can extend into the ventricular septum, the ventricular surface of the anterior mitral valve leaflet (AMVL) and are associated with mitral annular calcification (MAC). Cusp motion becomes restricted and aortic stenosis (AS) ensues. Ulcerations and thrombi may form, being a potential mimicker of IE [16, 32], and may form a nidus for infective endocarditis. There is a paucity of data on IE occurring with aortic sclerosis, although empirically, the risk is very small. Endocarditis of calcific trileaflet AS is relatively uncommon. According to Delahaye [33] 27/366 cases of native valve IE were pure AS. Risk is higher in patients with BAV and/or AR. In a study from the Mayo clinic [10], 310 native valves were excised for IE and it was reported 59% had no calcification. Mild-moderate and severe calcification was present in 37% and 5%, respectively. The most common underlying cardiac structural abnormalities were BAV (38% of 170 aortic valves) and MVP (43% of 120 mitral valves). This finding would suggest that IE is less common in severely calcified valves [10]. Another study with pathologic correlation found pre-existing calcification present in 27% of valves with IE, though numbers in the study were small [11].

Acquired degenerative changes of the AV leaflets can occur secondarily in the context of conditions leading to annuloaortic dilatation. In this pathology, the leaflets come together at the free edges rather than the zone of coaptation, leading to focal thickening, and increased risk of NBTE and IE [17].

6.1.1.3. Fenestrations

Acquired age-related fenestrations form within the lunular region of the aortic semilunar cusps, adjacent to the commissures, often in association with myxomatous AV disease.

Fenestrations are found in approximately 5% of females and 10–20% of males, mostly present from the age of <45 years with a minor increase in prevalence over time, in males [28]. They are not routinely identified on echo because of their location above the line of closure. Fenestrations result in valvular regurgitation in the following circumstances: (i) spontaneous rupture resulting in a flail cusp, (ii) fenestration enlarges to extend below the zone of coaptation and/or (iii) reduced leaflet coaptation, such as prolapse or root dilatation, when the fenestration is no longer 'sealed-off' within the cusp closure zone [34, 35]. The risk of IE associated with fenestrations or valvular perforations is unknown.

6.1.1.4. Lambl's excrescences

Lambl's excrescences increase in prevalence with age and may become incorporated into the noduli arantii [28]. They are located along the lines of cusp closure of left-sided (high pressure) valves. They are composed of a fibro-elastic core with an endothelial layer covering the surface. There is associated turbulence and relative stasis of blood flow, which predisposes to formation of NBTE and IE [34]. Although the risk of IE is unknown, empirically it is uncommon. Occasionally Lambl's excrescences can mimic vegetation and lead to a false-positive diagnosis of IE. However, Lambl's are usually identified as thin single or multiple filamentous strands on echo, which help differentiate them from typical vegetations and papillary fibroelastomas.

6.1.2. Myxomatous degeneration

Primary myxomatous degeneration (PMD) of the AV is less common than of the MV. In cases of significant 'pure' AS, it has been said to be the primary underlying pathology in up to 10–36% of subjects [38], however other pathological studies examining excised regurgitant aortic valves have reported much lower rates of PMD, at 2% [36] and in a more recent clinicopathological correlation study from China, 3% (35 of 1080 excised aortic valves) [37]. Histological findings include degeneration of the fibrosa layer, disruption of collagen fibres and deposition of mucopolysaccharides [37]. The cusps are susceptible to developing fenestrations adjacent to the commissures and with time, the prolapsing cusps develop thickening of the free margin, thought secondary to chronic trauma from the regurgitant jet [38]. The incidence of endocarditis with this pathology is unknown, however empirically, high velocity regurgitant jets increase the risk of IE.

6.2. Degenerative disease of the mitral valve

6.2.1. Mitral valve sclerosis and age-related changes

Mitral valve sclerosis is commonly encountered in the elderly and characterised by leaflet thickening. In patients >60 years, the leaflets are at least twice the thickness compared to early adulthood [22]. The following changes are frequently noted on the anterior leaflet: (i) senile sclerosis - nodular thickening on the atrial surface of the closing edge, up to age of 65 years, (ii) atheromatosis—age-related lipoid deposition (yellow plaque) on the ventricular aspect of the base of the leaflets extending towards and sometimes involving the chordal apparatus [28]. The following changes may be noted at the posterior leaflet: (i) puckered scars—infrequent at 3–5%, > 65 years, (ii) fibro-elastic hyperplasia (mitral opacity) of the atrial surface in ~20%, >65 years and, (iii) mucoid or myxomatous degeneration (~ 5–10%) ± prolapse, with increased proteoglycans in the spongiosa layer [28]. The condition shows a slight increase with age in the milder forms. Severe forms of mucoid change were not related to age [28]. Fibroelastic deficiency (FED) is seen more commonly in the elderly and can lead to leaflet prolapse and/or chordal rupture.

Mitral annular calcification (MAC) is common in the elderly though can occur prematurely in certain other conditions such as hypertrophic cardiomyopathy (HCM), PMD, diabetes and renal disease. MAC commonly involves the posterior annulus and parallels AV calcification, with a sharp rise >55 years [28]. Normal sphincteric action of the annulus is altered and MR ensues [17]. Inflammation accompanies MAC and complications such as ulcerative erosion, thrombus formation, systemic embolic, liquefaction necrosis, infected vegetations and abscess formation occur with increased frequency [34, 39]. With large protruding MAC deposits, it is theorised there is alteration of local blood flow, predisposing to NBTE and IE [39]. Mitral stenosis can also occur as calcium encroaches on the leaflets. Vegetations form at the base of the mitral leaflet [39] rather than the leaflet closure line, as seen with typical regurgitant lesions [17] and are localised accurately with 3-D echo. Although MAC predisposes to IE, the exact risk is unknown.

6.2.2. Myxomatous mitral valve disease and prolapse

Mitral valve prolapse (MVP) most commonly occurs due to PMD. Secondary myxomatous degeneration can occur in other conditions, such as RHD and age-related degeneration. Additional causes of prolapse include congenital and papillary muscle dysfunction. The 'middle' tissue layer of healthy valves, the spongiosa, normally thickenings towards the leaflet/cusp margins and this is not a pathological finding [16]. With pathological myxomatous changes, there is diffuse increase in deposition of glycosaminoglycans in leaflets, cusps, chords and annuli and thrombi may form [16]. In a study from China, echocardiography (either TTE or TOE) correctly identified valve prolapse and thickening in 85% of patients in which myxomatous disease was confirmed pathologically [37].

6.2.2.1. Prevalence of mitral prolapse and regurgitation in healthy individuals

In a landmark study, data was collected from a healthy population comprising the offspring of the original Framingham study group [40]. Echocardiographic criteria (2-D) used in the study were as follows: (i) prolapse - superior displacement of the mitral leaflet(s) >2 mm above the atrioventricular annular plane in the long-axis window, (ii) classic MVP - at least 2 mm prolapse with leaflet thickness ≥5 mm and, (iii) non-class MVP – ≥2 mm prolapse with leaflet thickness <5 mm [40]. A total of 2.4% met criteria for prolapse. Classic MVP was found in 1.3% of persons and non-classic MVP in 1.1% [40], with mean age mid 50s and a slight female preponderance. Mean MR volume was mild in the classic group and a trace in the non-classic and control groups. Severe MR was only found in the classic groups and comprised 7% of cases [40].

6.2.2.2. Prevalence and risk of mitral prolapse in endocarditis

Mitral valve prolapse occurs in 7–30% of cases of native valve IE, nearly always in the presence of MR and associated with redundant leaflets. Of note, NBTE forms on atrial aspect of thickened, redundant leaflets [17]. In a large clinicopathological correlation study of 120 native mitral valves excised due to IE, 43% had a history of prolapse [10]. The estimated risk of IE is shown in **Table 1**. Recent data published by Katan et al. [41] found a higher incidence of IE in MVP compared to earlier publications, thought in part due to the previous overestimation of true MVP in healthy individuals using less stringent diagnostic methods [41].

6.2.2.3. Mitral prolapse — echocardiographic predictors of endocarditis risk

Mitral regurgitation confirmed on echo and/or typical murmur, has been shown to be a predictor of risk in studies that have specifically assessed this variable (**Table 1**). In the study by Katan et al. [41], no cases of IE occurred in patients without a history of MR during follow-up. Nishimura et al. [47], found redundant leaflets (i.e. M-mode thickness $\geq$5 mm) were associated with IE, though numbers were small. Marks et al. [48] also confirmed classic MVP with leaflet thickening $\geq$5 mm (2-D echo) and redundancy was associated with IE risk over non classic MVP.

6.3. Degenerative disease of the right-sided cardiac valves

Gross degenerative changes of the right-sided valves are uncommon compared to the higher-pressure environment of left-sided valves. The TV often undergoes only minimal change, with nodular thickening along the closing edge of the anterior valve leaflet. Mild diffuse leaflet thickening may occur in middle age; though in a minority of patients (>65 years), may become moderate or severe [28]. Myxoid degeneration of TV leaflets occurs occasionally [49], with TV prolapse (TVP) and PMD occurring in about 4% of cases [37, 40] . The risk of IE in TVP is unknown.

The pulmonary valve (PV) remains translucent and thin in the vast majority. Nodular thickening (noduli Morgani) along the centre part of the closing margin occurs in <50% of subjects,

	Overall incidence of IE in MVP (risk per 1000 patient-years)	MVP with regurgitation (risk per 1000 patient-years)	Overall incidence of IE in MVP with murmur (risk odds ratio – 'OR')
Katan et al. [41]	0.87	0.63[1]; 2.9[2]; 7.16[3]	
Clemens et al. [42] and Tay and Yip [43]	0.38	n/a	15.1
Retchin et al. [44]	0.3	n/a	n/a
Hickey et al. [45]	0.14	n/a	5.3
Danchin et al. [46]	n/a	n/a	14.5

[1]Less than moderate MR.
[2]At least moderate MR.
[3]Flail leaflet.

Table 1. Risk of infective endocarditis associated with mitral valve prolapse and regurgitation.

increasing gradually with age [28]. The mild age-related degenerative changes of the PV are not typically associated with IE.

7. Congenital heart disease

7.1. Overall incidence of endocarditis in congenital heart disease

Recently published research estimates the incidence of adult congenital heart disease (ACHD)-associated IE is 1.0–1.33 cases per 1000 patient-years and in children (0–18 years), 0.41 cases per 1000 patient-years. Cumulative first incidence of IE, from birth to 18 years, was shown to be 6.1/1000 [5, 50, 51]. According to published data from the USA, the estimated incidence in children is lower, at 0.05–0.12 cases per 1000 patient-years [52, 53]. Interestingly, Marom et al. found 18% of children with IE had no underlying structural heart disease and no identifiable risk factors, compared to earlier published rates, ranging from 2.5–19% [54].

7.2. Incidence of endocarditis in complex congenital heart disease

Incidence rate in complex CHD has recently been published by Kuijpers et al. [5], 2017. Incidence of IE (per 1000 patient-years) reported according to lesion-specific pathology include: pulmonary atresia (PA) with ventricular septal defect (VSD), 7.84; double outlet right ventricle (DORV), 3.59; Marfans, 2.35; univentricular heart (UVH), 1.9; Tetralogy of Fallot (ToF), 1.8; congenitally corrected transposition (cTGA), 0.93; transposition, 0.89; and Ebstein's anomaly, 0.7.

7.3. Endocarditis in simple shunts

7.3.1. Ventricular septal defect

Overall estimated incidence of IE with a VSD in ACHD is 1.0–1.33 and for children, 0.41 per 1000 patient-years (**Table 2**). In another study, the incidence was reported at 1.86 in adults and 1.06 in children, per 1000 patient-years (p = 0.06) [55]. The majority of studies have identified the following risk factors: i) unrepaired VSD ii) co-existent AR and, iii) residual defect at site of VSD repair. It has not been unequivocally proven a restrictive defect carries a higher risk. A VSD associated with AR carries a 2x relative risk (incidence increase from 1.25 up to 3.48/1000) [55], whilst a VSD that has undergone secondary aneurysmal transformation to form a Gerbode defect (LV-LA shunt) carries a risk of 5 per 1000 patient-years [56]. In one study, non-operated VSD's carried a 2.6x risk (0.73 versus 1.87/1000 patient-years) [55].

7.3.2. Atrial septal defect

Secundum ASD IE incidence is estimated at 0.23 for children and 0.28–0.64/1000 patient-years in adults (**Table 2**). A higher than expected risk was likely due to concomitant valve disease or misdiagnosed primum defects [50]. Isolated ASD is rarely associated with infective endocarditis [57]. The risk in adults with atrioventricular septal defect (AVSD) is estimated at 0.89 per 1000 patient-years (**Table 2**).

		CHD	ASD; VSD; AVSD; PDA	Left-sided[1] Right-sided[2]	Cyanotic (complex/conotruncal)[3] Cyanotic (conotruncal/single ventricle)[4]
Kuijpers et al. [5] (ACHD; Included prosthetic valves)	Incidence (per 1000 pt. years)	1.33	0.64; 0.82; 0.89; 0.0	1.89; 0.57	1.94 n/a
	Adjusted HR (95% CI)	n/a	n/a n/a n/a n/a	n/a n/a	n/a n/a
Mylotte et al. [51] (ACHD; Excluded prosthetic valves; Included conduits and repairs)	Incident IE (per 1000 pt. years)	1.0	0.28; 0.65; n/a; 0.24	1.61; 0.35	n/a 1.17
	Adjusted OR[5,] (95% CI)	n/a	n/a; 2.81 (1.87–4.21); n/a; n/a	5.11 (3.6–7.25); n/a	n/a 4.82 (3.12–7.46)
Rushani et al. [50], (Paediatric)	Incidence (per 1000 pt. years)	0.41	0.23; 0.24; n/a; 0.35	0.44; 0.29	n/a 2.07
	Adjusted Rate Ratio (95% CI)	n/a	n/a; 0.97 (0.56–1.66); n/a; 1.25 (0.5–3.13)	1.88 (1.01–3.49); 1.22 (0.52–2.86)	n/a 6.44 (3.95–10.5)

[1]Left-sided includes: coarctation, aortic and mitral disease (Mylotte et al. and Rushani et al.); or LVOTO (left ventricular outflow tract obstruction), Marfan, BAV, CoA, MV defect, other LVOT (Kuijpers et al).

[2]Right-sided includes: Ebstein, anomaly of pulmonary artery/valve, TV disease (Mylotte et al. and Rushani et al); or Ebstein, RVOTO (right ventricular outflow tract obstruction), other (Kuijpers et al).

[3]Cyanotic (complex/conotruncal) includes: PA + VSD, DORV, UVH, ToF, TGA, Other (Kuijpers et al).

[4]Cyanotic (conotruncal/single-ventricle): ToF, TGA, truncus, hypoplastic left heart and univentricular heart (Mylotte et al. and Rushani et al.)

[5]Odds ratio when referenced to ASD, PDA, R-sided groups.

Table 2. Contemporary estimates of incidence and risk hazard ratios for infective endocarditis in children and adults with congenital heart disease, across selected lesion-specific groups.

7.3.3. Ductus arteriosus

The estimated risk of IE with patent ductus arteriosus (PDA) is 0.24 and 0.35 per 1000 patient-years in adults and children, respectively, whilst other data have shown for an unrepaired PDA, the IE risk is 0.35–1.4 per 1000 patient-years, in a mixed adult and paediatric cohort [12, 50]. According to one study, the risk of IE was only present <4 years of age, likely due to ligation procedure essentially eliminating IE occurrence in older children [50].

7.3.4. Echocardiography

Echo assessment of a VSD should include identification of vegetations or other IE complications, whether involving the defect, the valves or mural endocardium. Also, imaging must define shunt anatomy, efficacy of closure (where present), cardiac chamber size and function, pulmonary artery pressure and haemodynamics. Aneurysmal formation and Gerbode defect should be excluded. Echo is fundamental in the routine and peri-procedural assessment of ASD and other shunts. It is also important to note the presence or absence of an ASD (or other shunt) in valvular endocarditis. For example, an infected TV may be a source of paradoxical embolism. The direction of the regurgitant jet and shunt, along with the size and mobility of a vegetation are important factors when assessing the risk of embolisation.

7.4. Bicuspid aortic valve and aortic coarctation

Bicuspid aortic valve (BAV) is a common congenital abnormality and undergoes accelerated degenerative change and dystrophic calcification [17]. Only a minority develop 'pure' regurgitation. Prevalence of BAV is as high as 1–2% of the population, more common in men and a pre-existing lesion in approximately 20% of cases of IE [12]. The estimated hazard ratio (HR) for adults with a BAV, of acquiring IE up to middle age is 6.3 (CI, 3.0–13.4), with an incidence of approximately 2 per 1000 patient-years [5, 58]. According to Kiyota et al. [59], BAV carries a relative risk (RR) of 23.1 times that of a tricuspid aortic valve for acquiring IE. With aortic coarctation (AoC), the incidence of IE is <1 per 1000 patient years [12, 58]. At 25 years out, the cumulative incidence of IE in another study was 3.5% (563 pts. with median age at time of surgery, 1.9 years) [60].

7.5. Congenital aortic stenosis

Incidence of IE in congenital aortic stenosis is estimated at 2.0–2.71 per 1000 patient-years [12, 61]. Echocardiographic predictors of risk of endocarditis include AV gradient and a non-statistically significant increase in the presence of regurgitation. In the Second Natural History Study (NHS-2), Gersony et al. [55], found patients with peak gradient (PG) across the aortic valve of <50 mmHg had an IE rate of 0.45 per 1000 person-years versus 5.44 per 1000 person-years in those with gradient ≥50 mmHg. When the stenotic valve was associated with aortic regurgitation (AR), rates of IE increased from 1.98 up to 3.43 per 1000 patient-years (not statistically significant, p = 0.105) [55]. In those managed medically and with a PG < 50 mmHg, the risk of IE was 0.27 per 1000 person-years and for patient with aortic valve replacement (AVR), follow-up rate of IE was 1.53 per 1000 person-years [55]. In a different study, the cumulative risk was 13.3% out to 25 years post-surgery (median age of surgery 7.0 years) in patients where follow-up was available. This equates to a higher annualised incidence of 7.2 per 1000 patient-years [60].

7.6. Pulmonary valve and tetralogy of Fallot

Pulmonary stenosis (PS) is usually related to congenital valve stenosis, sometimes in association with genetic syndromes. Pulmonary regurgitation (PR) due to congenital disease is mostly seen following previous repair of ToF or valvotomy [62]. Endocarditis of the PV is relatively uncommon both pre and post-surgery [55, 57, 60], except in palliative shunts [60]. In PS, a rate of 0.09 per 1000 person-years has been reported [55]. Tetralogy of Fallot carries a risk of approximately 1–2.3 per 1000 patient-years [12, 58].

7.7. Post-surgical and catheter intervention

In the Kuijpers et al. study [5], the following were noted: (i) 8 cases of IE with closed ASD, but of those, 6/8 were associated with a valve abnormality; (ii) 13 cases of IE with VSD, where 9/13 were open, and (iii) no cases of IE with PDA (83.6% were closed). A large population-based registry study of children who underwent surgical repair of congenital heart lesions reported no patient developed IE after surgical repair of PDA (620 patients, median age 2.6 years) and likewise in an ACHD population, no IE was reported [58]. The annualised risk of IE post repair of AoC has been estimated at 1.2 per 1000 patient-years [60]. Very uncommonly, early (<6 months) IE occurs after closure. Late onset IE is very rare and is usually due to delayed endothelialisation [63–65]. In fact, in a surgical follow-up study by Morris et al. [60], no children who underwent repair of an isolated secundum ASD developed IE following surgery. Small numbers were seen with primum ASD and complete AVSD. After 6 months post-surgical closure of ASD, VSD and PDA, the risk of IE is virtually eliminated. The same holds true for transcatheter closure, although with residual defects, the risk is not eliminated [52]. After definitive surgical repair of ToF, the risk is estimated at 0.7 per 1000 patient years but is much higher for a palliative shunt, at 8.2 per 1000 patient-years [60].

In a study by Rushani et al. [50], from the age of 0–6 months, unoperated cyanotic disease had an adjusted rate ratio (using ASD as a reference) for IE of 7.56, compared with the operated group at 9.22. For unoperated left-sided cardiac lesions, the rate ratio of IE was 2.35, though data was insufficient in the operated group to calculate the ratio [50].

In one study, the risk of IE was 5x increased early (<6 months) after any cardiac surgery in children [50] and 9.07x increased in adults up to 6 months after any non-valvular cardiac surgery [51]. Kuijpers et al. [5] reported valved-prosthetics in ACHD carry a hazard ratio (HR) of 17.29 (at 6 months), 15.91 (6-12 months) and 5.26 (>12 months) post-surgery. Non-valve containing prosthetics and repairs were associated with a HR of 3.34 at 0–6 months but no increase risk >6 months. The current European endocarditis prophylaxis guidelines (referred to elsewhere in this chapter) and US guidelines, accordingly recommend antibiotic prophylaxis for 6 months after complete closure of a defect with prosthetic material, regardless of whether it be percutaneously or surgically treated [57, 61].

8. Hypertrophic cardiomyopathy

8.1. Pathophysiology and diagnosis

Hypertrophic cardiomyopathy (HCM) is an inherited genetic disorder characterised by myocardial thickening. Often this is asymmetric with marked involvement of the ventricular septum. In this setting, increased gradients are generated through the left ventricular outflow tract (LVOT) and if sufficient, result in systolic motion of the anterior mitral leaflet (SAM). Repeated trauma from contact between endocardial surfaces, results in formation of plaques on the ventricular septum, at the point of contact with the MV leaflet. There are altered mechanical and haemodynamic forces acting on the MV, AV and LVOT. This predisposes to endothelial trauma and inflammation, with the potential formation of NBTE and IE at multiple sites [17].

8.2. Echocardiographic diagnosis and predictors of endocarditis risk

Modern echocardiography is readily utilised to diagnose hypertrophic obstructive cardiomyopathy (HOCM). Typical criteria include an unexplained septal thickness of ≥15 mm and LVOT obstruction as a resting or provoked gradient of ≥30 mmHg. In one study [66], the incidence of IE was 1.4 per 1000 patient-years. Echocardiographic predictors of IE risk included: (i) resting LVOT obstruction with incidence of 3.0 per 1000 patient-years, and (ii) marked left atrial dilatation (in presence of resting LVOT obstruction) with incidence of 9.2 per 1000 patient-years. Left ventricular wall thickness was not associated with increased risk [66].

There is overall conflicting data, with some studies finding IE is related to LVOT gradient and a propensity for MV infection, whilst other studies have found the contrary, with no particular relation to LVOT gradient or predilection for AV or MV [67].

9. Postinflammatory valve disease

9.1. Background and pathologic changes

The most common type of postinflammatory valve disease occurs as a sequela of rheumatic fever, leading to RHD. As discussed earlier in this chapter, the incidence has dramatically reduced in high-income countries, except in certain indigenous populations and remains a major global health burden across middle and low-income countries. In Australia, the estimated rate of ARF in young indigenous Australians aged 5–14 years is 150–380 per 100,000 person-years [68].

Rheumatic AV changes include thickening of the cusps, extending to the free margins and associated with commissural fusion. Calcification may eventually develop and occurs predominantly at the commissures and cusp margins. Concomitant changes at the MV are usual and involve thickening and retraction of the leaflets and chords along with commissural fusion. With 'pure' aortic regurgitation, there is cusp fibrosis with leaflet retraction. Fusion of the cusps may mimic a congenital BAV and a 'fish mouth' appearance of the MV on echo. Systemic lupus erythematosus and other inflammatory and autoimmune conditions can mimic rheumatic changes [16]. Rheumatic heart disease may involve all cardiac valves, but the mitral is most commonly affected. Stenosis is more commonly present at the mitral valve and regurgitation involving the aortic [49].

9.2. Echocardiographic diagnosis of rheumatic heart disease

The revised Jones Criteria [69] for diagnosis of ARF, importantly has now incorporated Doppler echo for both acute and chronic valvulitis. In the previous guideline (1992), cardiac involvement was based on clinical auscultation. Modern-era echo has been validated for diagnosis of subclinical carditis. Echo may either help confirm or exclude carditis when a murmur is present, or it may detect subclinical carditis. The most common cardiac changes are cardiac valve involvement (valvulitis) and may be accompanied by a pancarditis with or without a myopericarditis [69].

9.2.1. Echocardiographic diagnosis: Doppler haemodynamics and 2D features

With acute rheumatic mitral and aortic valvulopathy, functional and haemodynamic changes are readily diagnosed by Doppler echocardiography. The regurgitation must be demonstrated in at least 2 views with a peak jet velocity of >3 m/s, a pan systolic or diastolic jet respectively and a jet length of ≥2 cm for MR and ≥1 cm for AR. Morphological changes may or may not be present early during infection [69]. The morphological change(s) seen at the MV during acute valvulitis/carditis include: (i) annular dilatation, (ii) chordal elongation/rupture, (iii) leaflet prolapse and/or (iv) beading/nodular thickening of the leaflet tips. Chronic changes of the mitral valve apparatus include: (i) thickening of the leaflets/chords, (ii) chordal fusion, (iii) restriction of leaflet motion and/or (iv) calcification [69]. Acute and chronic aortic valve changes of rheumatic valvulitis/carditis demonstrated with 2-D echo include: (i) irregular and/or focal thickening of the leaflets, (ii) leaflet retraction/restriction with or without coaptation defects and/or (iii) leaflet prolapse [69].

9.2.2. Risk of endocarditis

Incidence of IE in persons with RHD is 3.8–440 per 1000 patient-years [61]. Data published from the National Health Service in England [70], revealed a marginally lower incidence of 3.05 cases per 1000 patient-years, compared with nonrheumatic valve disease at 2.73 per 1000 patient-years in the same study. The incidence of IE in rheumatic mitral stenosis is estimated at 0.17 per 1000 patient-years. Severity of valvular haemodynamics in RHD and risk of IE is not well described.

10. Intravenous drug use

Intravenous drug use (IVDU), along with cardiac-devices, CHD and vascular access catheters, are the major risk factors for RSIE. Right-sided IE constitutes 5–10% of IE cases and approximately 90% of RSIE involves the TV [71]. Overall, IVDU use accounts for 5–10% of all cases of IE [3, 72]. The median age at time of infection is 30–40 years, not infrequently seen in patients with human immunodeficiency virus (HIV). The majority of cases (right-sided > left-sided) are thought to involve structurally normal cardiac valves [8, 72]. Staphylococcus is the usual microorganism however infections are not infrequently polymicrobial [57]. Various fungi and pseudomonas are noteworthy for severe cases of IVDU-associated IE [8]. Interestingly, streptococci and enterococci more commonly affect left-sided valves, often with underlying structural abnormalities [73, 74].

According to Mathew et al. [75], the overall incidence of left-sided cardiac involvement was similar to right-sided IE, with a minority involving both right and left-sided valves [75]. Others have reported a predominance of right-sided lesions in patients with IVDU [72, 76]. The overall incidence of IE in IVDU is estimated at 0.7–20 cases per 1000 patient-years [74, 77].

The increased risk of IVDU patients acquiring IE is likely attributable to a multitude of factors. Proposed explanations include: (i) particulate matter injury to endothelium from substance injection, (ii) drug-induced thrombus formation and vasospasm, (iii) immune complex deposition on valves, (iv) altered host immune function, (v) frequent exposure to high volume bacterial inoculation, (v) increased prevalence of staphylococcal skin carriage, and (vi) sympathomimetic -induced PHTN resulting in an increase in valvular regurgitation velocity and endothelial trauma. A preference for right-sided involvement of structurally normal valves may also be related to altered host and microorganism factors [71, 74, 78]. It is theorised particulate matter up to 8–10 μm in size can transit across the normal pulmonary vasculature and potentially traumatise left-sided valvular endothelium [75]. However, the relatively high prevalence of left-sided valve involvement in the IVDU cohort without apparent underlying valve disease, may not be completely explained by the above theories and warrants further research.

Transthoracic echocardiography is often very useful in IVDU patients for excluding predisposing underlying structural heart disease and providing confirmation of IE, especially for TV endocarditis. Patients with IVDU are often younger and with satisfactory acoustic windows. In addition, the TV is located anteriorly within chest, being in close proximity to the imaging transducer. The use of TOE is preferred for complicated cases of right and left-sided IE, such as periannular extension, prosthetic valves, nondiagnostic TTE, CHD and for excluding infection at other sites within the right heart, such as the Eustachian valve, atrial wall or vena cavae.

11. Prosthetic cardiac valves, devices and risk of endocarditis

11.1. Surgical valves

The estimated risk of prosthetic valve endocarditis (PVE) overall is 0.3–1.2% per patient year (3–12 per 1000 patient-years) [57]. Recent study data from the National Health Service in England [70] reported an incidence of 4.64 cases per 1000 patient-years. In a landmark early study from the 1980s, the risk for mechanical valve IE was shown to be higher in first 3 months post-surgery, whilst for porcine valves, the IE risk was higher >12 months. The cumulative risk by 5 years was not significantly different between mechanical and porcine [79].

A large study recently published, incorporating contemporary valve data, has found bio-prosthetic valves do carry a higher risk for IE than mechanical valves, with a multivariable-adjusted hazard ratio of 1.65 (CI, 1.16–2.37) for early (<12 month) and 1.53 (CI, 1.25–1.86) for late (>12 months) IE. The crude incidence rates were 11.7 vs. 7 per 1000 patient-years for early IE and 6.0 vs. 4.3 per 1000 patient-years at 1–5 years (post-surgery) for bioprosthetic and mechanical valves, respectively. Similar rates were seen out to 15 years of follow-up in both groups. The overall combined incidence for PVE was 0.57% (5.7/1000) per patient-year [80]. It was suggested structural deterioration of prosthetic valves is a contributing risk factor, but this requires further investigation. Another study found a higher risk of IE with bioprosthetic over mechanical AVR, where the incidence of re-hospitalisation for IE was at 2.2% versus 1.4%, over 12 years follow-up, with adjusted hazard ratio of 1.6 (CI, 1.31–1.94). This difference was seen across all groups, except those aged 75–80 years and patients with renal failure [80].

11.2. Valve repairs

Valve repairs with prosthetic material carry a reported incidence of 4.71 cases per 1000 patient years [70]. In a pooled analysis (24 studies), recurrence of IE after mitral valve repair versus surgical replacement was 1.8% compared to 7.3% (p 0.0013), with a mean follow-up of approximately 50 months [81].

11.3. Transcatheter valves

The incidence of IE in transcatheter aortic valve replacement (TAVR) is similar to surgically placed prosthetic valves. There is no reported significant difference between self-expanding and balloon-expanding IE rates. Residual moderate or severe regurgitation was associated with higher rates of IE at 16.3 per 1000 patient-years versus 9.3 per 1000 patient-years for mild or no aortic regurgitation [82].

For pulmonary transcatheter valve (Medtronic Melody™), one study [83] reported a rate of IE of 3% per patient-year for a median follow-up of approximately 2 years. With regard to valved-conduits, the incidence of IE with RVOT homografts was lower at 0.8% per patient-year compared to Contegra-Melody conduit rate of 2.7–3.0% per patient-year. In patients with an infected Melody valve, 4/8 had a peak gradient >40 mmHg, whilst only 5/99 in the non-IE group had a similar gradient (p < 0.05) [83]. This suggests a possible increased risk of IE with residual post-procedural gradients, but numbers are insufficient and further studies are required to confirm or refute this assertion.

11.4. Device-related endocarditis

Ventricular assist devices (VADs) carry an incidence of IE of 5.8 cases per 1000 patient-years [70]. In one study investigating VAD infections, the following rates (cases per 100 LVAD-years) were found: i) all infection types –32.8 (CI, 26.7–39.9), ii) IE 1.6 (CI, 0.5–3.8) and iii) bloodstream – VAD-related, 7.5 (CI, 4.7–11.2) [84].

Implantable pacemakers (PPM) and cardiac defibrillators (ICD) have a reported incidence of IE ranging from 0.68–1.9 cases per 1000 patient-years [57, 70]. Cardiac device-related infective endocarditis accounts for 10–23% of device infections [85]. Numerous risk factors have been identified, including previous device-related infection, however information on risk related to underlying structural cardiac or TV pathology is uncertain. From the ICE-PICS data [86], 6.4% of all cases of IE were CDRIE. Over one-third of cases had associated valvular involvement, most commonly the tricuspid valve.

11.5. Recurrent native and prosthetic valve infective endocarditis

One of the most important cardiac risk factors for endocarditis is a prior history of IE. In the ICE- PCS cohort, recurrent IE occurred in 4.8% of patients, given an odds ratio of 2.8 (CI, 1.5–5.1) [87]. This is concordant with findings from other published studies with rates between 3.3 and 11.7% [88, 89]. In a recent study, the risk for recurrent IE was 14.36 per 1000 patient-years [70]. In a different study, the risk of recurrence (in patient-years) was estimated as follows: (i) history of previous IE, 7.4 per 1000, (ii) prosthetic valve surgery for native valve IE, 6.3 per 1000 and, (iii) prosthetic valve surgery for prosthetic valve IE, 21.6 per 1000 [61]. In a meta-analysis comparing biological versus mechanical valve for IE surgery, recurrence of IE in mechanical valves was 3–9% and for biological valves 7–29% [90] . Other studies have found equal rates of reinfection of bioprosthetic and mechanical valves.

Renzulli et al. [91], interestingly reported there was no association with previous perivalvular extension and recurrent risk [91]. In a study focussing on aortic homografts, Flameng et al. [92] found the recurrence rate of IE was relatively low at 7% at a mean follow-up of 8 ± 5 years. A significant downside is the high rate of structural deterioration of aortic homografts, with a rate of 40% at 10 years [92].

Shimokawa et al. [93] reviewed long term outcomes of mitral valve repair following IE in patients with prolapse and found good outcomes when compared with repair for degenerative MVP without IE. In this study, there were no recurrences of IE [93]. In another meta-analysis, comparing MV replacement with MV repair in the setting of IE, the 5 year risk of recurrent IE was favourable in the repair group with OR 0.39 (0.10–1.58) [94].

12. Conclusion

The three main categories of cardiac disease predisposing to infective endocarditis are degenerative valve disease, congenital heart disease and less commonly in high-income countries, rheumatic heart disease. The changing epidemiology has been associated with an ageing population, increased prevalence of prosthetic valves, devices and shunts, and health-care exposure. This chapter has outlined the underlying pathology, risks and echocardiographic predictors for IE associated with a selection of lesion-specific cardiac pathologies. The chapter also addressed the observation of structurally 'normal' cardiac valves accounting for a rising proportion of IE cases. Whether this relates to microorganism virulence, host factors, early structural and functional changes associated with degenerative valve disease, or a combination of all of the above, is unproven. Only further focused research using modern-era high resolution imaging and clinicopathological correlation, will provide new insight into this interesting question.

Author details

John F. Sedgwick[1,2]* and Gregory M. Scalia[1,2]

*Address all correspondence to: sedgwick.j@hotmail.com

1 Department of Echocardiography, Cardiology Program, The Prince Charles Hospital, Brisbane, Australia

2 The University of Queensland, Brisbane, Australia

References

[1] Cherubin CE, Neu HC. Infective endocarditis at the Presbyterian Hospital in New York City from 1938-1967. The American Journal of Medicine. 1971;**51**(1):83-96

[2] McKinsey DS, Ratts TE, Bisno AL. Underlying cardiac lesions in adults with infective endocarditis: The changing spectrum. The American Journal of Medicine. 1987;**82**(4):681-688

[3] Murdoch DR et al. Clinical presentation, etiology, and outcome of infective endocarditis in the 21st century: The international collaboration on endocarditis–prospective cohort study. Archives of Internal Medicine. 2009;**169**(5):463-473

[4] Cahill TJ, Prendergast BD. Infective endocarditis. The Lancet. 2016;**387**(10021):882-893

[5] Kuijpers JM et al. Incidence, risk factors, and predictors of infective endocarditis in adult congenital heart disease: Focus on the use of prosthetic material. European Heart Journal. 2017;**38**(26):2048-2056

[6] Di Filippo S et al. Current patterns of infective endocarditis in congenital heart disease. Heart. 2006;**92**(10):1490

[7] Habib G et al. ESC guidelines for the management of infective endocarditisThe task force for the Management of Infective Endocarditis of the European Society of Cardiology (ESC)endorsed by: European Association for Cardio-Thoracic Surgery (EACTS), the European Association of Nuclear Medicine (EANM). European Heart Journal. 2015;**36**(44):3075-3128

[8] Karl W et al. Mechanisms of infective endocarditis: Pathogen–host interaction and risk states. Nature Reviews Cardiology. 2013;**11**(1):35

[9] Baddour LM, FWK, Suri RM, Wilson WR. Cardiovascular Infections. In: Braunwald's Heart Disease A Textbook of Cardiovascular Medicine. 10th ed. Philadelphia, PA: Elsevier Philadelphia, PA: Elsevier Saunders; 2014

[10] Castonguay MC et al. Surgical pathology of native valve endocarditis in 310 specimens from 287 patients (1985-2004). Cardiovascular Pathology. 2013;**22**(1):19-27

[11] Collins JA, Zhang Y, Burke AP. Pathologic findings in native infective endocarditis. Pathology, Research and Practice. 2014;**210**(12):997-1004

[12] Michel P, Acar J. Native cardiac disease predisposing to infective endocarditis. European Heart Journal. 1995;**16**:2-6

[13] Rodbard S. Blood velocity and endocarditis. Circulation. 1963;**27**:18-28

[14] Ferrieri P et al. Unique features of infective endocarditis in childhood. Pediatrics. 2002;**109**(5):931

[15] Rodbard S. Blood velocity and endocarditis. Circulation. 1963;**27**:18

[16] Vaideeswar P, Butany J. Chapter 12 - Valvular heart disease. In: Cardiovascular Pathology. 4th ed. San Diego: Academic Press; 2016. pp. 485-528

[17] Thiene G, Basso C. Pathology and pathogenesis of infective endocarditis in native heart valves. Cardiovascular Pathology. 2006;**15**(5):256-263

[18] Sun BJ et al. Infective endocarditis involving apparently structurally normal valves in patients without previously recognized predisposing heart disease. Journal of the American College of Cardiology. 2015;**65**(3):307-309

[19] Castillo FJ et al. Changes in clinical profile, epidemiology and prognosis of left-sided native-valve infective endocarditis without predisposing heart conditions. Revista Española de Cardiología. 2015:445-448

[20] Olmos C et al. Comparison of clinical features of left-sided infective endocarditis involving previously normal versus previously abnormal valves. American Journal of Cardiology. 2014;**114**(2):278-283

[21] Que Y-A, Moreillon P. Infective endocarditis. Nature Reviews. Cardiology. 2011;**8**(6):322-336

[22] Sahasakul Y et al. Age-related changes in aortic and mitral valve thickness: Implications for two-dimensional echocardiography based on an autopsy study of 200 normal human hearts. The American Journal of Cardiology. 1988;**62**(7):424-430

[23] Crawford MH, Roldan CA. Quantitative assessment of valve thickness in normal subjects by transesophageal echocardiography. The American Journal of Cardiology. 2001;**87**(12):1419-1423

[24] Okura H et al. Prevalence and correlates of physiological valvular regurgitation in healthy subjects - a color Doppler echocardiographic study in the current era. Circulation Journal. 2011;**75**(11):2699-2704

[25] Dodo H et al. Are high-velocity tricuspid and pulmonary regurgitation endocarditis risk substrates? American Heart Journal. 1998;**136**(1):109-114

[26] López JJ et al. Age-dependent profile of left-sided infective endocarditis: A 3-center experience. Circulation. 2010;**121**(7):892-897

[27] Durante-Mangoni E et al. Current features of infective endocarditis in elderly patients: Results of the international collaboration on endocarditis prospective cohort study. Archives of Internal Medicine. 2008;**168**(19):2095-2103

[28] Pomerance A. Ageing changes in human heart valves. British Heart Journal. 1967;**29**(2):222

[29] Robicsek F, Thubrikar MJ, Fokin AA. Cause of degenerative disease of the trileaflet aortic valve: Review of subject and presentation of a new theory. The Annals of Thoracic Surgery. 2002;**73**(4):1346-1354

[30] Otto CM et al. Association of aortic-valve sclerosis with cardiovascular mortality and morbidity in the elderly. The New England Journal of Medicine. 1999;**341**(3):142-147

[31] Gharacholou SM et al. Aortic valve sclerosis and clinical outcomes: Moving toward a definition. The American Journal of Medicine. 2011;**124**(2):103-110

[32] Aikawa E, Schoen FJ. Chapter 9 - calcific and degenerative heart valve disease A2 - Willis, Monte S. In: Homeister JW, Stone JR, editors. Cellular and Molecular Pathobiology of Cardiovascular Disease. San Diego: Academic Press; 2014. pp. 161-180

[33] Delahaye JP et al. Infective endocarditis on stenotic aortic valves. European Heart Journal. 1988;**9**(Suppl E):43

[34] Chan K-L, Veinot JP. Anatomic Basis of Echocardiographic Diagnosis Kwan-Leung Chan, John P. Veinot. London: London: Springer; 2010

[35] Blaszyk H, Witkiewicz AK, Edwards WD. Acute aortic regurgitation due to spontaneous rupture of a fenestrated cusp: Report in a 65-year-old man and review of seven additional cases. Cardiovascular Pathology. 1999;**8**(4):213-216

[36] Waller BF, Howard J, Fess S. Pathology of aortic valve stenosis and pure aortic regurgitation: A clinical morphologic assessment — Part II. Clinical Cardiology. 1994;**17**(3):150-156

[37] He Y et al. Echocardiographic determination of the prevalence of primary Myxomatous degeneration of the cardiac valves. Journal of the American Society of Echocardiography. 2011;**24**(4):399-404

[38] Komiya T. Aortic valve repair update. General Thoracic and Cardiovascular Surgery. 2015;**63**(6):309-319

[39] Pressman GS et al. Mitral annular calcification as a possible Nidus for endocarditis: A descriptive series with bacteriological differences noted. Journal of the American Society of Echocardiography. 2017;**30**(6):572-578

[40] Freed LA et al. Prevalence and clinical outcome of mitral-valve prolapse. The New England Journal of Medicine. 1999;**341**(1):1-7

[41] Katan O et al. Incidence and predictors of infective endocarditis in mitral valve prolapse: A population-based study: A population-based study. Mayo Clinic Proceedings. 2016;**91**(3):336-342

[42] Clemens JD et al. A controlled evaluation of the risk of bacterial endocarditis in persons with mitral-valve prolapse. The New England Journal of Medicine. 1982;**307**(13):776-781

[43] Tay J, Yip W. Risk of bacterial endocarditis in persons with mitral-valve prolapse. The New England Journal of Medicine. 1983;**308**(5):282

[44] Retchin SM, Fletcher RH, Waugh RA. Endocarditis and mitral valve prolapse: What is the "risk"? International Journal of Cardiology. 1984;**5**(5):653-659

[45] Hickey AJ, Macmahon SW, Wilcken DEL. Mitral valve prolapse and bacterial endocarditis: When is antibiotic prophylaxis necessary? American Heart Journal. 1985;**109**(3):431-435

[46] Danchin N et al. Mitral valve prolapse as a risk factor for infective endocarditis. The Lancet. 1989;**333**(8641):743-745

[47] Nishimura RA et al. Echocardiographically documented mitral-valve prolapse. Long-term follow-up of 237 patients. The New England Journal of Medicine. 1985;**313**(21):1305

[48] Marks AR et al. Identification of high-risk and low-risk subgroups of patients with mitral-valve prolapse. The New England Journal of Medicine. 1989;**320**(16):1031

[49] Seki A, Fishbein MC. Chapter 2 - age-related cardiovascular changes and diseases A2 - Buja, L. Maximilian. In: Butany J, editor. Cardiovascular Pathology. 4th ed. San Diego: Academic Press; 2016. pp. 57-83

[50] Rushani SD et al. Infective endocarditis in children with congenital heart disease: Cumulative incidence and predictors. Circulation. 2013;**128**(13):1412-1419

[51] Mylotte D et al. Incidence, predictors, and mortality of infective endocarditis in adults with congenital heart disease without prosthetic valves. The American Journal of Cardiology. 2017;**120**(12):2278-2283

[52] Baltimore RS et al. Infective endocarditis in childhood: 2015 update. Circulation. 2015

[53] Pasquali SK et al. Trends in endocarditis hospitalizations at US children's hospitals: Impact of the 2007 American Heart Association antibiotic prophylaxis guidelines. American Heart Journal. 2012;**163**(5):894-899

[54] Marom D et al. Infective endocarditis in previously healthy children with structurally normal hearts. Pediatric Cardiology. 2013;**34**(6):1415-1421

[55] Gersony WM et al. Bacterial endocarditis in patients with aortic stenosis, pulmonary stenosis, or ventricular septal defect. Circulation. 1993;**87**(2 Suppl):I121

[56] Wu M-H et al. Ventricular septal defect with secondary left ventricular-to-right atrial shunt is associated with a higher risk for infective endocarditis and a lower late chance of closure. Pediatrics. 2006;**117**(2):e262

[57] Habib G et al. ESC guidelines for the management of infective endocarditis: The task force for the management of infective endocarditis of the European Society of Cardiology (ESC). Endorsed by: European Association for Cardio-Thoracic Surgery (EACTS), the European Association of Nuclear Medicine (EANM). European Heart Journal. 2015, 2015;**36**(44):3075

[58] Verheugt CL et al. Turning 18 with congenital heart disease: Prediction of infective endocarditis based on a large population. European Heart Journal. 2011;**32**(15):1926-1934

[59] Kiyota Y et al. Risk and outcomes of aortic valve endocarditis among patients with bicuspid and tricuspid aortic valves. Open Heart. 2017;**4**(1)

[60] Morris CD, Reller MD, Menashe VD. Thirty-year incidence of infective endocarditis after surgery for congenital heart defect. JAMA. 1998;**279**(8):599-603

[61] Wilson AW et al. Prevention of infective endocarditis: Guidelines from the American Heart Association: A guideline from the American Heart Association rheumatic fever, endocarditis, and Kawasaki disease committee, council on cardiovascular disease in the young, and the council on clinical cardiology, council on cardiovascular surgery and anesthesia, and the quality of care and outcomes research interdisciplinary working group. Circulation. 2007;**116**(15):1736-1754

[62] Bruce CJ, Connolly HM. Valvular heart disease: Changing concepts in disease management: Right-sided valve disease deserves a little more respect.(vascular medicine) (report). Circulation. 2009;**119**(20):2726-2734

[63] Zahr F et al. Late bacterial endocarditis of an amplatzer atrial septal defect occluder device. The American Journal of Cardiology. 2010;**105**(2):279

[64] Slesnick TC et al. Images in cardiovascular medicine. Incomplete endothelialization and late development of acute bacterial endocarditis after implantation of an Amplatzer septal occluder device. Circulation. 2008;**117**(18):e326-e327

[65] Amedro P, Soulatges C, Fraisse A. Infective endocarditis after device closure of atrial septal defects: Case report and review of the literature. Catheterization and Cardiovascular Interventions. 2017;**89**(2):324-334

[66] Spirito P et al. Infective endocarditis in hypertrophic cardiomyopathy: Prevalence, incidence, and indications for antibiotic prophylaxis. Circulation. 1999;**99**(16):2132-2137

[67] Sims JR et al. Clinical, radiographic, and microbiologic features of infective endocarditis in patients with hypertrophic cardiomyopathy. The American Journal of Cardiology. 2018;**121**(4):480-484

[68] Parnaby MG, Carapetis JR. Rheumatic Fever in Indigenous Australian Children. Melbourne. Journal of Paediatrics and Child Health. Australia; Sept 2010;**46**(7):527-533

[69] Gewitz HM et al. Revision of the Jones criteria for the diagnosis of acute rheumatic fever in the era of Doppler echocardiography: A scientific statement from the American Heart Association. Circulation. 2015;**131**(20):1806-1818

[70] Thornhill MH et al. Quantifying infective endocarditis risk in patients with predisposing cardiac conditions. European Heart Journal. 2017:ehx655-ehx655

[71] Hussain ST et al. Tricuspid valve endocarditis. Annals of Cardiothoracic Surgery. 2017;**6**(3):255-261

[72] Ortiz-Bautista C et al. Current profile of infective endocarditis in intravenous drug users: The prognostic relevance of the valves involved. International Journal of Cardiology. 2015;**187**:472-474

[73] Colville T, Sharma V, Albouaini K. Infective endocarditis in intravenous drug users: A review article. Postgraduate Medical Journal. 2016;**92**(1084):105

[74] Frontera JA, Gradon JD. Right-side endocarditis in injection drug users: Review of proposed mechanisms of pathogenesis. Clinical Infectious Diseases. 2000;**30**(2):374-379

[75] Mathew J et al. Clinical features, site of involvement, bacteriologic findings, and outcome of infective endocarditis in intravenous drug users. Archives of Internal Medicine. 1995;**155**(15):1641-1648

[76] Moss R, Munt B. Injection drug use and right sided endocarditis. (valve disease). Heart. 2003;**89**(5):577

[77] Axelsson A et al. Echocardiographic findings suggestive of infective endocarditis in asymptomatic Danish injection drug users attending urban injection facilities. American Journal of Cardiology. 2014;**114**(1):100-104

[78] Akinosoglou K et al. Native valve right sided infective endocarditis. European Journal of Internal Medicine. 2013;**24**(6):510-519

[79] Calderwood BS et al. Risk factors for the development of prosthetic valve endocarditis. Circulation. 1985;**72**(1):31-37

[80] Glaser JN et al. Prosthetic valve endocarditis after surgical aortic valve replacement. Circulation. 2017;**136**(3):329-331

[81] Feringa HHH et al. Mitral valve repair and replacement in endocarditis: A systematic review of literature. The Annals of Thoracic Surgery. 2007;**83**(2):564-570

[82] Regueiro A et al. Association between Transcatheter aortic valve replacement and subsequent infective endocarditis and in-hospital death. JAMA. 2016;**316**(10):1083-1092

[83] Van Dijck I et al. Infective endocarditis of a transcatheter pulmonary valve in comparison with surgical implants. Heart. 2015;**101**(10):788

[84] Nienaber JJC et al. Clinical manifestations and management of left ventricular assist device-associated infections. Clinical infectious diseases: an official publication of the Infectious Diseases Society of America. 2013;**57**(10):1438

[85] Arif S, Baddour LM, Sohail MR. Cardiac Device Related Endocarditis. Gilbert H. Infective Endocarditis. Epidemiology, Diagnosis, Imaging, Therapy, and Prevention. Cham: Springer International Publishing: Imprint, Springer; 2016. pp. 187-205

[86] Athan E et al. Clinical characteristics and outcome of infective endocarditis involving implantable cardiac devices. JAMA. 2012;**307**(16):1727-1735

[87] Alagna L et al. Repeat endocarditis: Analysis of risk factors based on the international collaboration on endocarditis – Prospective cohort study. Clinical Microbiology and Infection. 2014;**20**(6):566-575

[88] Shih C-J et al. Long-term clinical outcome of major adverse cardiac events in survivors of infective endocarditis: A Nationwide population-based study. Circulation. 2014;**130**(19):1684-1691

[89] Mansur AJ et al. Relapses, recurrences, valve replacements, and mortality during the long-term follow-up after infective endocarditis. American Heart Journal. 2001;**141**(1):78-86

[90] Newton S, Hunter S. What type of valve replacement should be used in patients with endocarditis? Interactive Cardiovascular and Thoracic Surgery. 2010;**11**(6):784-788

[91] Renzulli A et al. Recurrent infective endocarditis: A multivariate analysis of 21 years of experience. The Annals of Thoracic Surgery. 2001;**72**(1):39-43

[92] Flameng W et al. Durability of homografts used to treat complex aortic valve endocarditis. The Annals of Thoracic Surgery. 2015;**99**(4):1234-1238

[93] Shimokawa T et al. Long-term outcome of mitral valve repair for infective endocarditis. The Annals of Thoracic Surgery. 2009;**88**(3):733-739

[94] Wang T, Wang M, Pemberton J. Surgery for mitral valve endocarditis: Meta-analysis of repair or replacement. European Heart Journal. 2016;**37**(s1):1238-1238

8

Septic Embolism in Endocarditis: Anatomic and Pathophysiologic Considerations

Vikas Yellapu, Daniel Ackerman, Santo Longo and
Stanislaw P. Stawicki

Abstract

Septic embolism is a relatively common and potentially severe complication of infective endocarditis (IE). Septic emboli (SE), most often described as consisting of a combination of thrombus and infectious material—either bacterial or fungal—can be caused by hematogenous spread from virtually any anatomic site; however, it most commonly originates from cardiac valves. During the past two decades there has been a confluence of various risk factors that, both alone and in combination, led to greater incidence of both IE and SE, including increasing population age, greater use of prosthetic valves, implantation of various intracardiac devices, escalating intravenous drug use, and the high incidence of healthcare associated infections with antibiotic resistant microorganisms. From a clinical standpoint, SE can present at any time during the course of IE and may even be the initial presenting sign. SE may affect virtually any location in the human body, but some organs (e.g., liver, spleen, brain) and anatomic regions (e.g., lower extremity) tend to be more frequently involved. The most important aspect of management involves prompt recognition and proactive therapeutic approach. Given the broad spectrum of clinical presentations, symptoms and complications, SE can be challenging to diagnose and treat. Following the identification of SE, appropriate antibiotic coverage should be immediately instituted followed by supportive and/or interventional management, depending on the severity of presentation and the associated complications. In this chapter we explore the pathophysiology, anatomic origins, diagnostic tools, therapeutic measures, and new developments in SE, focusing predominantly on bacterial infections of cardiac origin.

Keywords: endocarditis, infective endocarditis, morbidity and mortality, septic embolism

1. Introduction

The collective understanding of infective endocarditis (IE) has changed significantly since its early characterization by Sir William Osler [1, 2]. In most low-and-middle income countries, rheumatic fever accounts for approximately two-thirds of all endocarditis cases [3–5], whereas in developed countries it is responsible for less than 10% of instances [6]. Over the past decade the incidence of IE has been increasing, with a recent study showing an overall increase of >30% between 2000 and 2011 [7]. The American Heart Association identified IE and associated complications as a major source of cardiovascular disability [8].

This surge in IE has been linked, in part, to recent medical advances, including increased use of implantable cardiac devices and a growing population of patients with chronic comorbidities [5, 9, 10]. Moreover, 10–35% of newly diagnosed cases of IE are thought to be healthcare associated infections, and hospital-acquired IE attributable to sources other than cardiac surgery is an emerging problem with mortality as high as 30–50% [11, 12]. The above observations can be explained, to some degree, by increases in antibiotic resistance including greater incidence of methicillin-resistant *Staphylococcus aureus* (MRSA), and higher prevalence of comorbidities in an increasingly aging population [2, 5, 12, 13].

In terms of intravenous drug use, injectable heroin has seen significant escalation [14, 15], with an associated incidence of IE growing by 58% between 2000 and 2013 [14]. In addition to the disease burden on individual patients and their families, the health-care system is further taxed with managing this difficult and expensive to treat population [14, 16]. Finally, it is important to recognize that recent years have seen IE presentations becoming more acute in nature, making diagnosis and treatment more challenging at times [5, 17, 18]. Among key complications of acute IE, the development of potentially devastating septic emboli (SE) may be seen. In this chapter, we will focus on the pathophysiology, diagnosis, and management of SE in the context of IE, using a systematic anatomic approach and outlining some of the most recent developments in this fast-changing area of cardiovascular infectious disease.

2. Pathophysiology of septic emboli

When discussing the pathophysiology of emboli of cardiac origin, one must consider both non-infective (Libman-Sacks or autoimmune, Marantic or related to wasting illnesses such as cancer) and infective (e.g., bacterial or fungal) endocarditis [19–21]. As an overarching theme, any condition that results in structural "damage or alteration" of cardiac valves has the potential to trigger an inflammatory reaction leading to the formation of valvular "vegetations" and thromboembolic complications [22]. In contrast to non-infectious valvular etiologies which lead to sterile emboli, IE has the potential to produce SE which typically are composed of a conglomerate of infectious organisms, inflammatory cells, platelets and fibrin [23]. In contrast to non-infectious emboli, SE have the potential to result in both vascular compromise and hematogenous spread of infection [24–26]. Evidence shows that as many as 50–82% of patients with IE may be affected by some form of SE, including both symptomatic and sub-clinical presentations [27–29]. In terms of valvular propensity for systemic (non-pulmonary) SE development, mitral valve is the most commonly involved [10, 30].

The genesis of SE is predicated on the appearance of a thrombus in a critical cardiac (usually valvular, **Figure 1**) location. This is usually associated with the presence of infected pacemaker leads, prosthetic valve, or some form of anatomic (acquired or congenital) abnormality of the native valve [30]. Bacterial species that feature specific adhesion matrix molecules are particularly likely to attach onto the damaged valvular surfaces, endocardium, or exposed prosthetic material [30–32]. Simultaneous presence of inflamed tissue and microorganisms leads to further accumulation of fibrin-platelet-microorganism complexes, contributing to the growth of infectious vegetations [33, 34]. If fragments of such vegetations—in whole or in part—are released into the circulation, SE is said to have occurred [5, 31, 32]. Microorganisms most often implicated include *Staphylococci, Beta-hemolytic Streptococci, Haemophilus, Actinobacteria, Caridobacterium, Eikenella,* and *Kingella.* The latter 5 are often listed under the acronym, "HACEK", and are less likely to cause IE than *Staphylococci* and *Streptococci* [10, 32, 35, 36]. Identifying the causative organism is critical to instituting prompt treatment with the most appropriate antibiotics. It is important to recognize that SE may affect any organ system or anatomic location, although certain patterns of involvement tend to be more common than others. This chapter will review key clinical evidence and developments regarding the diagnosis and management of SE. The authors will organize the current discussion according to regional/anatomic considerations in order to systematize and simplify the review process.

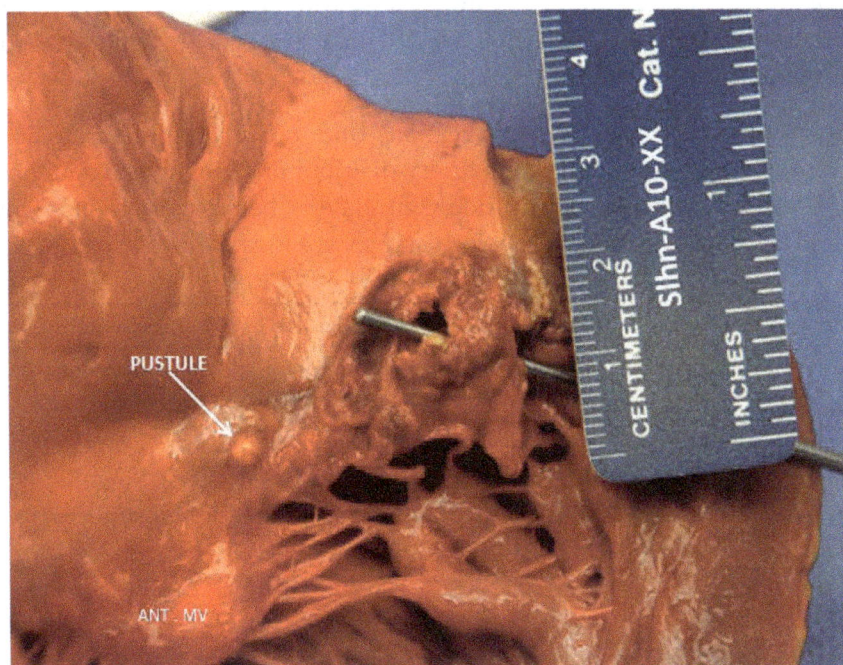

Figure 1. An example of a large necrotic bacterial vegetation, leading to the replacement of the entire posterior mitral valve leaflet. A pustule can be seen in the immediate vicinity of the vegetation. Also note the normal-appearing leaflet, chorda tendinea, and papillary muscles of the anterior leaflet (labeled as ANT. MV).

3. Head and neck

3.1. Brain

It is well known that there are many different central nervous system (CNS) manifestations of SE [37]. However, proving direct cause-and-effect relationship has been more challenging. Evidence suggests that septic cerebral embolic events may complicate as many as 40% of cases of IE, with recurrence rates for SE reaching 50% [38]. Cumulatively, manifestations of SE within the cerebral circulation can be divided into cerebral infarction (purely ischemic, purely hemorrhagic, or combined), CNS infection (encephalitis, meningitis, and abscess formation); and vasculopathy (vasculitis, mycotic aneurysm formation), with widely varied clinical presentations [38]. Summary of potential CNS manifestations of IE is provided in **Table 1**.

Involvement of SE within the CNS can be broadly categorized into cerebrovascular and non-cerebrovascular event types. Given that approximately 20% of cardiac output is dedicated to supplying the cerebrovascular system, it is no surprise that the brain is among the most commonly involved organs in IE. In fact, it is not uncommon for a cerebrovascular event to precede the formal diagnosis of IE, and to be the trigger for subsequent cardiac work-up [39]. Consistent with the above information, the greatest risk factor for a cerebral SE is left-sided IE, especially when due to *Staphylococcus aureus* infection. For embolic strokes, symptomatology heavily depends on the final resting point of the embolus. In one extreme case, complete cortical blindness followed the rupture of bilateral occipital mycotic aneurysms [40]. Even among patients with a limited duration of initial clinical symptoms, the risk of recurrent brain infarction may be as high as 80% [41]. **Figure 2** demonstrates septic embolism to the brain originating from mitral valve endocarditis.

Among patients experiencing CNS complications due to SE, approximately 50–60% have ischemic lesions, with the middle cerebral artery distribution being most commonly affected [42, 43]. Associated symptoms may include contralateral hemiplegia, homonymous hemianopia, dysarthric or aphasic speech, neglect, and sensory loss. It is difficult to differentiate

Cerebrovascular	Infections	Secondary complications	Rare complications
Ischemic stroke	Meningoencephalitis	Toxic-metabolic encephalopathy	Myeloradiculitis
Intracerebral hemorrhage	Cerebritis	Seizure	Spinal cord infarction
Subarachnoid hemorrhage	Abscess formation	Headache	Discitis/osteomyelitis
Mycotic aneurysm formation	Ventriculitis		Cranial neuropathies
	Ependymitis		Mononeuritis multiplex
			Myalgia

Adopted from Ref. [6].

Table 1. Central nervous system manifestations of infective endocarditis.

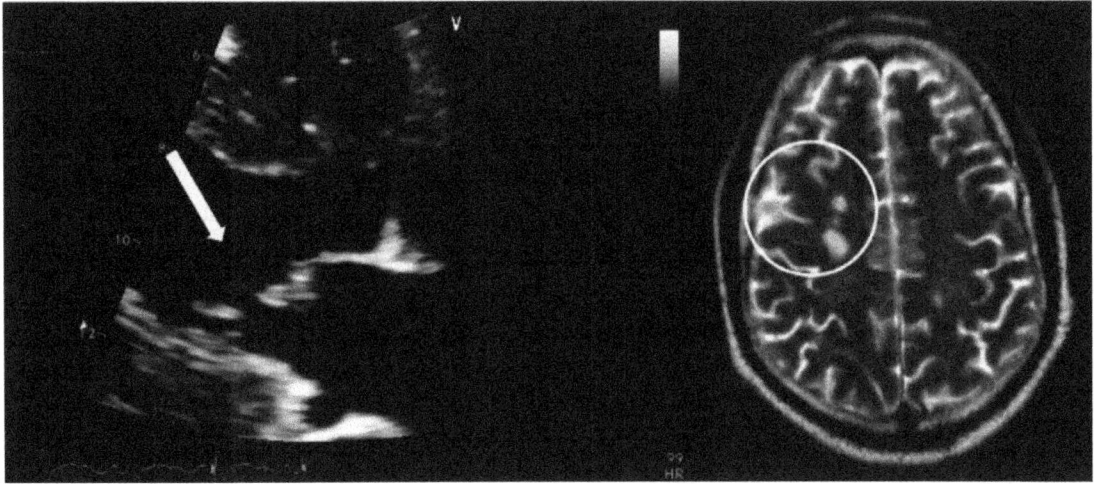

Figure 2. An example of septic embolization to the brain (circled) originating from an infected vegetation on the mitral valve (arrow) (source: Ref. [29]. Image used under the terms of the Creative Commons Attribution-Noncommercial-Share Alike 3.0 Unported license).

between intracerebral hemorrhage and ischemic infarction based on clinical symptoms alone, and importantly, the American Stroke Association recommends against the use of intravenous Alteplase in cases of suspected ischemic stroke due to SE because of elevated potential for hemorrhagic conversion [23]. At the time of this publication there is no specific recommendation for or against intra-arterial intervention (e.g., thrombectomy) in the setting of SE causing large vessel occlusion and cerebral infarction, and cases should be evaluated on an individual basis.

Risk factors for mortality in stroke caused by SE include MRSA infection, older patient age, and larger vegetation size [44]. Patients with right-sided IE can also experience cerebral SE although it is very uncommon and occurs through the so-called "paradoxical embolus" pathway [45, 46]. Prompt evaluation for cerebral SE is critical in any patient presenting with focal neurologic symptoms, and usually starts with computed tomography (CT) of the brain to rule out bleeding, and potentially CT-Angiography to evaluate the cerebral circulation for patency. One must keep in mind that, regardless of clinical symptoms, the majority of patients with IE have some evidence of cerebral SE on magnetic resonance imaging (MRI) [47, 48].

Patients with cerebral SE have elevated mortality rates compared to patients presenting with stroke from other etiologies. In fact, baseline mortality of approximately 8–9% may reach nearly 40% in the presence of meningitis, hemorrhage, or brain abscess [39]. In the setting of mild cerebral ischemia, immediate antibiotic therapy combined with valve surgery within 48 h results in improved outcomes, including fewer systemic embolic events and more favorable mortality profile [49]. Recent studies also suggest that an ischemic stroke secondary to IE is unlikely to transform into a hemorrhagic stroke [50]. Primary indications for surgery in the setting of IE include the emergence of heart failure, uncontrolled infection, and embolism prevention [49]. Note that antithrombotic therapy is somewhat controversial in this setting. The American Heart Association guidelines for surgical intervention state that in the absence of severe neurological deficits, cardiac surgery should be considered urgently [50, 51]. In cases of severe ischemic stroke, it is recommended to delay surgery by at least 4 weeks, and with hemorrhagic stroke (usually a more severe complication) at least 4 weeks are recommended prior to proceeding with cardiac surgery [50].

3.2. Eyes

Septic embolization involving ocular and facial structures is extremely rare. There is, however, fragmentary case-based evidence for such occurrences. In one example, Dadu et al. [52], described SE involving the ophthalmic artery and the inferior muscular artery, resulting in diplopia due to medial rectus muscle paralysis. In that particular case, IE of the mitral valve was causative. In another rare occurrence, Cumurcu et al. [53], describe a case of a septic metastasis to the iris, resulting in iris abscess and endophthalmitis.

3.3. Thyroid

The possibility of SE to the thyroid has been proposed in 1959 by Richie while describing acute suppurative thyroiditis in a child [54]. Cabizuca et al. [55], reported an unusual case of IE leading to acute thyroiditis, presumably due to septic embolization. Although undoubtedly uncommon, the paucity of literature reports in this area is likely due to limited awareness and under-recognition of similar clinical presentations.

4. The thorax

Given the pathophysiologic factors discussed earlier in the chapter, SE of cardiac origin tend to follow the pattern of "cardiac output." Consequently, a generalization can be made that the higher the blood flow to a specific organ or anatomic region, the higher the chance of SE traveling there. Within the thorax, there are two commonly described types of septic emboli — those originating on the "left side" of the heart and involving the coronary arterial circulation or thoracic aorta [56, 57], and those originating from the "right side" and involving the pulmonary arterial circuit [58–60].

4.1. Coronary circulation

First described in the 1910s and 1920s, septic coronary embolism continues to be under-recognized as a cause of acute coronary ischemia [56]. These types of emboli predominantly originate from bacterial valvular vegetations [61]. A high index of clinical suspicion is required because electrocardiographic (ECG) and laboratory changes characteristic of myocardial ischemia can easily be misinterpreted as being due to more typical coronary artery thrombosis [29]. The diagnosis is established through the performance of a comprehensive work-up, including trans-thoracic and trans-esophageal echocardiography (TEE), with subsequent angiography as indicated [62, 63]. Management may include a variety of both non-interventional and interventional procedures, up to and including surgical cardiac revascularization at the time of valve replacement [29].

4.2. Thoracic aorta

Mycotic aneurysms of the aorta have been described as a consequence of septic emboli from infective endocarditis [64]. Clinical management of these lesions is challenging, partly due to the presence of active infection within the aneurysm itself, and partly due to the associated inflammatory changes and altered (e.g., diminished) structural integrity of the involved aorta [65]. Mycotic aortic aneurysms are associated with significant mortality and complications, including the potential for the development of aortoesophageal or aortotracheobronchial fistula [66, 67].

4.3. Pulmonary artery

Pulmonary artery aneurysms (PAA) of infectious etiology are among less frequently seen complications of endocarditis [68, 69]. They are similar to mycotic aneurysms, with the main difference being the location of occurrence [70]. PAAs (also referred to as Rasmussen's aneurysms) can be seen in patients with tuberculosis. However, there have been recent cases with PAAs being associated with endocarditis [70, 71]. These aneurysms require prompt surgical treatment given published mortality rates of approximately 50% [72]. Patients with aneurysms that are symptomatic or >6 centimeters in size are candidates for surgery [73]. Data regarding surgical treatment are limited; however, recent studies have shown that steel coil embolization may be applicable in this setting [70, 74–76]. While PAAs are uncommon in endocarditis, they should be considered in patients with IE that present with pulmonary symptoms.

4.4. Pulmonary circulation

Pulmonary SE are relatively common complications of right-sided IE (RSIE). As outlined in previous sections, any areas through which large volume of blood transits will be inherently susceptible to SE. The pulmonary arterial circuit is no exception in this regard. From an anatomic standpoint, evidence suggests that septic pulmonary emboli (SPE) involve both upper and lower lobes, with bilateral upper lobes involved in >70% of patients, and peripheral or subpleural zones involved in >90% of cases [58]. Centrally located lesions were noted in only about 25% of instances [58]. SPE are distinct from other types of pulmonary emboli because of their tendency to form cavitary lesions with air-fluid levels [77]. A significant proportion of patients with RSIE are intravenous drug users [78, 79], although there is an increasing number of patients with SPE who present with IE due to implanted cardiac devices [80, 81]. SPE in intravenous drug users can manifest with empyema, and is most likely to be associated with endocarditis due to *S. aureus* infection [82]. Other common complications of SPE include pulmonary abscess and pulmonary nodules [77]. If patients with either empyema or a pulmonary abscess are identified, it is crucial to continue intravenous antibiotics and preform an incision and drainage prior to any required valve surgery [83]. Waiting is not recommended as a strategy in these patients, mainly because of the risk of further complications associated with therapeutic delays [83, 84]. Pulmonary and perivalvular abscess should be suspected in intravenous drug users who fail to respond to antibiotic administration [84].

As with any other type of pulmonary embolism (PE), SPE can be life threatening [85–87]. It is important to note that it may be initially difficult to differentiate between the two types of PE. Consequently, diagnosis and management requires high levels of clinical suspicion, appropriate diagnostics (e.g., TEE), and immediate treatment (antibiotics, with surgery if indicated). Most SPE patients present with constitutional symptoms, dyspnea, chest pain, and cough (including hemoptysis) [58]. CT imaging may show the presence of cavitary lesions with an associated "feeding vessel sign," representing a pulmonary artery coursing directly into the infected area [88].

5. Abdomen and retroperitoneum

5.1. The spleen

Septic embolism to the spleen is well described as a complication of IE [10]. In fact, after SE to the central nervous system (>50%), spleen appears to be the second most commonly involved organ in terms of frequency (approximately 30%), with some variability across sources of reported data [18, 28, 89]. One of most common presentations of SE to the spleen is the appearance of single or multiple abscesses [90], including microscopic lesions that were difficult-to-detect until the advent of advanced CT imaging [89]. Abdominal CT and MRI are the gold standard for diagnosing splenic abscesses [8]. Infected splenic artery aneurysms attributed to embolic sequelae of IE have also been reported [91]. Clinical management involves splenectomy in about 50% of cases, with percutaneous drainage indicated for large isolated abscesses and patients who are poor surgical candidates [29]. In cases of splenic arterial aneurysm and infarction, prompt surgical intervention is recommended. Patients should undergo drainage of the abscess or splenectomy prior to any cardiac surgery. This may help prevent further propagation and/or distant spread of the systemic infectious process [8, 91]. An example of splenic SE is shown in **Figure 3** [92].

5.2. The liver

Septic emboli to the liver are relatively common, occurring in >10% of cases of IE [10]. Similar to SE to the spleen, SE to the liver have the potential to evolve over time, coalescing from smaller "micro-abscesses" into larger collections [10]. Hepatic abscesses can be present in association with either right-sided or left-sided endocarditis [93, 94]; however, it may be difficult to determine whether the origin of the infection is cardiac or extra-cardiac, especially when the involved microorganism has known affinity for both locations [94]. Clinical management should follow established guidelines and practices for the treatment of IE and hepatic abscesses [29]. Similar to splenic abscess management, hepatic abscess should be drained as soon as possible in order to prevent worsening and/or further spread of the systemic infectious process [95].

5.3. The pancreas

Due to its vague clinical presentation, SE to the pancreas has the potential to go unrecognized. This is partially because SE to the pancreas often co-occurs with SE to other organs, potentially leading to "clinical masking" of organ-specific symptoms and/or signs [96]. Clinically, septic emboli to the pancreas may result in a picture resembling acute pancreatitis, and are

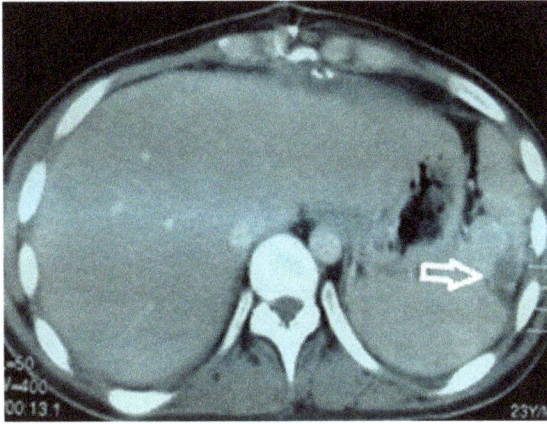

Figure 3. An example of septic embolus to the spleen. In this particular case, the embolus originated from *Corynebacterium diphtheriae* endocarditis (source: Ref. [92]. Image used under the terms of Creative commons Attribution-Noncommercial-NoDerivs Unported license).

usually characterized by leukocytosis, elevated pancreatic enzymes, peri-pancreatic "stranding" on CT scan, and acute abdominal pain [29]. Most often, pancreatic involvement in the setting of IE and SE tends to be self-limited [10]. At times, the finding of pseudoaneurysms involving adjacent arterial structures may provide a hint that the origin of the observed clinical syndrome is a result of SE [97].

5.4. The kidneys

Similar to the pancreas, SE to the kidneys is most often described in the setting of multi-visceral involvement [29]. Overall, renal SE are relatively frequent in the setting of IE, and their manifestations include infarcts in 31% of cases and glomerulonephritis in 26% [98]. Of interest, glomerulonephritis seen in association with IE has been shown not to feature immune complex deposition [98]. The co-occurrence of SE to other organs with arterial "high-flow" characteristics is exemplified by cases involving simultaneous cerebral, splenic, renal, and intestinal emboli [96]. Clinically, patients with renal SE may be found to have hematuria, glomerulonephritis, and evidence of renal failure [10]. Management focuses on preservation of renal function and is generally supportive, including antibiotic treatment, end-organ support (if required), and percutaneous or open interventions (in cases where abscess drainage is indicated) [98–100].

Etiology of renal injury in patients with IE is not always obvious, especially given the combined effect of cardiac dysfunction, sepsis, and concurrent treatment with potentially nephrotoxic antibiotics [98, 101]. Systemic infection can lead to acute tubular necrosis, while antibiotic treatment can lead to acute interstitial nephritis [102]. It is important to differentiate these conditions from the glomerulonephritis that is seen in IE, with an outline of important differentiating factors provided in **Table 2**.

5.5. The intestines including mesenteric involvement

Given its large surface area and rich vasculature, the bowel receives a significant amount of cardiac output and is highly susceptible to SE originating from IE [10, 29]. Fortunately, when compared to other organs and organ systems outlined above, arterial distribution to the

Type of kidney injury→	Glomerular	Interstitial	Tubular	Vascular
Typical causes	Bacterial endocarditis and vasculitis	Antibiotics	Sepsis and hypovolemia	Renal ischemia
Cast type	Red blood cell casts	White blood cell casts	Granular casts	Tubular epithelial cell casts
Clinical management	Treatment of underlying etiology	Remove inciting substance	Hydration and treatment of underlying condition	Surgical correction of underlying pathology

Table 2. Types of kidney injury, including their associated differentiating characteristics [102].

bowel appears to be less commonly affected (e.g., superior mesenteric artery in 3%, inferior mesenteric in <1%) [103]. This may be, at least in part, due to the presence of some degree of redundancy within the mesenteric vasculature, as opposed to a lack of such redundancy in the kidney or spleen. Occlusion of the superior mesenteric artery by SE is relatively well described in the setting of mitral valve endocarditis [104]. Mesenteric pseudoaneurysm attributable to SE has also been described [105]. In cases of acute arterial occlusion, bowel infarction may follow without prompt restoration of adequate blood flow to the involved segment(s) of bowel [106].

5.6. Reproductive organs

The involvement of reproductive organs in septic embolic complications is very uncommon. However, the authors believe that at least a brief overview of this under-recognized topic is warranted. In terms of testicular involvement, symptomatic presentation, including swelling, has been reported in conjunction with right-sided endocarditis [107]. It is thought that the this unusual clinical picture may result from SE [52, 107]. In another case, pneumococcal pulmonary valve endocarditis has been circumstantially linked to epididymo-orchitis and a scrotal abscess [108], although the directionality of causation may be difficult to prove except for the fact that *Streptococcus pneumoniae* isolated from the epididymo-orchitis is seldom a primary cause of scrotal infection. Equally uncommon, ovarian involvement has also been reported. In an exceedingly rare case, a female patient presented with a giant pyomyoma suggestive of ovarian neoplasm [109]. The origin of this presentation, however, was traced to *Streptococcus agalactiae* endocarditis and deep vein thrombosis of the right external iliac and femoral veins [109].

6. Extremities and musculoskeletal system

In general terms, extremity involvement in association with IE represents approximately one-third of all cases of SE, with clinical manifestations involving the musculature in approximately 40% cases and bones/joints in >10% of instances [10, 110]. Other than massive embolic events involving acute occlusion of arterial flow to an extremity producing significant ischemia, symptoms tend to be more "nebulous" in terms of clinical presentation, more self-limited in nature, and easily overlooked by clinicians [10, 100]. Pathognomonic signs such as Osler nodes

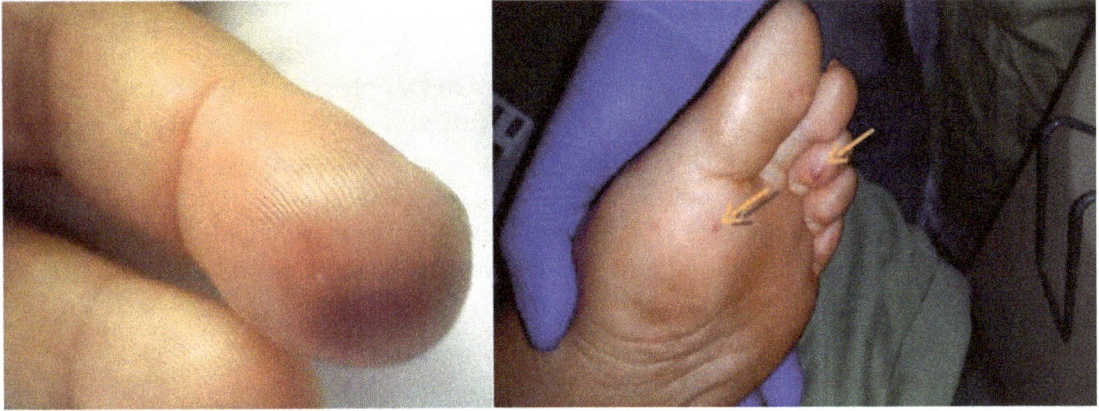

Figure 4. (A, left) An example of an Osler node in a patient with infective endocarditis (source: Ref. [112], image used in accordance with the terms of the CC BY 4.0 License); (B, right) Janeway lesions (see arrows) in a patient with aortic valve vegetation (source: Ref. [113], image used under the terms of the Creative Commons Attribution-NonCommercial 4.0 International License).

and Janeway lesions are rare (2.7 and 1.6% cases, respectively) but highly suggestive of endocarditis [111]. **Figure 4A** shows an example of an Osler node, while **Figure 4B** demonstrates a Janeway lesion [112, 113].

6.1. Acute extremity ischemia

This potentially devastating presentation has been reported in the setting of more severe cases of IE, often involving valve replacement [114–116], with some patients experience multiple/recurring embolic events [114, 115]. In terms of clinical presentation, patients may exhibit a broad spectrum of complaints including pain, pallor, poikilothermia, and paresthesias with extreme cases threatening the viability of the limb itself [114]. Both surgical and thrombolytic management options have been reported [117, 118]. Prompt recognition of the cardiac source of SE is critical in preventing further embolic events.

6.2. Septic arthritis

Due to their non-specific nature and general commonality, joint-related complaints can be challenging to diagnose and easily misinterpreted. Not infrequently, multiple diagnostic tools must be utilized to successfully identify the cardiac source of the patient's original symptoms (and thus the proximal source of infection) [119]. In one case, it was the complaint of septic arthritis which led to the ultimate diagnosis of streptococcal endocarditis [120]. Similar to other embolic phenomena associated with IE, septic arthritis tends to be a manifestation of multi-focal metastases of infectious material [119, 121].

7. Uncommon neurologic presentations

This section will discuss a heterogeneous group of less common manifestations of SE affecting the CNS, including extracranial involvement. The paucity of published literature in this broad topic area is likely due to limited awareness and under-recognition of such clinical presentations. Within the microcosm of SE associated with IE, approximately 30–40% of events involve neurological manifestations [10, 122]. Beyond the more commonly seen complaints (e.g., stroke, transient ischemic attack, meningitis, brain abscess) within this subset, less frequently reported clinical manifestations may include visual loss, seizures, acute mononeuropathy, and even spinal cord involvement [122–124]. Septic emboli can migrate to the spinal cord, causing segmental infarction [122, 123]. These exceedingly rare events have the potential to result in severe disability and often accompany additional, simultaneous SE to other anatomic regions [10].

8. Miscellaneous considerations

During the past two decades, significant increases have been noted in the number of valvular repairs, valve replacements, intracardiac devices and hemodialysis catheter placements [125–128]. Collectively, these procedures inherently create a small, but significant risk of IE, especially in patients with chronic comorbid conditions such as renal insufficiency, diabetes and autoimmune diseases [129–131]. Given the potential for major morbidity and mortality associated with IE in the setting of indwelling intravascular/intracardiac devices, the primary focus should be on prevention. Within this context, efforts include more selective device implantation policies and better modulation of known post-implantation risks [132].

In terms of general diagnostic considerations, numerous guidelines and recommendations have been published to date. Although beyond the scope of the current discussion, certain aspects of these recommendations warrant a brief mention [133, 134]. One very important highlight is the emphasis on prompt echocardiography in cases of suspected IE, with TEE recommended if the initial TTE is negative and clinical suspicion remains high [8]. Echocardiographic imaging can then be repeated in 3–5 days if clinical symptoms/suspicion persist [8]. It is also suggested that patients with vegetations >10 mm in size, embolic events while on antibiotic treatment, and patients with >2 embolic events should be evaluated for surgical intervention [8]. One unique diagnostic consideration is the inability to use magnetic resonance imaging (MRI) in patients with certain types of intravascular devices/implants. Amraoui et al. recently described the use of positron emission tomography (PET) as an alternative method of identifying foci of SE in patients with implantable cardiac devices, with limited success [135].

Treatment options start with intravenous antibiotics, however in certain cases prompt surgical treatment is necessary. The American Heart Association developed guidelines to assist with identification of patients who require prompt surgical intervention [136]. Patients with IE who develop decreased left ventricular ejection fraction (LVEF) or a new aortic or mitral valve murmur require prompt surgery [50, 136, 137]. Patients with preserved LVEF that are stable and adequately managed on medical therapy do not need an immediate corrective surgery [138]. However, a recent study demonstrated that surgical intervention in the setting of CHF can reduce mortality from approximately 60–85% to 15–35% when compared to medical therapy alone [139, 140]. Patients who present with valvular vegetations >10 mm in size, or with multiple vegetations on imaging, are likely to benefit from surgery [136]. Another important indication for surgery is lack of improvement after 7 days of appropriate antibiotic therapy [136]. Any SE to end organs or associated arterial aneurysms also warrant immediate surgical evaluation and prompt intervention. As mentioned earlier in the chapter, emboli to different anatomic regions may require distinct plans and different timing in terms of surgical intervention [50]. The diagnosis of prosthetic valve endocarditis constitutes another major indication for surgical intervention. Patients who present within 60 days of discharge following the placement of a new prosthetic valve with persistent fevers should be evaluated for the presence of IE, and if proven to harbor such infection should undergo operative management. It is important to remember that roughly 25% of prosthetic valve patients may be at risk of IE [136, 141].

9. Conclusions

Despite significant clinical research and advances in clinical management, septic embolism associated with infectious endocarditis continues to be a diagnostic and therapeutic challenge. Given the increasing number of intravascular and intracardiac device implantations, as well as the greater prevalence of chronic comorbid conditions, it is not surprising that the incidence of both infectious endocarditis and septic embolism has followed suit. In this chapter, we outlined general pathophysiologic and anatomic considerations with which all physicians should be familiar. This important knowledge should serve to assist providers in maintaining a high level of clinical suspicion for potential IE and/or SE. Given the continued high rates of associated disability and mortality, more research is needed to better understand and treat these "low-frequency, high-impact" events.

Author details

Vikas Yellapu[1], Daniel Ackerman[2], Santo Longo[3] and Stanislaw P. Stawicki[1]*

*Address all correspondence to: stawicki.ace@gmail.com

1 Department of Research and Innovation, St. Luke's University Health Network, Bethlehem, Pennsylvania, USA

2 Center for Neurosciences, St. Luke's University Health Network, Bethlehem, Pennsylvania, USA

3 Department of Pathology, St. Luke's University Health Network, Bethlehem, Pennsylvania, USA

References

[1] Osler W. Gulstonian lectures on malignant endocarditis. The Lancet. 1885;**125**(3210):415-418

[2] Alpert JS, Klotz SA. Infective endocarditis. In: Fuster V et al., editors. Hurst's the Heart. 14th ed. New York, NY: McGraw-Hill Education; 2017

[3] Carapetis JR et al. The global burden of group A streptococcal diseases. The Lancet Infectious Diseases;**5**(11):685-694

[4] Marijon E et al. Prevalence of rheumatic heart disease detected by echocardiographic screening. New England Journal of Medicine. 2007;**357**(5):470-476

[5] Cahill TJ, Prendergast BD. Infective endocarditis. The Lancet. 2016;**387**(10021):882-893

[6] Klaas JP. Neurologic complications of cardiac and aortic disease. Continuum: Lifelong Learning in Neurology. 2017;**23**(3, Neurology of Systemic Disease):654-668

[7] Pant S et al. Trends in infective endocarditis incidence, microbiology, and valve replacement in the United States from 2000 to 2011. Journal of the American College of Cardiology. 2015;**65**(19):2070-2076

[8] Baddour LM et al. Infective Endocarditis in Adults: Diagnosis, Antimicrobial Therapy, and Management of Complications. A Scientific Statement for Healthcare Professionals From the American Heart Association. Circulation. 2015;**132**(15):1435-1486

[9] Stawicki SP et al. Comorbidity polypharmacy score and its clinical utility: A pragmatic practitioner's perspective. Journal of Emergencies, Trauma, and Shock. 2015;**8**(4):224-231

[10] Wojda TR et al. Septic embolism: A potentially devastating complication of infective endocarditis. In: Contemporary Challenges in Endocarditis. Rijeka, Croatia: InTech; 2016

[11] Fernandez-Guerrero ML et al. Hospital-acquired infectious endocarditis not associated with cardiac surgery: An emerging problem. Clinical Infectious Diseases. 1995;**20**(1):16-23

[12] Benito N et al. Health care-associated native valve endocarditis: Importance of non-nosocomial acquisition. Annals of Internal Medicine. 2009;**150**(9):586-594

[13] Murdoch DR et al. Clinical presentation, etiology, and outcome of infective endocarditis in the 21st century: The international collaboration on endocarditis-prospective cohort study. Archives of Internal Medicine. 2009;**169**(5):463-473

[14] Wurcel AG et al. Increasing infectious endocarditis admissions among young people who inject drugs. Open Forum Infectious Diseases. 2016;**3**(3):ofw157

[15] Hedden SL. Behavioral Health Trends in the United States: Results from the 2014 National Survey on Drug Use and Health. Substance Abuse and Mental Health Services Administration, Department of Heath & Human Services; 2015

[16] Chakraborty K, Basu D. Physical complications of intravenous drug abuse: A comprehensive review. Eastern Journal of Psychiatry. 2009;**12**(1):49

[17] Cabell CH et al. Changing patient characteristics and the effect on mortality in endocarditis. Archives of Internal Medicine. 2002;**162**(1):90-94

[18] Hoen B et al. Changing profile of infective endocarditis: Results of a 1-year survey in France. JAMA. 2002;**288**(1):75-81

[19] Hennerici MG et al. Case Studies in Stroke: Common and Uncommon Presentations. Cambridge, UK: Cambridge University Press; 2006

[20] Rooth E. Hemostatic disturbances in acute ischemic stroke. 2011. Available from: https://openarchive.ki.se/xmlui/bitstream/handle/10616/40820/Elisabeth_Rooth_Thesis. pdf?sequence=1. [Last accessed on April 24, 2018]

[21] Hanna J, Furlan A. 20. Cardiac Disease and Embolic Sources. Brain Ischemia: Basic Concepts and Clinical Relevance. London, UK: Springer; 2012. p. 299

[22] Katsouli A, Massad MG. Current issues in the diagnosis and management of blood culture-negative infective and non-infective endocarditis. The Annals of Thoracic Surgery. 2013;95(4):1467-1474

[23] Demaerschalk B et al. On behalf of the American Heart Association Stroke Council and Council on Epidemiology and Prevention. Scientific rationale for the inclusion and exclusion criteria for intravenous alteplase in acute ischemic stroke: A statement for healthcare professionals from the American Heart Association/American Stroke Association [published online ahead of print December 22, 2015]. Stroke. DOI: 10.1161/STR.0000000000000086. Available from: https://professional.heart.org/professional/ScienceNews/UCM_479831_Putting-the-Patient-First-Comments-on-Scientific-Rationale-for-the-Inclusion-a.jsp

[24] Kannoth S, Thomas SV. Intracranial microbial aneurysm (infectious aneurysm): Current options for diagnosis and management. Neurocritical Care. 2009;11(1):120

[25] Olaison L, Pettersson G. Current best practices and guidelines: Indications for surgical intervention in infective endocarditis. Cardiology Clinics. 2003;21(2):235-251

[26] Peters PJ, Harrison T, Lennox JL. A dangerous dilemma: Management of infectious intracranial aneurysms complicating endocarditis. The Lancet Infectious Diseases. 2006;6(11):742-748

[27] Snygg-Martin U et al. Cerebrovascular complications in patients with left-sided infective endocarditis are common: A prospective study using magnetic resonance imaging and neurochemical brain damage markers. Clinical Infectious Diseases. 2008;47(1):23-30

[28] Millaire A et al. Incidence and prognosis of embolic events and metastatic infections in infective endocarditis. European Heart Journal. 1997;18(4):677-684

[29] Stawicki SP et al. Septic embolism in the intensive care unit. International Journal of Critical Illness and Injury Science. 2013;3(1):58

[30] Anguera I et al. Staphylococcus lugdunensis infective endocarditis: Description of 10 cases and analysis of native valve, prosthetic valve, and pacemaker lead endocarditis clinical profiles. Heart. 2005;91(2):e10

[31] Karchmer AW. Infective endocarditis. In: Kasper D et al., editors. Harrison's Principles of Internal Medicine. 19th ed. New York, NY: McGraw-Hill Education; 2015

[32] Crawford MH, Doernberg S. Infective endocarditis. In: Crawford MH, editor. Current Diagnosis and Treatment: Cardiology. 5th ed. New York, NY: McGraw-Hill Education; 2017

[33] Werdan K et al. Mechanisms of infective endocarditis: Pathogen–host interaction and risk states. Nature Reviews Cardiology. 2014;**11**(1):35

[34] Kerrigan SW. Platelet bacterial interactions in the pathogenesis of infective endocarditis—Part II: The staphylococcus. In: Recent Advances in Infective Endocarditis. Rijeka, Croatia: InTech; 2013

[35] Duzenli AE, Dwyer J, Carey J. Haemophilus parainfluenzae endocarditis associated with maxillary sinusitis and complicated by cerebral emboli in a young man. Journal of Investigative Medicine High Impact Case Reports. 2017;**5**(2):2324709617704003

[36] Dunn JJ, Hindiyeh IY. Clinical microbiology in pediatrics. Perspectives in Pediatric Pathology. 2011;**28**:80-103

[37] Molinari GF. Septic cerebral embolism. Stroke. 1972;**3**(2):117-122

[38] Ruttmann E et al. Neurological outcome of septic cardioembolic stroke after infective endocarditis. Stroke. 2006;**37**(8):2094-2099

[39] Heiro M et al. Neurologic manifestations of infective endocarditis: A 17-year experience in a teaching hospital in Finland. Archives of Internal Medicine. 2000;**160**(18):2781-2787

[40] Lawrence-Friedl D, Bauer KM. Bilateral cortical blindness: An unusual presentation of bacterial endocarditis. Annals of Emergency Medicine. 1992;**21**(12):1502-1504

[41] Horstkotte D et al. Emergency heart valve replacement after acute cerebral embolism during florid endocarditis. Medizinische Klinik (Munich, Germany: 1983). 1998;**93**(5):284-293

[42] Derex L, Bonnefoy E, Delahaye F. Impact of stroke on therapeutic decision making in infective endocarditis. Journal of Neurology. 2010;**257**(3):315-321

[43] Purves D, Augustine G, Fitzpatrick D. The blood supply of the brain and spinal cord. Neuroscience. 2nd ed. Sunderland, MA: Sinauer Associates; 2001

[44] Leitman M et al. Vegetation size in patients with infective endocarditis. European Heart Journal-Cardiovascular Imaging. 2011;**13**(4):330-338

[45] Sancetta SM, Zimmerman HA. Congenital heart disease with septal defects in which paradoxical brain abscess causes death: A review of the literature and report of two cases. Circulation. 1950;**1**(4):593-601

[46] Hart RG et al. Stroke in infective endocarditis. Stroke. 1990;**21**(5):695-700

[47] Bakshi R et al. Cranial magnetic resonance imaging findings in bacterial endocarditis: The neuroimaging spectrum of septic brain embolization demonstrated in twelve patients. Journal of Neuroimaging. 1999;**9**(2):78-84

[48] Cooper HA et al. Subclinical brain embolization in left-sided infective endocarditis: Results from the evaluation by MRI of the brains of patients with left-sided intracardiac solid masses (EMBOLISM) pilot study. Circulation. 2009;**120**(7):585-591

[49] Kang D-H. Timing of surgery in infective endocarditis. Heart. 2015;**101**(22):1786-1791

[50] Yanagawa B et al. Surgical management of infective endocarditis complicated by embolic stroke: Practical recommendations for clinicians. Circulation. 2016;**134**(17):1280-1292

[51] Baddour LM et al. Infective endocarditis in adults: Diagnosis, antimicrobial therapy, and management of complications: A scientific statement for healthcare professionals from the American Heart Association. Circulation. 2015;**132**(15):1435-1486

[52] Dadu RT, Dadu R, Zane S. Unusual presentation of endocarditis with nutritional variant streptococci. Clujul Medical. 2013;**86**(2):153

[53] Cumurcu T, Demirel S, Doganay S. Iris abscess as an unusual presentation of endogenous endophthalmitis after intramuscular injection. Ocular Immunology and Inflammation. 2010;**18**(3):190-191

[54] Richie JL. Acute suppurative thyroiditis in a child. AMA Journal of Diseases of Children. 1959;**97**(4):493-494

[55] Cabizuca C et al. Acute thyroiditis due to septic emboli derived from infective endocarditis. Postgraduate Medical Journal. 2008;**84**(994):445-446

[56] Brunson JG. Coronary embolism in bacterial endocarditis. The American Journal of Pathology. 1953;**29**(4):689

[57] Caraballo V. Fatal myocardial infarction resulting from coronary artery septic embolism after abortion: Unusual cause and complication of endocarditis. Annals of Emergency Medicine. 1997;**29**(1):175-177

[58] Cook RJ et al. Septic pulmonary embolism: Presenting features and clinical course of 14 patients. Chest. 2005;**128**(1):162-166

[59] Kuhlman JE, Fishman EK, Teigen C. Pulmonary septic emboli: Diagnosis with CT. Radiology. 1990;**174**(1):211-213

[60] MacMillan J, Milstein S, Samson P. Clinical spectrum of septic pulmonary embolism and infarction. The Journal of Thoracic and Cardiovascular Surgery. 1978;**75**(5):670-679

[61] Whitaker J et al. Successful treatment of ST elevation myocardial infarction caused by septic embolus with the use of a thrombectomy catheter in infective endocarditis. BMJ Case Reports. 2011;**2011**:bcr0320114002

[62] Kessavane A et al. Septic coronary embolism in aortic valvular endocarditis. The Journal of Heart Valve Disease. 2009;**18**(5):572-574

[63] Taniike M et al. Acute myocardial infarction caused by a septic coronary embolism diagnosed and treated with a thrombectomy catheter. Heart. 2005;**91**(5):e34

[64] Pasic M. Mycotic aneurysm of the aorta: Evolving surgical concept. The Annals of Thoracic Surgery. 1996;**61**(4):1053-1054

[65] Knosalla C et al. Using aortic allograft material to treat mycotic aneurysms of the thoracic aorta. The Annals of Thoracic Surgery. 1996;**61**(4):1146-1152

[66] van Doorn RC et al. Aortoesophageal fistula secondary to mycotic thoracic aortic aneurysm: Endovascular repair and transhiatal esophagectomy. Journal of Endovascular Therapy. 2002;**9**(2):212-217

[67] MacIntosh EL, Parrott JC, Unruh HW. Fistulas between the aorta and traceobronchial tree. The Annals of Thoracic Surgery. 1991;**51**(3):515-519

[68] Ungaro R et al. Solitary peripheral pulmonary artery aneurysms. Pathogenesis and surgical treatment. The Journal of Thoracic and Cardiovascular Surgery. 1976;**71**(4):566-571

[69] Deterling Jr RA, Clagett OT. Aneurysm of the pulmonary artery: Review of the literature and report of a case. American Heart Journal. **34**(4):471-499

[70] Theodoropoulos P et al. Pulmonary artery aneurysms: Four case reports and literature review. The International Journal of Angiology: Official Publication of the International College of Angiology Inc. 2013;**22**(3):143-148

[71] Wells I et al. Pulmonary mycotic aneurysm secondary to left-sided infective endocarditis treated with detachable coils. Clinical Radiology Extra. 2004;**59**(5):37-39

[72] Benveniste O, Bruneel F, Bédos JP, Wolff M, Lesèche G, Leport C, Vildé JL, Vachon F, Régnier B. Ruptured mycotic pulmonary artery aneurysm: An unusual complication of right-sided endocarditis. Scandinavian Journal of Infectious Diseases, 1998; **30**(6):626-628

[73] Ferretti GR et al. False aneurysm of the pulmonary artery induced by a Swan-Ganz catheter: Clinical presentation and radiologic management. AJR. American Journal of Roentgenology. 1996;**167**(4):941-945

[74] Caralps JM et al. True aneurysm of the main pulmonary artery: Surgical correction. The Annals of Thoracic Surgery. 1978;**25**(6):561-563

[75] Hamawy AH, Cartledge RG, Girardi LN. Graft repair of a pulmonary artery aneurysm. The Heart Surgery Forum. 2002;**5**(4):396-398

[76] Sakuma M et al. Peripheral pulmonary artery aneurysms in patients with pulmonary artery hypertension. Internal Medicine. 2007;**46**(13):979-984

[77] Wong K et al. Clinical and radiographic spectrum of septic pulmonary embolism. Archives of Disease in Childhood. 2002;**87**(4):312-315

[78] Rossi SE, Goodman PC, Franquet T. Nonthrombotic pulmonary emboli. American Journal of Roentgenology. 2000;**174**(6):1499-1508

[79] Hecht SR, Berger M. Right-sided endocarditis in intravenous drug users: Prognostic features in 102 episodes. Annals of Internal Medicine. 1992;**117**(7):560-566

[80] Graziosi M et al. Role of 18 F-FDG PET/CT in the diagnosis of infective endocarditis in patients with an implanted cardiac device: A prospective study. European Journal of Nuclear Medicine and Molecular Imaging. 2014;**41**(8):1617-1623

[81] Grammes JA et al. Percutaneous pacemaker and implantable cardioverter-defibrillator lead extraction in 100 patients with intracardiac vegetations defined by transesophageal echocardiogram. Journal of the American College of Cardiology. 2010;**55**(9):886-894

[82] Ye R et al. Clinical characteristics of septic pulmonary embolism in adults: A systematic review. Respiratory Medicine. 2014;**108**(1):1-8

[83] Horstkotte D et al. Guidelines on prevention, diagnosis and treatment of infective endocarditis executive summary; the task force on infective endocarditis of the European society of cardiology. European Heart Journal. 2004;**25**(3):267-276

[84] Olaison L, Pettersson G. Current best practices and guidelines: Indications for surgical intervention in infective endocarditis. Infectious Disease Clinics of North America. 2002;**16**(2):453-475

[85] Rockoff MA, Gang DL, Vacanti JP. Fatal pulmonary embolism following removal of a central venous catheter. Journal of Pediatric Surgery. 1984;**19**(3):307-309

[86] Sheu C-C et al. Spontaneous pneumothorax as a complication of septic pulmonary embolism in an intravenous drug user: A case report. The Kaohsiung Journal of Medical Sciences. 2006;**22**(2):89-93

[87] Goswami U et al. Associations and outcomes of septic pulmonary embolism. The Open Respiratory Medicine Journal. 2014;**8**:28

[88] Dodd JD, Souza CA, Müller NL. High-resolution MDCT of pulmonary septic embolism: Evaluation of the feeding vessel sign. American Journal of Roentgenology. 2006;**187**(3):623-629

[89] Ting W et al. Splenic septic emboli in endocarditis. Circulation. 1990;**82**(5 Suppl):IV105-IV109

[90] Chulay JD, Lankerani MR. Splenic abscess: Report of 10 cases and review of the literature. The American Journal of Medicine. 1976;**61**(4):513-522

[91] McCready RA et al. Infected splenic artery aneurysm with associated splenic abscess formation secondary to bacterial endocarditis: Case report and review of the literature. Journal of Vascular Surgery. 2007;**45**(5):1066-1068

[92] Patris V et al. Corynebacterium diphtheriae endocarditis with multifocal septic emboli: Can prompt diagnosis help avoid surgery? The American Journal of Case Reports. 2014;**15**:352

[93] Yang W, Lin H-D, Wang L-M. Pyogenic liver abscess associated with septic pulmonary embolism. Journal of the Chinese Medical Association. 2008;**71**(9):442-447

[94] Tran MP et al. Streptococcus intermedius causing infective endocarditis and abscesses: A report of three cases and review of the literature. BMC Infectious Diseases. 2008;**8**(1):154

[95] Rashid RM, Salah W, Parada JP. "Streptococcus milleri" aortic valve endocarditis and hepatic abscess. Journal of Medical Microbiology. 2007;**56**(2):280-282

[96]   Hart RG, Kagan-Hallet K, Joerns SE. Mechanisms of intracranial hemorrhage in infective endocarditis. Stroke. 1987;**18**(6):1048-1056

[97]   Nwafor I et al. Giant pseudoaneurysm of a splanchnic artery: A case report. Journal of Vascular Medicine and Surgery. 2015;**3**(208):2

[98]   Majumdar A et al. Renal pathological findings in infective endocarditis. Nephrology Dialysis Transplantation. 2000;**15**(11):1782-1787

[99]   Townell NJ et al. Community-associated methicillin-resistant staphylococcus aureus endocarditis "down under": Case series and literature review. Scandinavian Journal of Infectious Diseases. 2012;**44**(7):536-540

[100] Colen TW et al. Radiologic manifestations of extra-cardiac complications of infective endocarditis. European Radiology. 2008;**18**(11):2433

[101] Gerlach AT et al. Risk factors for aminoglycoside-associated nephrotoxicity in surgical intensive care unit patients. International Journal of Critical Illness and Injury Science. 2011;**1**(1):17

[102] Cannon DC. The identification and pathogenesis of urine casts. Laboratory Medicine. 1979;**10**(1):8-11

[103] Kirkwood ML et al. Mycotic inferior mesenteric artery aneurysm secondary to native valve endocarditis caused by coagulase-negative Staphylococcus. Annals of Vascular Surgery. 2014;**28**(5):1312.e13-1312.e15

[104] Misawa S-i et al. Septic embolic occlusion of the superior mesenteric artery induced by mitral valve endocarditis. Annals of Thoracic and Cardiovascular Surgery. 2011; **17**(4):415-417

[105] Cassada DC et al. Mesenteric pseudoaneurysm resulting from septic embolism. Annals of Vascular Surgery. 1998;**12**(6):597-600

[106] Edwards MS et al. Acute occlusive mesenteric ischemia: Surgical management and outcomes. Annals of Vascular Surgery. 2003;**17**(1):72-79

[107] Muthukumaran CS, Govindaraj PR, Vettukattil J. Testicular swelling with pneumonia and septicaemia: A rare presentation of right-sided endocarditis. Cardiology in the Young. 2005;**15**(5):532-533

[108] Vrettos A et al. Pneumococcal pulmonary valve endocarditis. Echo Research and Practice. 2017;**4**(3):K1-K5

[109] Genta PR et al. Streptococcus agalactiae endocarditis and giant pyomyoma simulating ovarian cancer. Southern Medical Journal. 2001;**94**(5):508-511

[110] Churchill MA, Geraci JE, Hunder GG. Musculoskeletal manifestations of bacterial endocarditis. Annals of Internal Medicine. 1977;**87**(6):754-759

[111] Bachmeyer C, Dubourdieu V, Poignet B. Do not disregard diagnostic clues of endocarditis: Comment on the article by Garg et al. Arthritis Care & Research. 2018. DOI:

https://doi.org/10.1002/acr.23526. Availabe from: https://onlinelibrary.wiley.com/doi/abs/10.1002/acr.23526 [ahead of print]

[112] Tsagaratos C, Taha FW. Recognizing infective endocarditis in the emergency department. The Western Journal of Emergency Medicine. 2012;**13**(1):92-93

[113] Fareedy SB, Rajagopalan P, Schmidt EC. Janeway lesions: A valuable clinical sign in patients with infective endocarditis. Journal of Community Hospital Internal Medicine Perspectives. 2016;**6**(2):30660

[114] Kitts D, Bongard FS, Klein SR. Septic embolism complicating infective endocarditis. Journal of Vascular Surgery. 1991;**14**(4):480-487

[115] Mandell GL et al. Enterococcal endocarditis: An analysis of 38 patients observed at the New York Hospital-Cornell medical Center. Archives of Internal Medicine. 1970; **125**(2):258-264

[116] Pessinaba S et al. Vascular complications of infective endocarditis. Médecine et Maladies Infectieuses. 2012;**42**(5):213-217

[117] Lozano P et al. Acute lower limb ischemia complicating endocarditis due toCandida parapsilosis in a drug abuser. Annals of Vascular Surgery. 1994;**8**(6):591-594

[118] Miroslav M et al. Rare forms of peripheral arterial embolism: Review of 11 cases. Vascular. 2005;**13**(4):222-229

[119] Bonfiglioli R et al. 18 F-FDG PET/CT diagnosis of unexpected extracardiac septic embolisms in patients with suspected cardiac endocarditis. European Journal of Nuclear Medicine and Molecular Imaging. 2013;**40**(8):1190-1196

[120] Good AE, Hague JM, Kauffman CA. Streptococcal endocarditis initially seen as septic arthritis. Archives of Internal Medicine. 1978;**138**:805-806

[121] Bossert M et al. Septic arthritis of the acromioclavicular joint. Joint, Bone, Spine. 2010;**77**(5):466-469

[122] Royden Jones Jr H, Siekert RG. Neurological manifestations of infective endocarditis: Review of clinical and therapeutic challenges. Brain. 1989;**112**(5):1295-1315

[123] Sandson TA, Friedman JH. Spinal cord infarction. Report of 8 cases and review of the literature. Medicine. 1989;**68**(5):282-292

[124] Siccoli M et al. Successful intra-arterial thrombolysis in basilar thrombosis secondary to infectious endocarditis. Cerebrovascular Diseases. 2003;**16**(3):295-297

[125] Premuzic V et al. Complications of permanent hemodialysis catheter placement; need for better pre-implantation algorithm? Therapeutic Apheresis and Dialysis. 2016;**20**(4): 394-399

[126] Falk V. Transcatheter aortic valve replacement indications should not be expanded to lower-risk and younger patients response to falk. Circulation. 2014;**130**(25):2332-2342

[127] Chaker Z et al. Sex differences in the utilization and outcomes of surgical aortic valve replacement for severe aortic stenosis. Journal of the American Heart Association. 2017;**6**(9):e006370

[128] Bradshaw PJ et al. Trends in the incidence and prevalence of cardiac pacemaker insertions in an ageing population. Open Heart. 2014;**1**(1):e000177

[129] Salvador VBD et al. Clinical risk factors for infective endocarditis in *Staphylococcus aureus* Bacteremia. Texas Heart Institute Journal. 2017;**44**(1):10-15

[130] Desai RJ et al. Risk of serious infections associated with use of immunosuppressive agents in pregnant women with autoimmune inflammatory conditions: Cohort study. BMJ. 2017;**356**:j895

[131] Polyzos KA, Konstantelias AA, Falagas ME. Risk factors for cardiac implantable electronic device infection: A systematic review and meta-analysis. EP Europace. 2015; **17**(5):767-777

[132] Nielsen JC, Gerdes JC, Varma N. Infected cardiac-implantable electronic devices: Prevention, diagnosis, and treatment. European Heart Journal. 2015;**36**(37):2484-2490

[133] Habib G et al. 2015 ESC guidelines for the management of infective endocarditis: The task force for the management of infective endocarditis of the European Society of Cardiology (ESC) endorsed by: European Association for Cardio-Thoracic Surgery (EACTS), the European Association of Nuclear Medicine (EANM). European Heart Journal. 2015;**36**(44):3075-3128

[134] Pappas PG et al. Clinical practice guideline for the management of candidiasis: 2016 update by the Infectious Diseases Society of America. Clinical Infectious Diseases. 2015;**62**(4):e1-e50

[135] Amraoui S et al. Contribution of PET imaging to the diagnosis of septic embolism in patients with pacing lead endocarditis. JACC: Cardiovascular Imaging. 2016;**9**(3):283-290

[136] Prendergast BD, Tornos P. Surgery for infective endocarditis: Who and when? Circulation. 2010;**121**(9):1141-1152

[137] Tornos P et al. Infective endocarditis in Europe: Lessons from the Euro heart survey. Heart. 2005;**91**(5):571-575

[138] Hasbun R et al. Complicated left-sided native valve endocarditis in adults: Risk classification for mortality. JAMA. 2003;**289**(15):1933-1940

[139] Croft CH et al. Analysis of surgical versus medical therapy in active complicated native valve infective endocarditis. American Journal of Cardiology. 1983;**51**(10):1650-1655

[140] Richardson JV et al. Treatment of infective endocarditis: A 10-year comparative analysis. Circulation. 1978;**58**(4):589-597

[141] Pansini S et al. Risk of recurrence after reoperation for prosthetic valve endocarditis. The Journal of Heart Valve Disease. 1997;**6**(1):84-87

9

Epidemiology of Infective Endocarditis

Fabian Andres Giraldo Vallejo

Abstract

Infective endocarditis is a rare disease, with an incidence of two to six episodes per 100,000 habitants/year. Incidence is higher in elderly people; besides, this group is often affected by many comorbidities. There is a clear and observable change in the spectrum of heart diseases predisposing to infective endocarditis in the last decades. Up to one-third of the patients acquire the disease on a health-care-associated environment. Despite advances in health-care logistics, infective endocarditis remains a big concern especially in low-income countries, where the main cause of infection is rheumatic fever. In-hospital mortality persists relatively high despite development in medical and surgical treatment. Patients with infective endocarditis need rapid response and prompt diagnosis from a multidisciplinary group including cardiologists, surgeons, infectologists, and radiologists.

Keywords: endocarditis, epidemiology, microbiology, outcome, incidence, mortality

1. Introduction

The term *infective endocarditis* (IE) denotes infection of the endocardial surface of the heart. Infection involves heart valves most commonly but may occur within a septal defect, chordae tendinae, or in the mural endocardium. Infections of arteriovenous shunts, arterioarterial shunts (patent ductus arteriosus), or coarctation of the aorta are clinically and pathologically similar to IE. The characteristic lesion of the IE, the vegetation, is a variably sized mass with inflammatory cells, platelets, fibrin, and abundant immerse microorganisms. The term *infective endocarditis,* first used by Thayer and later popularized by Lerner and Weinstein,is preferable to the former term bacterial endocarditis, because chlamydiae, rickettsiae, mycoplasmas, fungi, and perhaps even viruses may be responsible for the syndrome [1].

Diagnostic criteria for IE were published in 1982 by von Reyn and colleagues (The Beth Israel criteria), but these criteria did not use echocardiographic findings in the case definitions [2]. Including the central role of echocardiography in the evaluation of suspected IE, new case definitions and diagnostic criteria (The Duke criteria) were proposed in 1994 [3], modified in 2000, and widely used since then (**Table 1**) [4]. Echocardiography utility in the diagnosis of IE is clearly recognized [5], transesophageal imaging has superior sensitivity and specificity, is cost-effective, and is recommended when transthoracic approach is negative and a high clinical suspicion is present. The utility of both modalities is diminished when used indiscriminately [6, 7]. Advances in imaging technology have had minimal impact at the day-to-day clinical level; the role of three-dimensional (3D) echocardiography and other modes of clinical imaging (magnetic resonance imaging, computed tomography, and technetium scintigraphy) are yet to be formally evaluated [8].

Definition of infective endocarditis (IE) according to modified Duke criteria

Definite infective endocarditis

Pathologic criteria

- Microorganisms demonstrated by culture or histologic examination of a vegetation, a vegetation that has embolized, or an intracardiac abscess specimen; *or*

- Pathologic lesions; vegetation or intracardiac abscess confirmed by histologic examination showing active endocarditis

Clinical criteria

- Two major criteria; *or*

- One major criterion and three minor criteria; *or*

- Five minor criteria

Possible infective endocarditis

- One major criterion and one minor criterion; *or*

- Three minor criteria

Rejected

- Firm alternate diagnosis explaining evidence of IE; *or*

- Resolution of IE syndrome with antibiotic therapy for ≤4 days; *or*

- No pathologic evidence of IE at surgery or autopsy, with antibiotic therapy for ≤4 days; *or*

- Does not meet criteria for possible IE, as above

Major criteria

Blood culture positive for IE

- Typical microorganisms consistent with IE from two separate blood cultures: viridans *Streptococci, Streptococcus bovis*, HACEK group, *Staphylococcus aureus*; *or*

- Community-acquired *Enterococci*, in the absence of a primary focus; *or*

- Microorganisms consistent with IE from persistently positive blood cultures, defined as follows:

- At least two positive cultures of blood samples drawn >12 h apart; *or*

- All of three or a majority of ≥ four separate cultures of blood (with first and last sample drawn at least 1 h apart)

- Single positive blood culture for *Coxiella burnetii* or antiphase I IgG antibody titer >1:800

Evidence of endocardial involvement

- Echocardiogram positive for IE (TEE recommended in patients with prosthetic valves, rated at least "possible IE" by clinical criteria, or complicated IE (paravalvular abscess); TTE as first test in other patients), defined as follows:

  ○ Oscillating intracardiac mass on valve or supporting structures, in the path of regurgitant jets, or on implanted material in the absence of an alternative anatomic explanation; *or*

  ○ Abscess; *or*

  ○ New partial dehiscence of prosthetic valve New valvular regurgitation (worsening or changing of preexisting murmur not sufficient)

Minor criteria

- Predisposition, predisposing heart condition or injection drug use

- Fever, temperature >38·C (100.4·F)

- Vascular phenomena, major arterial emboli, septic pulmonary infarcts, mycotic aneurysm, intracranial hemorrhage, conjunctival hemorrhages, and Janeway lesions

- Immunologic phenomena: glomerulonephritis, Osler's nodes, Roth's spots, and rheumatoid factor

- Microbiologic evidence: positive blood culture but does not meet a major criterion as noted above* or serologic evidence of active infection with organism consistent with IE

- Echocardiographic minor criteria eliminated

TEE, transesophageal echocardiography; TTE, transthoracic echocardiography. Modified from [4].

Table 1. HACEK, *Hemophilus* spp., *Aggregatibacter* spp., *Cardiobacterium hominis, Eikenella corrodens,* and *Kingella* spp.

The challenges associated with IE are of increasing importance. The patients affected are older and sicker than those in the past, often with many comorbidities [9]. *Staphylococcus aureus* has surpassed penicillin-sensitive *Streptococci* as the most common cause in many high-income countries [10]. The population at risk is growing and health-care-associated *Staphylococcal bacteremia,* a conditioning of IE, is a major problem around the world [11].

In the last 30 years, the overall incidence of IE has remained between two and six per 100,000 individuals per year in the general population [12–14], whereas associated mortality has remained between 10 and 30% depending on the type of pathogen [15], the site of infection (native or prosthetic valve), and the underlying condition [16]. This quiescent trends in mortality and incidence are due to a continuing evolution of epidemiological features and risk factors rather to a lack of medical progress. The variability of disease presentation and course represents a challenge for the physician [8]. Even though clinical practices are clearly explained by international guides, they are derived mainly from observational cohort studies rather than randomized trials [17, 18]. Chronic rheumatic heart disease was considered a primary risk factor for IE until the widespread introduction of antibiotics; nevertheless, this finding prevails for low-income countries [14]. Current behavior in industrialized countries portraits different risk groups including prosthetic valve recipients, intravenous (IV) drug users, individuals with intravenous catheters, patients undergoing hemodialysis, and elderly people with degenerative valve lesions. Oral *Streptococci* are the main cause of IE in the general population [14, 19, 20], whereas *S. aureus* and coagulase-negative *Staphylococci* (e.g., *S. epidermidis*) are more frequently found in intravenous drug users, individuals with prosthetic-valve IE and in those with health-care-related IE [12, 21–23] and group *D Streptococci* (e.g. *S. gallolyticus*) are increasingly prevalent in elderly patients [12, 14, 19, 24, 25]. Patients with IE require opportune diagnosis and prompt response from a multidisciplinary group including cardiologists, cardiac surgeons, infectious disease specialists, and radiologists. The logistics of high-level patient care remains difficult even in developed countries and is frequently unobtainable in low-income countries.

2. Epidemiology

The incidence of IE is difficult to determine, because the diagnosis criteria and reporting methods vary with different series [2, 26]. The annual incidence of IE reported in Olmsted County, MN, was five to seven cases per 100,000 person-years, from 1970 to 2000, with practically no change in this period interval [27]. Parallel results of 1.7 per 100,000 person-years were reported from a survey in Louisiana [28], similar to reports from France (2.4/100,000 person-year) [19, 29] and United Kingdom [30]. But these results are less than incidence reports from the Delaware river Valley region (11.6/100,000 population) [31]. Several series have reported considerable increments in hospitalizations for IE, with most of the increase ascribable to *S. aureus* [32]. The proportion of acute cases of IE has increased from approximately 20% in the pre-antibiotic era, to more than 75% in the majority of high-income countries today [9].

When investigating at IE history, it can be seen that it affected children and young adults as a result of chronic rheumatic heart disease [33]; nevertheless, this remains the first key factor for IE in developing countries representing up to two-thirds of cases [34, 35] and infection is caused predominantly by community-acquired, penicillin-sensitive *Streptococci* entering via the oral cavity. The mean age of patients with IE has increased gradually in the antibiotic era. In 1926, the median age was younger than 30 years [36]; by 1943, it was 39 years [25], 50 years in the 1980s, and 55–60 years in the 1990s and 2000s [2, 12, 13, 19]. In a recent report including 58 centers in 25 countries, covering more than 2700 patients with definite IE by modified Duke criteria, the median age was 57.9 year [9]. In the period from 1993 to 2003, including 3784 patients with IE, the incidence of infection was <5 per 100,000 patients per year in individuals aged 50 years or less and >15 per 100,000 patients per year in those older than 65 years [12]. In a recent review comprising 3477 patients, the mean age of individuals with IE in 1980s was 45.3 years versus 57.2 years in 2000s [37]. These increasing rates of IE in the elderly could be the accumulation of factors such as improved living standards, which indirectly increase the population with degenerative valve disease hence leading to increasingly prosthetic valve surgeries in older patients. More men are affected than women; 58.6% in 1970s versus 66.3% in 2000s [37]. In a French study, the incidence of IE increased in patients older than 50 years and peaked at 194 infected per million habitants in men aged 75–79 years (**Figure 1**) [10].

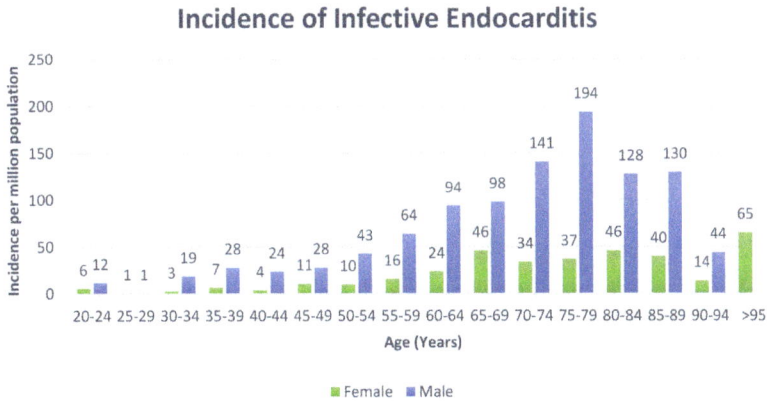

Figure 1. Incidence of infective endocarditis according to age and sex in a French population study of 497 patients. Zenith at 194 cases per million in men aged 75–79 years. Adapted from Selton-Suty et al. [10].

The causative agent has not changed much over time: *Staphylococci* spp., *Streptococci* spp., and *Enterococci* spp. still comprising more than 80% of all cases. Among these, *S. aureus* exceeds *Streptococci* spp. by 12% (**Figure 2**) [9].

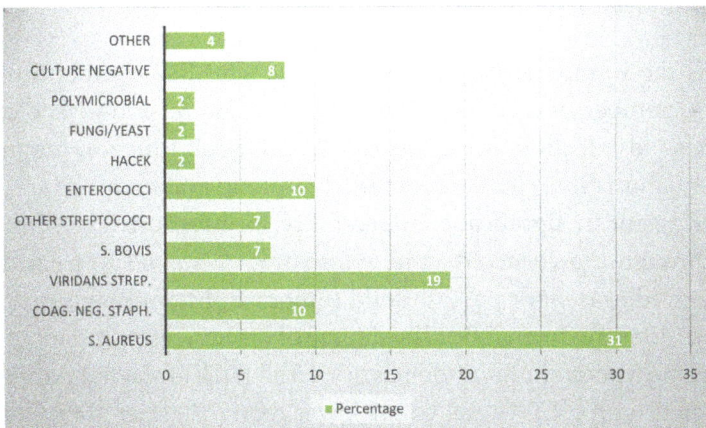

Figure 2. Microbiologic etiology of endocarditis in 1558 patients. Fifty-eight hospitals in 25 countries between June 2000 and September 2005. Data from Murdoch DR, Corey CR, Hoen B., et al. [9]

2.1. Health-care-associated endocarditis

Owing to introduction of new therapeutic modalities (e.g., pacemakers, intravenous catheters, hyperalimentation lines, and dialysis shunts), health-care-associated IE, a relatively new form of the disease, has emerged [2, 9, 22, 23, 38–40]. Health-care-associated endocarditis includes nosocomial IE as well as community IE after a recent hospitalization or as a consequence of long-term indwelling devices. In a recent prospective, multinational cohort study from 61 hospitals in 28 countries comprising 1622 patients with native valve endocarditis (NVE), and no intravenous drug abuse, 34% of patients had health-care-associated endocarditis with nearly half being community acquired [40]. Infection may compromise normal valves, including the tricuspid valve, as well as implanted intracardiac devices and valves [9, 21, 40–43]. The heart valve involved by infection varies considerably according to the different series. For mitral valve alone, the distribution ranges from 28 to 45%, aortic valve alone 5–36%, and aortic and mitral combined 0–35%. The tricuspid valve rarely is involved ranging from 0 to 6% and even less the pulmonary valve (<1%) [9, 44]. Health-care-associated IE accounts for 24 to 34% of cases not related to current cardiac surgery, and it involves an even larger proportion of cases in the United States [9, 23, 40]. Proportion of health-care-associated native valve endocarditis is 54% for nosocomial cases and 46% for community-based cases [40]. Mortality rates among these patients are high, ranging from 27 to 38%; aggravating factors include older patients and complex comorbidities [40, 41]. Among patients with health-care-associated IE, the largest subgroup belongs to individuals undergoing hemodialysis [22, 45]. Chronic hemodialysis has been identified as an independent risk factor for this type of IE [22, 40]. Patients undergoing hemodialysis have a higher risk of *S. aureus* infection causing IE [40, 45, 46]. The two most common pathogens related to health-care-associated IE are *Staphylococci* and *Enterococci*; the infection usually originates in the urinary tract or skin and intravenous lines or invasive procedures are often identified [40]. The risk of IE can be as high as 10% in cases of catheter-induced *S. aureus* bacteremia [39, 47, 48].

2.2. Immunocompromised patient IE

A special group is the immunocompromised patient who has a suboptimally functioning immune system. A number of conditions alter the immune response. The elderly has weak bactericidal response to infection. Impaired B-cell and T-cell function may develop in poor nutrition status or malnutrition. Hematologic and lymphoid malignancies and the medications used to treat them result in significant vulnerability to infection. The immune response is further reduced through the corticoids and cytotoxic drugs used to treat these conditions. Radiation therapy used to treat or palliate solid tumors and lymphoma suppresses antibody formation for weeks after treatment [49]. The degree of immunosuppression plays a major role in the outcome among human immunodeficiency virus (HIV)-infected patients with IE. Poor outcome is associated with a CD4+ cell count lower than 0.200 per 10(9)/L and left-sided or mixed IE [50, 51]. Common organisms associated with IE in HIV-infected patients are *S. aureus* and *Salmonella* [52]. Fungal microorganisms such as *Candida albicans*, *Aspergillus*, and *Cryptococcus neoformans* are more common in IV drug abusers with HIV. These patients possess a greater risk of developing IE on the right-sided heart valves [52]. Infection with HIV should not preclude cardiac surgery.

2.3. Prosthetic valve endocarditis.

Different series suggest that prosthetic valve endocarditis (PVE) accounts for 10–30% of cases of IE in the developed world [23, 41, 53, 54]. In patients undergoing valve surgery between 1965 and 1995, the cumulative incidence of PVE ranged from 1.4 to 3.1% at 12 months and 3 to 5.7% at 5 years [42]. Associated risks for the development of PVE include male sex, previous native valve compromise, and long cardiopulmonary bypass for prosthetic valve placement [55]. Microbial seeding may occur in the early postimplantation period, before endothelialization has established. The incidence is greatest in the first 6 months after valve surgery, then declines to a lower but stable rate (0.2–0.35% per year) [56–58]. The range of age of PVE patients varies from 50 to 74 years [19, 43, 53, 59–62]. The risk of PVE is higher when valve replacement is performed during active IE, especially with unknown pathogen or incomplete antibiotic treatment [58, 63–66]. Mechanical prostheses seem to have a slightly higher risk for PVE in the first 3 months after implantation and bioprosthetic valves have a higher risk after 1 year of replacement [56, 64, 65], maybe as a result of degeneration of bioprosthetic leaflets. Although the cumulative risk comparing mechanical with biological prosthesis is similar [42, 67, 68], the weighted mean incidence for infections of bioprostheses calculated from different series is 0.49% per patient-year for mitral valves and 0.91% per patient-year for aortic valves. For mechanical prostheses, the incidence is 0.18% per patient-year for mitral, 0.27% per patient-year for aortic, and 0.29% per patient-year for multiple implants [63]. PVE has been called *early* when infection occurred within 2 months of valve surgery and *late* when onset was >2 months. These terms were established to help distinguish PVE that instituted early as a complication of valve surgery from tardy infection that was likely to be community acquired [58, 69, 70]. However, in 2007, a study demonstrated a major shift according to the biological profile at 12 months after surgery, indicating that a more appropriate cutoff time to distinguish early from late PVE was 1 year [71]. Moreover, the European guidelines use this limit to classify the condition [17]. The causative pathogens involved in early PVE usually are methicillin-resistant *Staphylococci*, whereas in late PVE the common pathogens found are coagulase-negative *Staphylococci* and *Enterococci* (**Table 2**) [53]. In a large series including 2572 patients who underwent transcatheter aortic valve replacement (TAVR) in 14 centers between January 2008 and April 2013, the incidence of TAVR PVE was 1.13% (29 patients); the incidence of TAVR PVE by transfemoral approach was 1.1%, transapical 1.98%. The incidence of IE was 1.93% for balloon-expandable (23 of 1191) and 0.45% (6 of 1343) for self-expandable transcatheter heart valves. Early-onset IE (within 60 days) was diagnosed in 28% (eight patients), intermediate-onset IE (between 60 and 265 days) was diagnosed in 52% (15 patients), and late-onset IE (>1 year) was diagnosed in 20% (six patients) resulting in 80% of incidence of IE within the first 12 months of implantation (higher rates), contrasting with surgical valve IE. In the early-onset group, *S. aureus* and coagulase-negative *Staphylococci* were the most prevalent (50%), in the intermediate-onset group *Staphylococcal*, *Enterococcal*, and *non-viridans Streptococcal* species were the predominant pathogens (20% each), and in the late-onset group *Staphylococci* and *Enterococci* were identified (33% each), which does not resemble the late-onset surgical PVE [72].

PATHOGEN	EARLY PVE* (%)	LATE PVE* (%)
	N = 53	N = 331
Staphylococcus aureus	36	18
Coagulase-negative Staphylococci	17	20
Enterococcus	8	13
Viridans streptococci	2	10
Streptococcus bovis	2	7
HACEK	0	2
Fungi	9	3
Other	6	14
Culture negative	17	12

Adapted from Wang et al. [53]. *Early refers to IE within 2 months and late after 2 months, according to Wang et al. HACEK: *Hemophilus, Aggregatibacter spp., Cardiobacterium hominis, Eikenella corrodens, Kingella kingae*. PVE: Prosthetic valve endocarditis.

Table 2. Causative organisms for early and late PVE.

2.4. Cardiovascular-implantable electronic devices infection

The most commonly used cardiovascular-implantable electronic device (CIED) are permanent pacemaker, cardiac resynchronization therapy, and implantable cardioverter-defibrillator. Most of these are implanted using transvenous leads. This practice had dramatically reduced the risk of infection associated with the procedure. Nevertheless, complication by infection remains a problem that can lead to significant morbidity, mortality, and elevated costs [73–75]. Reports of CIED infection vary according to different series and range from 0.13 to 19.9% [76–78]. In a 16-year survey of Nationwide Inpatient Sample (NIS) from 1993 to 2008, the rate of CIED implantation increased 4.7% annually. The incidence of CIED infection remained stable until 2004, but increased almost twice in a 4-year period (2004–2008) from 1.53 to 2.41%, respectively [75]. The rate of infection associated with implantable cardioverter-defibrillator surpasses greatly that of the pacemaker [79–81].

2.5. Ventricular-assist devices infection

Patients who receive ventricular-assist devices (VADs) usually have various comorbidities, including a state of immune compromise. The risk of infection varies depending on the duration of VAD support [82]. Higher rates of infection are observed in the destination therapy group compared with the group where VAD is used as a bridge to transplantation [82]. Hravnak reported that registry patients with implant duration longer than 60 days were twice as likely to develop infection than those patients supported for less than 30 days [83]. The reported rates of infection in patients with VAD range from 13 to 80% and depend on multiple factors, including comorbidities, type of device implanted, and duration of VAD support [84]. Infection of VAD can present as three different syndromes: driveline infection (most frequent) presenting with local inflammatory changes and drainage at exit site, pocket site infection is the second syndrome presenting with local inflammatory changes, and the third (least frequent) is endocarditis comprising valves and/or internal lining of the device [84].

2.6. Infection of closure devices (atrial septal defect, patent ductus arteriosus, and ventricular septal defect)

Minimally invasive procedures are increasingly accepted as an option for cardiovascular congenital diseases [85–87]. Fortunately, complications derived from implantation of such devices are very rare, including infection (<1%) [85, 88–90].

2.7. Infective endocarditis in children

As in adults, trends in children IE are related to the evolution of care in the sick child, particularly children born with congenital heart disease. The incidence of children IE provides limited data, mostly based on inpatient admission which could not represent accurately the general population. In a report between 1933 and 1972, the incidence was 0.22–0.55 cases per 1000 pediatric hospital admissions [91]. A retrospective review between 1972 and 1982 found an incidence of 1/1280 pediatric admissions [92]. Later, in a multicenter study, the incidence of IE slightly decreased, ranging from 0.005 to 0.12 cases per 1000 pediatric admissions [93]. In other report including 47,518 patients, from 1998 to 2010, congenital heart disease was found as the major underlying condition associated to IE in children in high-income countries, with a cumulative incidence of 6.1 per 1000 children [94]. The distribution of IE between boys and girls is balanced in contrast with series in adults in whom men have a higher tendency to suffer the condition [94, 95]. Rheumatic fever is rare in developed countries, nevertheless is commonly found in low-income countries. In the presurgical era, the proportion of IE in children with rheumatic heart disease ranged from 30 to 50% [96]. A single center report covering seven decades found that IE occurred in 31% of rheumatic heart disease patients in presurgical era, compared to era 3 (1992–2004) with only 1.1% of patients having the condition [97]. Approximately 50% of cases of pediatric IE complicating congenital heart disease have had previous cardiac surgery, especially palliative shunts of complex cardiac repair [98]. Risk of postoperative IE in children depends greatly on the type of surgery; for example, a study from Oregon found a relatively low incidence of IE after tetralogy of Fallot repair (1.3%), ventricular septal repair (2.7%), atrial septal repair (2.8%), and aortic coarctation repair (3.5%). Nevertheless, a high incidence of IE was found in aortic stenosis (valve replacement) with a cumulative incidence at 25 years of 13.3% [99]. The rate of IE in structurally normal hearts is lower than those with a predisposing condition (22 vs. 78%), respectively [100]. A major risk factor to develop IE in an anatomically normal heart is an indwelling vascular catheter [101].

2.8. Infective endocarditis in adults

An important condition related to IE in the elderly is the congenital bicuspid aortic valve. In a prospective multicenter study, it was present in 16% of cases of native valve endocarditis [102]. Degenerative cardiac lesions assume an important role in the development of IE without underlying valve disease. In one study, degenerative lesions were present in 50% of patients with native valve IE older than 60 years [103]. Calcified mitral annulus is a common finding in elderly women but rarely complicate with IE (3.8%) [104]. Even not a classical condition related to IE, idiopathic hypertrophic subaortic stenosis may represent up to 5% of incidence of the infection [105]. And there is a higher mortality rate correlation if a murmur is present (up to 36% of patients with hypertrophic aortic stenosis and IE) [105]. Another condition associated with IE is the mitral prolapse syndrome. In different series, the range of IE in those patients with mitral valve prolapse can go from 11 to 23% [106, 107]. In another study, 8.6% of patients with mitral valve prolapse who were monitored prospectively for 9–22 years developed IE [108]. This syndrome must be suspected in patients with mid-systolic click with or without a late systolic murmur. This condition is not uncommon and has been found in 0.5–20% of otherwise healthy people, especially young women. It has become apparent that a significant proportion of patients with mitral valve prolapse have an anthropometrically distinct habitus, suggesting that this condition is only an element of a generalized developmental syndrome [109]. It may be useful to have in mind these characteristics to help identify patients with a high risk of developing IE. Having valvular redundancy and thickened leaflets may increase the risk of IE [103]. The combination of mitral valve prolapse and men older than 45 years also may increase the risk of IE [110]. In a detailed case-control study, 25% of patients with IE had mitral valve prolapse; the odds ratio (8.2 of 95% confidence interval, 2.4–28.4) indicated a substantially higher risk for IE in patients with mitral valve prolapse than for those without it [111]. Another study found that mitral valve prolapse IE presented with more subtle symptoms, less mortality, and responded better to antimicrobial therapy than other types of left-sided IE, even though recognition of the infection was delayed [112].

2.9. Infective endocarditis in drug abusers

All estimations of IE incidence in drug abusers are hindered because there are no enough data reporting the exact number of victims of illicit drug-abuse epidemic. Reports from the United States present an incidence of IE in intravenous drug abusers that range from 2 to 5% per year [113] or 1.5–2 cases per 1000 years of IV drug abuse with men more commonly affected [114]. Although congenital cardiac disease and right-sided heart instrumentation are associated with IE, IV drug abusers retain the majority of cases. Intravenous drug users and those with HIV primarily consist of relatively young adults [115]. Acute infection accounts for approximately 60% of hospital admissions among drug abusers and IE is responsible of 5–15% of these episodes [116]. The presence of IE in a drug addict is difficult to predict, especially from history and physical examination findings alone [117, 118]. More than 60% of IV drug abusers with IE do not have an underlying preexisting valvular disease [119]. Although cocaine use by an intravenous drug abuser should raise the suspicion of IE infection [120], the most credible predictors of IE in febrile intravenous drug users are visualization of vegetations by echocardiography and the presence of embolic phenomena [118]. Up to 13% of cases of IV drug abusers with febrile episodes have an echocardiographically demonstrated IE [118]. Although left-sided native valve endocarditis may be present in this group of patients, the tricuspid valve is more commonly affected in intravenous drug users [121, 122]. Only two-third of patients with proven IE diagnostic presented with heart murmurs on admission [116]. The frequency of valvular involvement is tricuspid alone or in combination with other valves, 52.2%; aortic alone, 18.5%; mitral alone 10.8%; and mitral and aortic combined, 12.5% [123]. Most of these patients are young (20–40 years old), and men are more commonly affected than women with a ratio of 4:1–6:1. Approximately 66% of the patients have extravalvular compromise which may help in the diagnosis [124–126]. Although there are studies reporting infection rate reductions (such as HIV, hepatitis, or abscess) with the implementation of a needle-exchange program [127, 128], to date, there are no conclusive evidence showing reduction in IE among this special group.

3. Conclusions

Much work remains to be completed. IE is a complex and challenging pathology with a high mortality rate despite current advancements in health care. Even though diagnostic and therapeutic modalities have progressed since the "rheumatic fever" era, there is still a concern in developing countries where rheumatic fever represents a major cause of IE and access to appropriate health care is not possible in large areas. Curiously, the changing epidemiology of IE depict us a disease that used to affect young patients, native valves, and had *Streptococci* as the main pathogen, to a disease that affect mainly older people with prosthetic valves implanted and *S. aureus* as the main pathogen. These changes occur alongside a better survival in older people but also with several comorbidities accompanying these patients. Imaging modalities such as echocardiography had greatly helped in the diagnosis of IE; the role of advanced imaging had yet to be clinically evaluated in a day-to-day basis. Chronic and immunosuppressive diseases play a major role as predisposing factors to develop IE. IV drug users comprise other group of patients severely affected by the disease. Adequate clinical analysis and high suspicion are necessary to help these "risk" patients and provide the right tools (multidisciplinary team) to detect and treat this limiting and deadly condition.

Author details

Fabian Andres Giraldo Vallejo

Address all correspondence to: fabiangiraldomd@gmail.com

Instituto del Corazón de Bucaramanga, Bucaramanga, Colombia

References

[1] Lerner PI, Weinstein L. Infective endocarditis in the antibiotic era. N Engl J Med. 1966;274(7):388–93 concl.

[2] Von Reyn CF, Levy BS, Arbeit RD, Friedland G, Crumpacker CS. Infective endocarditis: an analysis based on strict case definitions. Ann Intern Med. 1981;94(4 pt 1):505–18.

[3] Durack DT, Lukes AS, Bright DK. New criteria for diagnosis of infective endocarditis: utilization of specific echocardiographic findings. Duke Endocarditis Service. Am J Med. 1994;96(3):200–9.

[4] Li JS, Sexton DJ, Mick N, Nettles R, Fowler VG, Ryan T, et al. Proposed modifications to the Duke criteria for the diagnosis of infective endocarditis. Clin Infect Dis Off Publ Infect Dis Soc Am. 2000;30(4):633–8.

[5] Evangelista A. Echocardiography in infective endocarditis. Heart. 2004;90(6):614–7.

[6] Greaves K. Clinical criteria and the appropriate use of transthoracic echocardiography for the exclusion of infective endocarditis. Heart. 2003;89(3):273–5.

[7] Vieira MLC. Repeated echocardiographic examinations of patients with suspected infective endocarditis. Heart. 2004;90(9):1020–4.

[8] Prendergast BD. The changing face of infective endocarditis. Heart Br Card Soc. 2006;92(7):879–85.

[9] Murdoch DR. Clinical presentation, etiology, and outcome of infective endocarditis in the 21st century: the International Collaboration on Endocarditis–Prospective Cohort Study. Arch Intern Med. 2009;169(5):463.

[10] Selton-Suty C, Celard M, Le Moing V, Doco-Lecompte T, Chirouze C, Iung B, et al. Preeminence of *Staphylococcus aureus* in infective endocarditis: a 1-year population-based survey. Clin Infect Dis. 2012;54(9):1230–9.

[11] Allegranzi B, Nejad SB, Combescure C, Graafmans W, Attar H, Donaldson L, et al. Burden of endemic health-care-associated infection in developing countries: systematic review and meta-analysis. The Lancet. 2011;377(9761):228–41.

[12] Moreillon P, Que Y-A. Infective endocarditis. The Lancet. 2004;363(9403):139–49.

[13] de Sa DDC, Tleyjeh IM, Anavekar NS, Schultz JC, Thomas JM, Lahr BD, et al. Epidemiological trends of infective endocarditis: a population-based study in Olmsted County, Minnesota. Mayo Clin Proc. 2010;85(5):422–6.

[14] Tleyjeh IM, Abdel-Latif A, Rahbi H, Scott CG, Bailey KR, Steckelberg JM, et al. A systematic review of population-based studies of infective endocarditis. Chest. 2007;132(3):1025–35.

[15] Hasbun R, Vikram HR, Barakat LA, Buenconsejo J, Quagliarello VJ. Complicated left-sided native valve endocarditis in adults: risk classification for mortality. JAMA. 2003;289(15):1933–40.

[16] Chirouze C, Cabell CH, Fowler VG, Khayat N, Olaison L, Miro JM, et al. Prognostic factors in 61 cases of *Staphylococcus aureus* prosthetic valve infective endocarditis from

the International Collaboration on Endocarditis merged database. Clin Infect Dis Off Publ Infect Dis Soc Am. 2004;38(9):1323–7.

[17] Endorsed by the European Society of Clinical Microbiology and Infectious Diseases (ESCMID) and by the International Society of Chemotherapy (ISC) for Infection and Cancer, Authors/Task Force Members, Habib G, Hoen B, Tornos P, Thuny F, et al. Guidelines on the prevention, diagnosis, and treatment of infective endocarditis (new version 2009): The Task Force on the Prevention, Diagnosis, and Treatment of Infective Endocarditis of the European Society of Cardiology (ESC). Eur Heart J. 2009;30(19): 2369–413.

[18] Nishimura RA, Otto CM, Bonow RO, Carabello BA, Erwin JP, Guyton RA, et al. 2014 AHA/ACC guideline for the management of patients with valvular heart disease: a report of the American College of Cardiology/American Heart Association Task Force on Practice Guidelines. Circulation. 2014;129(23):e521–643.

[19] Hoen B, Alla F, Selton-Suty C, Béguinot I, Bouvet A, Briançon S, et al. Changing profile of infective endocarditis: results of a 1-year survey in France. JAMA. 2002;288(1):75–81.

[20] Letaief A, Boughzala E, Kaabia N, Ernez S, Abid F, Ben Chaabane T, et al. Epidemiology of infective endocarditis in Tunisia: a 10-year multicenter retrospective study. Int J Infect Dis IJID Off Publ Int Soc Infect Dis. 2007;11(5):430–3.

[21] Hill EE, Herijgers P, Claus P, Vanderschueren S, Herregods M-C, Peetermans WE. Infective endocarditis: changing epidemiology and predictors of 6-month mortality: a prospective cohort study. Eur Heart J. 2007;28(2):196–203.

[22] Cabell CH, Jollis JG, Peterson GE, Corey GR, Anderson DJ, Sexton DJ, et al. Changing patient characteristics and the effect on mortality in endocarditis. Arch Intern Med. 2002;162(1):90–4.

[23] Fowler VG, Miro JM, Hoen B, Cabell CH, Abrutyn E, Rubinstein E, et al. *Staphylococcus aureus* endocarditis: a consequence of medical progress. JAMA. 2005;293(24):3012–21.

[24] Lopez J, Revilla A, Vilacosta I, Sevilla T, Villacorta E, Sarria C, et al. Age-dependent profile of left-sided infective endocarditis: a 3-center experience. Circulation. 2010;121(7):892–7.

[25] Durante-Mangoni E. Current features of infective endocarditis in elderly patients: results of the International Collaboration on Endocarditis Prospective Cohort Study. Arch Intern Med. 2008;168(19):2095.

[26] Steckelberg JM, Melton LJ, Ilstrup DM, Rouse MS, Wilson WR. Influence of referral bias on the apparent clinical spectrum of infective endocarditis. Am J Med. 1990;88(6):582–8.

[27] Tleyjeh IM, Steckelberg JM, Murad HS, Anavekar NS, Ghomrawi HMK, Mirzoyev Z, et al. Temporal trends in infective endocarditis: a population-based study in Olmsted County, Minnesota. JAMA. 2005;293(24):3022–8.

[28] King JW, Nguyen VQ, Conrad SA. Results of a prospective statewide reporting system for infective endocarditis. Am J Med Sci. 1988;295(6):517–27.

[29] Delahaye F, Goulet V, Lacassin F, Ecochard R, Selton-Suty C, Hoen B, et al. Characteristics of infective endocarditis in France in 1991. A 1-year survey. Eur Heart J. 1995;16(3): 394–401.

[30] SHULMAN ST. Infective endocarditis: 1986. Pediatr Infect Dis J [Internet]. 1986;5(6). Available from: http://journals.lww.com/pidj/Fulltext/1986/11000/Infective_endocarditis__1986_.18.aspx.

[31] Berlin JA, Abrutyn E, Strom BL, Kinman JL, Levison ME, Korzeniowski OM, et al. Incidence of infective endocarditis in the Delaware Valley, 1988-1990. Am J Cardiol. 1995;76(12):933–6.

[32] Federspiel JJ. Increasing US rates of endocarditis with *Staphylococcus aureus*: 1999-2008. Arch Intern Med. 2012;172(4):363.

[33] Normand J, Bozio A, Etienne J, Sassolas F, Le Bris H. Changing patterns and prognosis of infective endocarditis in childhood. Eur Heart J. 1995;16(Suppl B):28–31.

[34] Carapetis JR, Steer AC, Mulholland EK, Weber M. The global burden of group A *Streptococcal* diseases. Lancet Infect Dis. 2005;5(11):685–94.

[35] Marijon E, Ou P, Celermajer DS, Ferreira B, Mocumbi AO, Jani D, et al. Prevalence of rheumatic heart disease detected by echocardiographic screening. N Engl J Med. 2007;357(5):470–6.

[36] Thayer WS. Studies on bacterial (infective) endocarditis. Johns Hopkins Hosp Rep. 1926;22(1):1–8.

[37] Slipczuk L, Codolosa JN, Davila CD, Romero-Corral A, Yun J, Pressman GS, et al. Infective endocarditis epidemiology over five decades: a systematic review. Schlievert PM, editor. PLoS ONE. 2013;8(12):e82665.

[38] Fernández-Guerrero ML, Verdejo C, Azofra J, de Górgolas M. Hospital-acquired infectious endocarditis not associated with cardiac surgery: an emerging problem. Clin Infect Dis Off Publ Infect Dis Soc Am. 1995;20(1):16–23.

[39] Gouëllo JP, Asfar P, Brenet O, Kouatchet A, Berthelot G, Alquier P. Nosocomial endocarditis in the intensive care unit: an analysis of 22 cases. Crit Care Med. 2000;28(2): 377–82.

[40] Benito N, Miró JM, de Lazzari E, Cabell CH, del Río A, Altclas J, et al. Health care-associated native valve endocarditis: importance of non-nosocomial acquisition. Ann Intern Med. 2009;150(9):586–94.

[41] Martín-Dávila P, Fortún J, Navas E, Cobo J, Jiménez-Mena M, Moya JL, et al. Nosocomial endocarditis in a tertiary hospital: an increasing trend in native valve cases. Chest. 2005;128(2):772–9.

[42] Karchmer AW, Longworth DL. Infections of intracardiac devices. Cardiol Clin. 2003;21(2):253–71, vii.

[43] Rivas P, Alonso J, Moya J, de Górgolas M, Martinell J, Fernández Guerrero ML. The impact of hospital-acquired infections on the microbial etiology and prognosis of late-onset prosthetic valve endocarditis. Chest. 2005;128(2):764–71.

[44] Come PC. Infective endocarditis: current perspectives. Compr Ther. 1982;8(7):57–70.

[45] Kamalakannan D, Pai RM, Johnson LB, Gardin JM, Saravolatz LD. Epidemiology and clinical outcomes of infective endocarditis in hemodialysis patients. Ann Thorac Surg. 2007;83(6):2081–6.

[46] Hoen B. Infective endocarditis: a frequent disease in dialysis patients. Nephrol Dial Transplant Off Publ Eur Dial Transpl Assoc Eur Ren Assoc. 2004;19(6):1360–2.

[47] Fowler VG, Sanders LL, Kong LK, McClelland RS, Gottlieb GS, Li J, et al. Infective endocarditis due to *Staphylococcus aureus*: 59 prospectively identified cases with follow-up. Clin Infect Dis Off Publ Infect Dis Soc Am. 1999;28(1):106–14.

[48] Chang F-Y, MacDonald BB, Peacock JE, Musher DM, Triplett P, Mylotte JM, et al. A prospective multicenter study of *Staphylococcus aureus* bacteremia: incidence of endocarditis, risk factors for mortality, and clinical impact of methicillin resistance. Medicine (Baltimore). 2003;82(5):322–32.

[49] Schell HM. The immunocompromised host and risk for cardiovascular infection. J Cardiovasc Nurs. 1999;13(2):31–48.

[50] Pulvirenti JJ, Kerns E, Benson C, Lisowski J, Demarais P, Weinstein RA. Infective endocarditis in injection drug users: importance of human immunodeficiency virus serostatus and degree of immunosuppression. Clin Infect Dis Off Publ Infect Dis Soc Am. 1996;22(1):40–5.

[51] Ribera E, Miró JM, Cortés E, Cruceta A, Merce J, Marco F, et al. Influence of human immunodeficiency virus 1 infection and degree of immunosuppression in the clinical characteristics and outcome of infective endocarditis in intravenous drug users. Arch Intern Med. 1998;158(18):2043–50.

[52] Fisher SD LS. Cardiovascular abnormalities in HIV-infected individuals. In: Braunwald E, editor. Heart disease: a textbook of cardiovascular medicine. 6th ed. Philadelphia: Saunders; 2001. pp. 2211–21.

[53] Wang A, Athan E, Pappas PA, Fowler VG, Olaison L, Paré C, et al. Contemporary clinical profile and outcome of prosthetic valve endocarditis. JAMA. 2007;297(12):1354–61.

[54] Habib G, Tribouilloy C, Thuny F, Giorgi R, Brahim A, Amazouz M, et al. Prosthetic valve endocarditis: who needs surgery? A multicentre study of 104 cases. Heart Br Card Soc. 2005;91(7):954–9.

[55] Hyde JA, Darouiche RO, Costerton JW. Strategies for prophylaxis against prosthetic valve endocarditis: a review article. J Heart Valve Dis. 1998;7(3):316–26.

[56] Calderwood SB, Swinski LA, Waternaux CM, Karchmer AW, Buckley MJ. Risk factors for the development of prosthetic valve endocarditis. Circulation. 1985;72(1):31–7.

[57] Glower DD, Landolfo KP, Cheruvu S, Cen YY, Harrison JK, Bashore TM, et al. Determinants of 15-year outcome with 1,119 standard Carpentier-Edwards porcine valves. Ann Thorac Surg. 1998;66(6 Suppl):S44–8.

[58] Ivert TS, Dismukes WE, Cobbs CG, Blackstone EH, Kirklin JW, Bergdahl LA. Prosthetic valve endocarditis. Circulation. 1984;69(2):223–32.

[59] Murashita T. Surgical results for active endocarditis with prosthetic valve replacement: impact of culture-negative endocarditis on early and late outcomes. Eur J Cardiothorac Surg. 2004;26(6):1104–11.

[60] Tornos P. Infective endocarditis in Europe: lessons from the Euro heart survey. Heart. 2005;91(5):571–5.

[61] Romano G, Carozza A, Della Corte A, De Santo LS, Amarelli C, Torella M, et al. Native versus primary prosthetic valve endocarditis: comparison of clinical features and long-term outcome in 353 patients. J Heart Valve Dis. 2004;13(2):200–8; discussion 208–9.

[62] Sohail MR, Martin KR, Wilson WR, Baddour LM, Harmsen WS, Steckelberg JM. Medical versus surgical management of *Staphylococcus aureus* prosthetic valve endo-carditis. Am J Med. 2006;119(2):147–54.

[63] Piper C. Valve disease: prosthetic valve endocarditis. Heart. 2001;85(5):590–3.

[64] Arvay A, Lengyel M. Incidence and risk factors of prosthetic valve endocarditis. Eur J Cardio-Thorac Surg Off J Eur Assoc Cardio-Thorac Surg. 1988;2(5):340–6.

[65] Hammermeister K, Sethi GK, Henderson WG, Grover FL, Oprian C, Rahimtoola SH. Outcomes 15 years after valve replacement with a mechanical versus a bioprosthetic valve: final report of the Veterans Affairs randomized trial. J Am Coll Cardiol. 2000;36(4):1152–8.

[66] Agnihotri A, Mcgiffin D, Galbraith A, Obrien M. The prevalence of infective endocar-ditis after aortic valve replacement. J Thorac Cardiovasc Surg. 1995;110(6):1708–24.

[67] Vongpatanasin W, Hillis LD, Lange RA. Prosthetic heart valves. N Engl J Med. 1996;335(6):407–16.

[68] Sidhu P, O'Kane H, Ali N, Gladstone DJ, Sarsam MA, Campalani G, et al. Mechanical or bioprosthetic valves in the elderly: a 20-year comparison. Ann Thorac Surg. 2001;71(5 Suppl):S257–60.

[69] Tornos P, Almirante B, Olona M, Permanyer G, González T, Carballo J, et al. Clinical outcome and long-term prognosis of late prosthetic valve endocarditis: a 20-year experience. Clin Infect Dis Off Publ Infect Dis Soc Am. 1997;24(3):381–6.

[70] Wilson WR, Jaumin PM, Danielson GK, Giuliani ER, Washington JA II, Geraci JE. Prosthetic valve endocarditis. Ann Intern Med. 1975;82(6):751–6.

[71] López J, Revilla A, Vilacosta I, Villacorta E, González-Juanatey C, Gómez I, et al. Definition, clinical profile, microbiological spectrum, and prognostic factors of early-onset prosthetic valve endocarditis. Eur Heart J. 2007;28(6):760–5.

[72] Latib A, Naim C, De Bonis M, Sinning JM, Maisano F, Barbanti M, et al. TAVR-associated prosthetic valve infective endocarditis. J Am Coll Cardiol. 2014;64(20):2176–8.

[73] Baddour LM, Cha Y-M, Wilson WR. Infections of cardiovascular implantable electronic devices. N Engl J Med. 2012;367(9):842–9.

[74] Sohail MR. Mortality and cost associated with cardiovascular implantable electronic device infections. Arch Intern Med. 2011;171(20):1821.

[75] Greenspon AJ, Patel JD, Lau E, Ochoa JA, Frisch DR, Ho RT, et al. 16-Year Trends in the infection burden for pacemakers and implantable cardioverter-defibrillators in the United States. J Am Coll Cardiol. 2011;58(10):1001–6.

[76] Sohail MR, Uslan DZ, Khan AH, Friedman PA, Hayes DL, Wilson WR, et al. Management and outcome of permanent pacemaker and implantable cardioverter-defibrillator infections. J Am Coll Cardiol. 2007;49(18):1851–9.

[77] Lai KK, Fontecchio SA. Infections associated with implantable cardioverter defibrillators placed transvenously and via thoracotomies: epidemiology, infection control, and management. Clin Infect Dis Off Publ Infect Dis Soc Am. 1998;27(2):265–9.

[78] Mela T, McGovern BA, Garan H, Vlahakes GJ, Torchiana DF, Ruskin J, et al. Long-term infection rates associated with the pectoral versus abdominal approach to cardioverter-defibrillator implants. Am J Cardiol. 2001;88(7):750–3.

[79] Voigt A, Shalaby A, Saba S. Rising rates of cardiac rhythm management device infections in the United States: 1996 through 2003. J Am Coll Cardiol. 2006;48(3):590–1.

[80] Sohail MR, Uslan DZ, Khan AH, Friedman PA, Hayes DL, Wilson WR, et al. Risk factor analysis of permanent pacemaker infection. Clin Infect Dis Off Publ Infect Dis Soc Am. 2007;45(2):166–73.

[81] Uslan DZ, Sohail MR, St Sauver JL, Friedman PA, Hayes DL, Stoner SM, et al. Permanent pacemaker and implantable cardioverter defibrillator infection: a population-based study. Arch Intern Med. 2007;167(7):669–75.

[82] Topkara VK, Kondareddy S, Malik F, Wang I-W, Mann DL, Ewald GA, et al. Infectious complications in patients with left ventricular assist device: etiology and outcomes in the continuous-flow era. Ann Thorac Surg. 2010;90(4):1270–7.

[83] Hravnak M, George E, Kormos RL. Management of chronic left ventricular assist device percutaneous lead insertion sites. J Heart Lung Transplant Off Publ Int Soc Heart Transplant. 1993;12(5):856–63.

[84] Baddour LM. Nonvalvular cardiovascular device-related infections. Circulation. 2003;108(16):2015–31.

[85] Allen HD, Beekman RH, Garson A, Hijazi ZM, Mullins C, O'Laughlin MP, et al. Pediatric therapeutic cardiac catheterization: a statement for healthcare professionals from the Council on Cardiovascular Disease in the Young, American Heart Association. Circulation. 1998;97(6):609–25.

[86] Rao PS, Sideris EB, Hausdorf G, Rey C, Lloyd TR, Beekman RH, et al. International experience with secundum atrial septal defect occlusion by the buttoned device. Am Heart J. 1994;128(5):1022–35.

[87] Pihkala J, Nykanen D, Freedom RM, Benson LN. Interventional cardiac catheterization. Pediatr Clin North Am. 1999;46(2):441–64.

[88] Zamora R, Rao PS, Lloyd TR, Beekman RH, Sideris EB. Intermediate-term results of Phase I Food and Drug Administration Trials of buttoned device occlusion of secundum atrial septal defects. J Am Coll Cardiol. 1998;31(3):674–6.

[89] Goldstein JA, Beardslee MA, Xu H, Sundt TM, Lasala JM. Infective endocarditis resulting from CardioSEAL closure of a patent foramen ovale. Catheter Cardiovasc Interv Off J Soc Card Angiogr Interv. 2002;55(2):217–20; discussion 221.

[90] Bullock AM, Menahem S, Wilkinson JL. Infective endocarditis on an occluder closing an atrial septal defect. Cardiol Young. 1999;9(1):65–7.

[91] Johnson DH, Rosenthal A, Nadas AS. A forty-year review of bacterial endocarditis in infancy and childhood. Circulation. 1975;51(4):581–8.

[92] Van Hare GF, Ben-Shachar G, Liebman J, Boxerbaum B, Riemenschneider TA. Infective endocarditis in infants and children during the past 10 years: a decade of change. Am Heart J. 1984;107(6):1235–40.

[93] Pasquali SK, He X, Mohamad Z, McCrindle BW, Newburger JW, Li JS, et al. Trends in endocarditis hospitalizations at US children's hospitals: impact of the 2007 American Heart Association Antibiotic Prophylaxis Guidelines. Am Heart J. 2012;163(5):894–9.

[94] Rushani D, Kaufman JS, Ionescu-Ittu R, Mackie AS, Pilote L, Therrien J, et al. Infective endocarditis in children with congenital heart disease: cumulative incidence and predictors. Circulation. 2013;128(13):1412–9.

[95] Day MD, Gauvreau K, Shulman S, Newburger JW. Characteristics of children hospitalized with infective endocarditis. Circulation. 2009;119(6):865–70.

[96] Stull TL LJ. Endocarditis in children. In: Kaye D, editor. Infective endocarditis. 2nd ed. New York, NY: Raven Press; pp. 313–27.

[97] Rosenthal LB, Feja KN, Levasseur SM, Alba LR, Gersony W, Saiman L. The changing epidemiology of pediatric endocarditis at a children's hospital over seven decades. Pediatr Cardiol. 2010;31(6):813–20.

[98] Saiman L, Prince A, Gersony WM. Pediatric infective endocarditis in the modern era. J Pediatr. 1993;122(6):847–53.

[99] Morris CD, Reller MD, Menashe VD. Thirty-year incidence of infective endocarditis after surgery for congenital heart defect. JAMA. 1998;279(8):599–603.

[100] Stockheim JA, Chadwick EG, Kessler S, Amer M, Abdel-Haq N, Dajani AS, et al. Are the Duke criteria superior to the Beth Israel criteria for the diagnosis of infective endocarditis in children? Clin Infect Dis Off Publ Infect Dis Soc Am. 1998;27(6):1451–6.

[101] Valente AM. Frequency of infective endocarditis among infants and children with *Staphylococcus aureus* bacteremia. PEDIATRICS [Internet]. 2004 December 15 [cited 2016 June 13]; Available from: http://pediatrics.aappublications.org/cgi/doi/10.1542/peds.2004-1152.

[102] Tribouilloy C, Rusinaru D, Sorel C, Thuny F, Casalta J-P, Riberi A, et al. Clinical characteristics and outcome of infective endocarditis in adults with bicuspid aortic valves: a multicentre observational study. Heart. 2010;96(21):1723–9.

[103] McKinsey DS, Ratts TE, Bisno AL. Underlying cardiac lesions in adults with infective endocarditis. The changing spectrum. Am J Med. 1987;82(4):681–8.

[104] Fulkerson PK, Beaver BM, Auseon JC, Graber HL. Calcification of the mitral annulus: etiology, clinical associations, complications and therapy. Am J Med. 1979;66(6):967–77.

[105] Chagnac A, Rudniki C, Loebel H, Zahavi I. Infectious endocarditis in idiopathic hypertrophic subaortic stenosis: report of three cases and review of the literature. Chest. 1982;81(3):346–9.

[106] Corrigall D, Bolen J, Hancock EW, Popp RL. Mitral valve prolapse and infective endocarditis. Am J Med. 1977;63(2):215–22.

[107] Yang L, Gu X, Zhang X. [Mitral valve prolapse and infective endocarditis]. Zhonghua Nei Ke Za Zhi. 1997;36(12):802–4.

[108] Jeresaty RM. Mitral valve prolapse–Click syndrome. Prog Cardiovasc Dis. 1973;15(6):623–52.

[109] Schutte JE, Gaffney FA, Blend L, Blomqvist CG. Distinctive anthropometric character-istics of women with mitral valve prolapse. Am J Med. 1981;71(4):533–8.

[110] Devereux RB, Kramer-Fox R, Kligfield P. Mitral valve prolapse: causes, clinical mani-festations, and management. Ann Intern Med. 1989;111(4):305–17.

[111] Clemens JD, Horwitz RI, Jaffe CC, Feinstein AR, Stanton BF. A controlled evaluation of the risk of bacterial endocarditis in persons with mitral-valve prolapse. N Engl J Med. 1982;307(13):776–81.

[112] Nolan CM, Kane JJ, Grunow WA. Infective endocarditis and mitral prolapse: a com-parison with other types of endocarditis. Arch Intern Med. 1981;141(4):447–50.

[113] Sande, M. A. LB, Mills J. CIH. Endocarditis in intravenous drug users. In: Kaye D, editor. Infective endocarditis. 2nd ed. New York, NY: Raven Press; 1992. pp. 345–9.

[114] Weinstein L, Brusch JL, editors. In: Infective endocarditis. New York, NY: Oxford University Press; 1996. pp. 194–209.

[115] Wilson LE, Thomas DL, Astemborski J, Freedman TL, Vlahov D. Prospective study of infective endocarditis among injection drug users. J Infect Dis. 2002;185(12):1761–6.

[116] Levine DP, Crane LR, Zervos MJ. Bacteremia in narcotic addicts at the Detroit Medical Center. II. Infectious endocarditis: a prospective comparative study. Rev Infect Dis. 1986;8(3):374–96.

[117] Marantz PR, Linzer M, Feiner CJ, Feinstein SA, Kozin AM, Friedland GH. Inability to predict diagnosis in febrile intravenous drug abusers. Ann Intern Med. 1987;106(6):823–8.

[118] Weisse AB, Heller DR, Schimenti RJ, Montgomery RL, Kapila R. The febrile parenteral drug user: a prospective study in 121 patients. Am J Med. 1993;94(3):274–80.

[119] Miró JM, Moreno A, Mestres CA. Infective endocarditis in intravenous drug abusers. Curr Infect Dis Rep. 2003;5(4):307–16.

[120] Chambers HF, Morris DL, Täuber MG, Modin G. Cocaine use and the risk for endo-carditis in intravenous drug users. Ann Intern Med. 1987;106(6):833–6.

[121] Moss R, Munt B. Injection drug use and right sided endocarditis. Heart Br Card Soc. 2003;89(5):577–81.

[122] Mathew J, Addai T, Anand A, Morrobel A, Maheshwari P, Freels S. Clinical features, site of involvement, bacteriologic findings, and outcome of infective endocarditis in intravenous drug users. Arch Intern Med. 1995;155(15):1641–8.

[123] Carozza A, De Santo LS, Romano G, Della Corte A, Ursomando F, Scardone M, et al. Infective endocarditis in intravenous drug abusers: patterns of presentation and long-term outcomes of surgical treatment. J Heart Valve Dis. 2006;15(1):125–31.

[124] Chambers HF, Korzeniowski OM, Sande MA. *Staphylococcus aureus* endocarditis: clinical manifestations in addicts and nonaddicts. Medicine (Baltimore). 1983;62(3): 170–7.

[125] Sklaver AR, Hoffman TA, Greenman RL. *Staphylococcal* endocarditis in addicts. South Med J. 1978;71(6):638–43.

[126] Thadepalli H, Francis CK. Diagnostic clues in metastatic lesions of endocarditis in addicts. West J Med. 1978;128(1):1–5.

[127] Braine N, Jarlais DCD, Ahmad S, Purchase D, Turner C. Long-term effects of syringe exchange on risk behavior and HIV prevention. AIDS Educ Prev. 2004;16(3):264–75.

[128] Vlahov D, Junge B. The role of needle exchange programs in HIV prevention. Public Health Rep Wash DC 1974. 1998;113(Suppl 1):75–80.

10

Blood Culture-Negative Endocarditis

Mio Ebato

Abstract

Blood culture-negative endocarditis is often severe and difficult to diagnose. Infective blood culture-negative endocarditis is classified into three main categories: (1) bacterial endocarditis with blood cultures sterilized by previous antibacterial treatment; (2) endocarditis related to fastidious microorganisms in which prolonged incubation is necessary; (3) true blood culture-negative endocarditis, due to intra-cellular bacteria that cannot be routinely cultured in blood with currently available. There are two major etiologies for noninfective endocarditis: (1) nonbacterial thrombotic endocarditis and (2) endocarditis related to systemic diseases (SLE and Behcet disease). Team approach including cardiologists, infection disease (ID) specialists, microbiologists, pathologist and immunologist is crucial for diagnosis and management of blood culture-negative endocarditis as it needs elegant and high-quality modern technics of histology, molecular analysis and essential epidemiological information.

Keywords: blood culture-negative endocarditis, fastidious microorganisms, intra-cellular bacteria, noninfective endocarditis

1. Introduction

Blood culture-negative IE (BCNIE) refers to infective endocarditis (IE) in which no causative microorganism can be grown using the usual blood culture methods. BCNIE accounts for 5–10% of all cases of endocarditis [1]. This variation is caused by differences in the diagnostic criteria and sampling strategies used. A European study included 820 cases indicated 20% of patients with confirmed IE had negative blood cultures [2]. BCNIE often produces considerable diagnostic and therapeutic dilemmas, which result in poor prognosis.

2. Main etiologies of BCNIE

There are three main causes for BCNIE.

1. Administration to antimicrobial agents before blood culture.

2. Endocarditis related to fastidious microorganisms in which prolonged incubation is necessary.

3. True blood culture-negative endocarditis, due to intra-cellular bacteria that cannot be detected by currently available routine blood culture system.

If all microbiological assays are negative, noninfective endocarditis is considered, and systematically differential diagnosis should be performed. Nonbacterial thrombotic endocarditis (marantic endocarditis) in patients with malignant tumor and systemic diseases such as SLE and Behçet are two main causes of noninfective endocarditis.

3. Diagnostic approach

Definitions of the terms used in the European Society of Cardiology 2015 [4] modified criteria adapted from modified Duke Criteria [3] were shown in **Table 1**. Diagnosis of IE is drawn as follows:

3.1. Definition

Pathological criteria: Microorganisms demonstrated by culture or on histological examination of a vegetation, a vegetation that has embolized, or an intracardiac abscess specimen; or pathological lesions; vegetation or intracardiac abscess by histological examination showing active endocarditis.

Clinical criteria: two major criteria; or one major criterion and three minor criteria or five minor criteria.

Possible IE: One major criterion and one minor criterion or three minor criteria.

Rejected IE: Firm alternate diagnosis; or Resolution of symptoms suggesting IE with antibiotic therapy for ≤4 days; or No pathological evidence of IE at surgery or autopsy, with antibiotic therapy for ≤4 days; or Does not meet criteria for possible IE, as above.

When blood culture is negative, systematic diagnostic approach should be performed for rapid and correct management of BCNIE. Diagnostic work-up in blood culture-negative endocarditis is shown in **Figure 1** [1, 4].

Major criteria

1. Blood cultures positive for IE

   a. Typical microorganisms consistent with IE from two separate blood cultures

   *Streptococcus viridance, Streptococcus bovis, HACEK group, *Staphylococcus aureus*

   **Community-acquired enterococci, in the absence of a primary focus

   b. Microorganisms consistent with IE from persistently positive blood cultures defined as follows

   **>2 positive blood cultures of blood samples drawn >12 h part; or

   **All of 3 or a majority of >4 separate cultures of blood (with first and last samples (drawn>1 h apart)

   c. Single positive blood culture for *Coxiella burnetii* or phase I IgG antibody titer>1:800

2. Imaging positive for IE

   a. Echocardiogram positive for IE: vegetation, abcess, pseudoaneurysm, intracardiac fistula, valvular perforation or aneurysma, new partial dehiscence of prosthetic valve

   b. Abnormal activity around the site of prosthetic valve implantation detected by 18F-FDG PET/CT (only if the prosthesis was implanted for 3 months) or radiolabeled leukocytes SPECT/CT.

   c. Definite paravalvular lesion by cardiac CT.

Minor criteria

1. Predisposition such as predisposing heart condition, or injection drug use.

2. Fever defined as temperature > 38°C

3. Valvular phenomena (including those detected by imaging only) major arterial emboli, septic pulmonary infarcts, infectious (mycotic) aneurysm, intracranial hemorrhages, conjunctival hemorrhages and Janeway's lesions.

4. Microbiological evidence: positive blood culture but does not meet a major criterion as noted above or serological evidence of active infection with organism consistent with IE

CT, computed tomography; FDG, fluorodeoxyglucose; HACEK, Haemophilus parainfluenzae, H. aphrophilus, H. paraphrophilus, H. influenzae, Actinobacillus actinomycetemcomitans, Cardiobacterium hominis, Eikenella corrodens, Kingella kingae, and K. denitrificans; IE, infective endocarditis; Ig, immunoglobulin; PET, positron emission tomography; SPECT, single photon emission computerized tomography.

Table 1. Definitions of the terms used in the European Society of Cardiology 2015 modified criteria adapted from modified Duke criteria.

3.2. Past history and clinical examination

A precise interview about epidemiological factors, history of prior infections, exposure to antimicrobials, should be made in all patients with suspected BCNIE [1, 4].

Previous exposure to antibiotics is the most common cause of BCNE, and even a short course of antibiotics can cause long-lasting suppression of bacterial activity. A history of animal exposures may predispose to certain microbiologic etiologies. Immunosuppression or prolonged antibiotic therapy suggests endocarditis due to fungi. The epidemiological clues for defining the etiology of BCNIE are shown in **Table 2** [1].

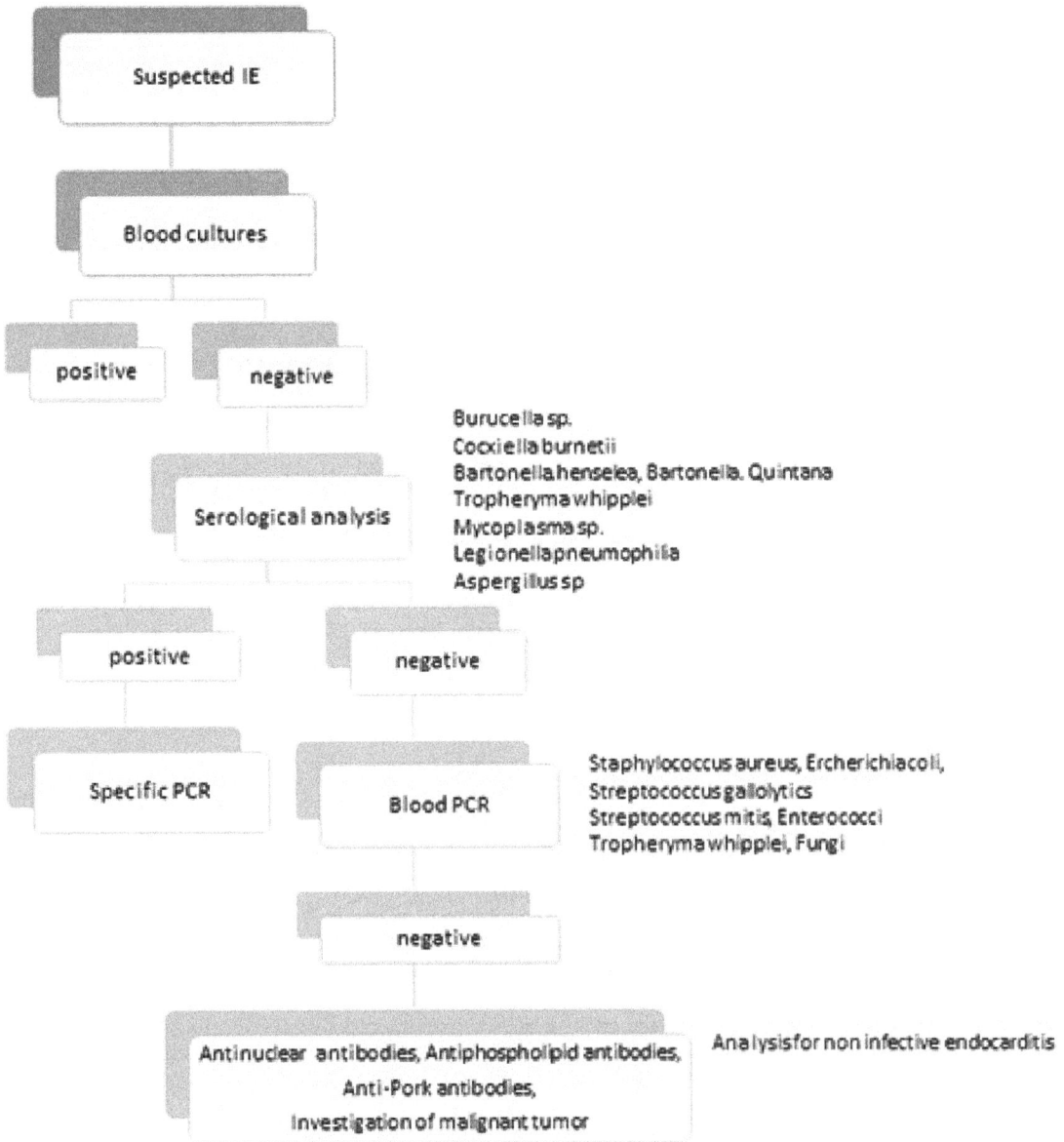

Figure 1. Diagnostic workup in blood culture-negative endocarditis.

3.3. Blood culture

BCNIE occurs frequently (45–60%) by common and easily grown staphylococci or streptococci in patients with preceding administration of antibiotics as it reduces the recovery rate of bacteria by 35–40% [5, 6]. In these cases, withdrawing antibiotics and repeating blood cultures are preferable methods to diagnose if the patient status allowed. The use of specific blood culture bottles for fastidious microorganisms is not recommended recently [1, 4, 5]. The extended incubation is applied only when cultures remain sterile after 48–72 h. Sophisticated automated systems allow isolating most pathogens that can grow slowly including Candida sp., deficient streptococci and HACEK group bacteria(Haemophilus, Aggregatibacter (previously

Epidemiological feature	Suspected microorganisms
Alcoholism, Cirrhosis	*Bartonella sp., Aeromnas sp., Listeria sp.*
Burn	*S. aureus*, Aerobic Gram-negative bacilli, Fungi
Chronic skin disorders	*S. aureus*, β-hemolytic streptococci
Genitourinary disorders	Enterococcus, GroupB streptococci, aerobic Gram-negative bacilli, *Neisseria gonorrhoeae*, Listeria monocytoogenes
Intravenous drug use, cardiovascular medical devices	*S. aureus*, CNS, Aerobic Gram-negative bacilli, β-Hemolytic streptococci, Fungi
Prosthetic valve replacement	Early(<1y): CNS, *S. aureus*, Aerobic Gram-negative bacilli, Fungi, *Corynebacterium sp., Legionella sp.*, Late(>1y): CNS, *S. aureus*, Viridance *Streptcoccus sp.*, Enterococcus sp., Fungi, Corynebacterium
Exposure to dog and/or cat	*Bartonella sp.,Pasteurella sp.*
Contact with contaminated milk or farm animal	*Brucella sp.*, Cociella bumetii
Homeless, body lice	*Bartonella sp.*
Gastrointestinal lesions	*S. gallolytics* (bovis), *Enterococcus sp.*, Clostridium spectrum
Dog or cat exposure	*Bartonella sp., Pasteurella sp., Capnocytophaga sp.*
Homeless, body lice	*Bartonella sp.*
Contact with contaminated milk or infected farm animals	*Brucella sp., Coxiella bumetii, Erysipelothrix sp.*
Diabetes mellitus	*S. aureus*, β-Hemolytic streptococci, *S. pneumoniae*
AIDS	*Salmonella sp., S. pneumoniae, S. aureus*
Organ transplantation	*S. aureus, Aspergillus fumigatus, Enterococcus sp., Candida sp.*

Table 2. Epidemiological clues for defining the etiology of blood culture-negative infective endocarditis *S. aureus*, Staphylococcus aureus; CNS, coagulase -negative staphylococci; *S. gallolytics*, Streptococcus gallolyticus; Streptococcus pneumonie.

Actinobacillus), Cardiobacterium, Eikenella, Kingella). Extending culture beyond 5 days is not contributive [1, 4–8]. The popular pathogens such as staphylococci, streptococci and entero-cocci are usually identified within 48 h. The European guidelines recommend that clinicians require prolonged incubation of vials only in the rare cases of cultures remaining negative at 48–72 h and if the diagnosis of IE remains plausible [4, 8].

3.4. Serology

The list of serological tests to be performed in case of blood culture-negative endocarditis used to include: *Legionella pneumophila*, *Mycoplasma hominis*, *Chlamydophila pneumoniae*, Brucella sp., *Coxiella burnetii* (*C. burnetii*), and Bartonella sp. Two major series showed that only Bartonella sp. and *C. burnetii* serological tests are contributive: 348 cases of suspected BCNIE were investigated between 1983 and 2001, the diagnosis was documented by serological tests in 268 cases (77%), including 266 cases of *C. burnetii* (n = 167) or Bartonella sp. (n = 99) [5]. The same team reported a second series of 745 patients presenting with suspected BCNIE having received a panel of serological tests between 2001 and 2009. They documented the predominance of Q fever and Bartonellosis. A total of 354 of the 356 cases documented by serological tests were positive for *C. burnetii* (n = 274) or Bartonella sp. (n = 80) [6]. In other words, if only Bartonella sp. and *C. burnetii* serological tests had been used, only 4 out of 624 diagnoses obtained by serological tests would have been missed. A review of endocarditis caused by fastidious pathogens shows that Mycoplasma sp. endocarditis is very rare (<10 reliable observations published to date, mostly due to M. hominis), as well as Legionella sp. endocarditis [7]. Moreover, most cases of endocarditis supposedly due to Chlamydophila sp. are probably cross-reactions with a Bartonella sp. In 2015, the only routinely recommended serological tests in case of negative blood cultures are tests for Q fever and Bartonellosis [4]. Brucellosis serological tests can be added in case of risk factors (living in endemic areas, occupational exposure, consumption of nonpasteurized dairy products). Serological tests for Mycoplasma sp. and Legionella sp. are still recommended in the 2015 ESC guidelines [4].

3.5. Evaluation of valve tissue

The more frequent use of valve replacement in the acute phase of infective endocarditis and the advent of molecular biology techniques have revolutionized the diagnosis of blood culture-negative endocarditis:

PCR systems based on universal bacterial 16S ribosomal RNA have demonstrated excellent sensitivity and specificity [8, 9], as well as PCR targeting bacteria specifically responsible for endocarditis with negative blood culture: Bartonella sp., *C. burnetii* [10] and *Tropheryma whipplei* (*T. whipplei*) [11].

Moreover, the microscopic examination of valves after Gram staining, and cultures on appropriate media provide important information not only for the identification of the pathogen involved when the data were not available preoperatively [12], but also information on its viability at the time of valve replacement, which will impact the duration of post-replacement treatment [11, 13]. The histological analysis of valves is not contributive to diagnose except some rare diagnoses such as porcine bioprosthesis endocarditis mediated by allergy to porcine proteins [22, 23]. Summary of diagnostic procedure of rare pathogens of BCNIE is shown in **Table 3**.

Pathogen	Diagnostic procedures
Brucella sp.	blood cultures, serology, immunohistology, PCR of surgical materials
Coxiella burnetii	serology (IgG phaseI >1:800, tissue culture, immunohistology, PCR of surgical materials
Bartonella sp.	blood cultures, serology, culture, immunohistology, PCR of surgical materials
Tropheryma whippplei	hystology and PCR of surgical materials
Mycoplasma sp.	serology, culture, immunohistology, PCR of surgical materials
Legionella sp.	blood cultures, serology, culture, immunohistology, PCR of surgical materials
Fungi	blood cultures, serology, immunohistology, PCR of surgical materials

Table 3. Summary of diagnostic procedure of rare pathogens of blood culture-negative infective endocarditis.

4. Treatment

4.1. Empirical therapy

Selection of medical therapy for patients with BCNIE is difficult. Some of the laboratory-based diagnostic techniques to define fastidious or rare pathogens are not available in most clinical laboratories. It consumed considerable time for completion of testing if specimens are sent to a referral laboratory. Patients with BCNIE are often treated empirically for the more common bacterial causes of IE during the waiting time. There is a need to provide empirical antimicrobials for all likely pathogens, though certain therapeutic agents, including aminoglycosides, have potentially toxic effects. Consultation with an ID specialist to define the most appropriate choice of therapy is recommended. Once additional clinical and laboratory data were brought, initial empirical therapy should be changed to more specific treatment. For patients with acute (days) clinical presentations of native valve infection, coverage for S aureus, β-hemolytic streptococci, and aerobic Gram-negative bacilli is reasonable. Empirical coverage could include vancomycin and cefepime as an initial regimen [1, 4, 14]. For patients with a subacute (weeks) presentation of native valve IE, empirical coverage of *S. aureus*, Viridance group streptococci (VGS), HACEK, and enterococci is reasonable. One treatment option could include vancomycin and ampicillin-sulbactam to provide some coverage for these organisms [1, 4, 14]. For patients with culture-negative prosthetic valve IE, coverage for staphylococci, enterococci, and aerobic Gram-negative bacilli is reasonable if the onset of symptoms is within 1 year of prosthetic valve placement. A regimen could include vancomycin, rifampin, gentamicin [1, 4, 14]. If symptom onset is >1 year after valve placement, then IE is more likely to be caused by staphylococci, VGS, and enterococci, and antibiotic therapy for these potential pathogens is reasonable [1, 4, 14]. One initial treatment option could include vancomycin and ceftriaxone. If subsequent blood culture results or other laboratory methodologies define a pathogen, then empirical therapy should be changed to focused therapy that is recommended for the specific pathogen identified.

4.2. Antibiotic treatment for fastidious microorganisms

HACEK Gram-negative bacilli are fastidious organisms, and the laboratory should be made aware that infection with these agents needs consultation to specialist. Because of slow growth, standard MIC tests may be difficult to interpret. Some HACEK-group bacilli produce beta-lactamases, and ampicillin is therefore no longer the first-line option. They are susceptible to ceftriaxone, other third-generation cephalosporins and quinolones; the standard treatment is ceftriaxone 2 g/day for 4 weeks in native valve endocarditis and for 6 weeks in prosthetic valve endocarditis. If they do not produce beta-lactamase, ampicillin (12 g/day i.v. in four or six doses) plus gentamicin (3 mg/kg/day) divided into two or three doses for 4–6 weeks is an option [1, 4, 13]. Ciprofloxacin (400 mg/8–12 h i.v. or 750 mg/12 h orally) is a less well-validated alternative. Clinical outcome of HACEK endocarditis is favorable.

In cases with fungi, mortality is very high, and treatment necessitates combined antifungal administration and surgical valve replacement. Antifungal therapy for Candida sp. includes liposomal amphotericin B with or without flucytosine or an echinocandin at high doses; and for Aspergillus spp., voriconazole is the drug of choice and some experts recommend the addition of an echinocandin or amphotericin B. Suppressive long-term treatment with oral azoles (fluconazole for Candida and voriconazole for Aspergillus) is recommended [1, 4, 14]. Consultation with an infectious doctor specialist in the Endocarditis Team is recommended.

4.3. Specific therapy for true culture-negative microorganisms

The recommended therapy for true culture-negative microorganisms in the European guidelines 2015 is shown in **Table 4** [4, 12]. Consultation with ID specialist is highly recommended for the treatment of these special organisms. This is an area with a very limited level of evidence. The treatment of *T. whipplei* endocarditis has not been standardized. Doxycycline + hydroxychloroquine for 12–18 months, with monitoring of plasma levels of these two agents (objective: achieving plasma concentrations of 0.8–1.2 mg/L for hydroxychloroquine, and < 5 mg/L for doxycycline), and of negativation of samples initially positive for *T. whipplei* was proposed. The treatment of Bartonella sp. endocarditis is a beta-lactam antibiotic (amoxicillin or ceftriaxone) or doxycycline for 4 weeks in combination with gentamicin for the first 2 weeks [1, 4, 14] the treatment of *C. burnetii* endocarditis, is doxycycline + hydroxychloroquine until a phase1 antibody rate <800 is reached for IgG, and <50 for IgM and IgA [1, 4, 14].

4.4. Surgical treatment of blood culture-negative IE

There is no specific recommendation for surgical treatment of BCNIE: cardiac surgery indications rely on the same criteria that apply for any type of endocarditis (heart failure, uncontrolled infection, risk of embolism [1, 4, 15]). However, an additional argument for the surgical treatment of BCNIE is the ability to harvest valve tissue, which often finally allows microbiological documentation.

Pathogens	Standard therapy	Treatment outcome
Brucella sp.	Doxycycline (200 mg/day) + contrimocazole (960 mg/12 h) + rifampicine (300~600 mg/day) for ≥3~6 months orally	Treatment success defined as IgG < 1:60
Bartonella sp.	Doxycycline (100 mg/12 h) orally for 4 weeks + gentamicin (3 mg/day) iv for 2 weeks	Success rate > 90%
Coxiella.burnetii (Q fever)	Doxycycline (200 mg/day) + hydroxychloroquine (200–600 mg/day) orally for ≥18 months	Treatment success defined as phase I IgG < 1:200 IgM, IgA < 1:50
Legionella sp.	Levofloxacin (500 mg/12 h) iv or orally for ≥6 weeks or clarithromycin (500 mg/12 h) iv for 2 weeks, then orally for 4 weeks + rifampin (300–1200 mg/24 h)	Optimal treatment unknown
Mycoplasma sp.	Levofloxacin (500 mg/12 h) iv or orally for ≥6 weeks	Optimal treatment unknown
Treaponema whipplei (Whipple's disease)	Doxycycline (200 mg/day) + hydroxychloroquine (200–600 mg/day) orally for ≥18 months	Long-term treatment, optical duration unknown

Table 4. Recommended therapy for true culture-negative microorganisms in the European guidelines 2015.

5. Noninfective endocarditis

When all microbiological assays are negative, the diagnosis of noninfectious endocarditis should systematically be considered (**Figure 1**).

5.1. Nonbacterial thrombotic endocarditis

Nonbacterial thrombotic endocarditis (marantic endocarditis, Trousseau syndrome) is observed in 1.2% of patients with active cancer at autopsy [16]. Usually, the single or multiple small vegetation-like lesions are observed predominantly on the mitral and aortic valves with no underlying valve diseases. These are associated with an underlying hypercoagulable state that justifies routine anticoagulation. Control of pathologically altered coagulation mechanism is essential for the treatment and the prognosis is poor without resolving the problem. The differential diagnosis with an infectious cause of BCNIE is often difficult, and the prognosis is poor [17]. The initial lesion is usually breast, lung, prostate, ovarian or colon cancer. However, it should not be forgotten that undiagnosed infective endocarditis is also common in cancer patients with sterile blood cultures and/or fastidious organisms that are difficult to identify by conventional methods.

5.2. Systemic diseases

Inflammatory diseases can cause endocarditis and produce a syndrome similar to culture-negative IE. Perhaps the one most often encounter is antiphospholipid antibody (APA) syndrome [18], which has been described as both a primary and a secondary syndrome of systemic lupus erythematosus(SLE) and malignancies. Sterile valvular vegetations form and often embolize, clinically mimicking in many respects with IE. The mitral valve is most often affected, and valvular regurgitation is the frequent functional abnormality. To complicate matters, the APA syndrome may also develop secondary to IE [19].

In patients with SLE, valve abnormalities are common (15–75% of autopsy series, depending on the severity of the disease), but rarely progress to a clinical stage of Libman-Sacks endocarditis [20]. The patients are usually young individuals with a very severe lupus poorly controlled by treatments. Immunological manifestations (Osler nodes) and embolism (stroke, often in combination with an antiphospholipid syndrome) may be observed. Valve lesions are mainly found in the left heart. Endocardium involvement may occur in Behçet's disease [21]. It is a disease of young ± male patients with a predominantly aortic involvement. Endocardium involvement in Behçet's disease is a poor prognostic factor. The treatment is of course should be targeted on the systemic disease (immune-suppressants, immune-modulators) with lifelong curative anticoagulation. Checkup for antinuclear antibodies as well as antiphospholipid antibody {anticardiolipin antibodies [immunoglobulin (Ig) G and anti-b2-glycoprotein 1 antibodies [IgG and IgM]} should be performed for the patients who are suspected to have noninfective endocarditis.

5.3. Allergy for porcine valve

When the patient has a porcine bioprosthesis implanted during last 6 months, anti-pork antibodies should be sought [22, 23] to consider allergy for the valve.

6. Conclusion

Blood culture-negative endocarditis is still a clinical challenge with heterogeneous pathology. Remarkable progress has been made in methodologies to evaluate the main etiologies in past two decades. Team approach including cardiologists, infectious disease specialists, microbiologists and immunologist is crucial for the correct diagnosis that is able to reach rapidly the new diagnostic microbiological techniques, and high-quality epidemiological information.

Conflict of interest

There is no conflict of interest for the theme.

Author details

Mio Ebato

Address all correspondence to: ippeiaki@med.showa-u.ac.jp

Division of Cardiology, Showa University Fujigaoka Hospital, Yokohama, Kanagawa, Japan

References

[1] Baddour LM, Wilson WR, Bayer AS, Fowler VG Jr, Tleyjeh IM, Rybak MJ, Barsic B, Lockhart PB, Gewitz MH, Levison ME, Bolger AF, Steckelberg JM, Baltimore RS, Fink AM, O'Gara P, Taubert KA. Infective endocarditis in adults: Diagnosis, antimicrobial therapy, and management of complications: A scientific statement for healthcare professionals from the American Heart Association. Circulation. 2015;**132**:1435-1486. DOI: 10.1161/CIR.0000000000000296

[2] Werner M, Andersson R, Olaison L, Hogevik H. A clinical study of culture-negative endocarditis. Medicine (Baltimore). 2003;**82**:263-273. DOI: 10.1097/01.md.0000085056.63483.d2

[3] Li JS, Sexton DJ, Mick N, Nettles R, Fowler VG Jr, Ryan T, Bashore T, Corey GR. Proposed modifications to the Duke criteria for the diagnosis of infective endocarditis. Clinical Infectious Diseases. 2000;**30**:633-638. DOI: 10.1086/313753

[4] Habib G, Lancellotti P, Antunes MJ, Bongiorni MG, Casalta JP, Del Zotti F, Dulgheru R, El Khoury G, Erba PA, Iung B, Miro JM, Mulder BJ, Plonska-Gosciniak E, Price S, Roos-Hesselink J, Snygg-Martin U, Thuny F, Tornos Mas P, Vilacosta I, Zamorano JL; Document Reviewers, Erol Ç, Nihoyannopoulos P, Aboyans V, Agewall S, Athanassopoulos G, Aytekin S, Benzer W, Bueno H, Broekhuizen L, Carerj S, Cosyns B, De Backer J, De Bonis M, Dimopoulos K, Donal E, Drexel H, Flachskampf FA, Hall R, Halvorsen S, Hoen B, Kirchhof P, Lainscak M, Leite-Moreira AF, Lip GY, Mestres CA, Piepoli MF, Punjabi PP, Rapezzi C,

Rosenhek R, Siebens K, Tamargo J, Walker DM. ESC Guidelines for the management of infective endocarditis: The Task Force for the Management of Infective Endocarditis of the European Society of Cardiology (ESC). Endorsed by: European Association for Cardio-Thoracic Surgery (EACTS), the European Association of Nuclear Medicine (EANM). European Heart Journal. 2015;36(44):3075-3128. DOI: 10.1093/eurheartj/ehv319. Epub 2015 Aug 29

[5] Houpikian P, Raoult D. Blood culture-negative endocarditis in a reference center: Etiologic diagnosis of 348 cases. Medicine (Baltimore) The Journal of Infectious Diseases. 2003;187(7):1097-1106. Epub 2003 Mar 14. PMID: 12660924

[6] Fournier PE, Thuny F, Richet H, Lepidi H, Casalta JP, Arzouni JP, et al. Comprehensive diagnostic strategy for blood culture-negative endocarditis: A prospective study of 819 new cases. Clinical Infectious Diseases. 2010;51(2):131-140. DOI: 10.1086/653675 PMID: 20540619

[7] Brouqui P, Raoult D. Endocarditis due to rare and fastidious bacteria. Clinical Micro-biology Reviews. 2001;14(1):177-207. Review. PMID: 11148009

[8] Baron EJ, Scott JD, Tompkins LS. Prolonged incubation and extensive sub-culturing do not increase recovery of clinically significant microorganisms from standard automated blood cultures. Clinical Infectious Diseases. 2005;41:1677-1680

[9] Vondracek M, Sartipy U, Aufwerber E, Julander I, Lindblom D, West-ling K. 16S rDNA sequencing of valve tissue improves microbiologicaldiagnosis in surgically treated patients with infective endocarditis. The Journal of Infection. 2011;62:472-478. DOI: 10.1016/j.jinf.2011.04.010 Epub 2011 May 1

[10] Marin M, Munoz P, Sanchez M, del Rosal M, Alcala L, Rodriguez-Creixems M, et al. Molecular diagnosis of infective endocarditis byreal-time broad-range polymerase chain reaction (PCR) and sequencing directly from heart valve tissue. Medicine (Baltimore). 2007;86:195-202. PMID: 17632260

[11] Fenollar F, Celard M, Lagier JC, Lepidi H, Fournier PE, Raoult D. Tropheryma whipplei endocarditis. Emerging Infectious Diseases. 2013;19:1721-1730

[12] Lamas Cda C, Ramos RG, Lopes GQ, Santos MS, Golebiovski WF, Weksler C, et al. Bartonella and Coxiella infective endocarditis in Brazil: Molecular evidence from excised valves from a cardiac surgery referral center in Riode Janeiro, Brazil, 1998 to 2009. International Journal of Infectious Diseases. 2013 Jan;17(1):e65-6. DOI: 10.1016/j. ijid.2012.10.009. Epub 2012 Dec 3

[13] Morris AJ, Drinkovic D, Pottumarthy S, Strickett MG, MacCulloch D, Lambie N, et al. Gram stain, culture, and histopathological examinationfindings for heart valves removed because of infective endocarditis. Clinical Infectious Diseases. 2003;36:697-704

[14] Gould FK, Denning DW, Elliott TS, Foweraker J, Perry JD, Prendergast BD, et al. Guidelines for the diagnosis and antibiotic treatment of endocarditis inadults: A report of the working Party of the British Society for Antimicrobial Chemotherapy. The Journal of Antimicrobial Chemotherapy. 2012;67:269-289

[15] Katsouli A, Massad MG. Current issues in the diagnosis and management of blood culture–negative infective and non-infective endocarditis. The Annals of Thoracic Surgery. 2013;**95**:1467-1474

[16] Fanale MA, Zeldenrust SR, Moynihan TJ. Some unusual complications of malignancies: Case 2. Marantic endocarditis in advanced cancer. Journal of Clinical Oncology. 2002;**20**: 4111-4114

[17] Eftychiou C, Fanourgiakis P, Vryonis E, Golfinopoulou S, Samarkos M, Kranidis A, et al. Factors associated with non-bacterial thrombotic endocarditis: Case report and literature review. The Journal of Heart Valve Disease. 2005;**14**:859-862

[18] Hojnik M, George J, Ziporen L, Shoenfeld Y. Heart valve involvement (Libman-sacks endocarditis) in the antiphospholipid syndrome. Circulation. 1996;**93**:1579-1587

[19] Kupferwasser LI, Hafner G, Mohr-Kahaly S, Erbel R, Meyer J, Darius H. The presence of infection-related antiphospholipid antibodies in infective endocarditis determines a major risk factor for embolic events. Journal of the American College of Cardiology. 1999; **33**:1365-1371

[20] Jain D, Halushka MK. Cardiac pathology of systemic lupus erythematosus. Journal of Clinical Pathology. 2009;**62**:584-592

[21] Geri G, Wechsler B, Thi Huong du L, Isnard R, Piette JC, Amoura Z, et al. Spectrum of cardiac lesions in Behcet disease: A series of 52 patients andreview of the literature. Medicine (Baltimore). 2012;**91**:25-34

[22] Fournier PE, Thuny F, Grisoli D, Lepidi H, Vitte J, Casalta JP, et al. Adeadly aversion to pork. Lancet. 2011;**377**:1542

[23] Loyens M, Thuny F, Grisoli D, Fournier PE, Casalta JP, Vitte J, et al. Link between endocarditis on porcine bioprosthetic valves and allergy to pork. International Journal of Cardiology. 2013;**167**(2):600

11

Prediction of Embolic Events in Infective Endocarditis Using Echocardiography

Luminita Iliuta

Abstract

Aim: Defining the echographic parameters which can help in identifying the high-risk groups for embolic events (EE) in patients with infective endocarditis (IE). *Material and method:* 236 patients with IE followed up 3 years with ECO parameters measured on the vegetations (VEG). *Results:* (1) the incidence rate of the EE was 51.27% without any significant differences for EE occurrence from the point of view of clinical parameters. (2) There was a significant correlation between the embolia occurrence and IE with staphylococcus, IE of the right heart, the length and mobility of VEG. The only independent predictors for EE were: the maximum length >15 mm and the increased mobility of VEG with the maximal angle >60.7. (3) In 23.14% of the patients with big and very mobile, EE occurred after starting the antibiotic treatment. *Conclusions:* (1) the VEG dimension and mobility determined by TEE are important predictors for the prognostic and are correlated with the embolic risk. (2) Significant ECO predictors of the EE occurrence were: VEG length >15 mm, neck/thickness ratio >0.69, and maximal angle of displacement of VEG in the cardiac cycle >60.7. (3) During the antibiotic treatment, the embolic risk depends only on VEG mobility and dimension.

Keywords: infective endocarditis, transesophageal echocardiography, embolic events, echocardiography, vegetation

1. Introduction

In general population, the infective endocarditis incidence has been estimated between 2 and 6 cases per 100,000 patient years, but it is significantly higher in patients with valvular heart disease and those with intravenous drug abuse. In 22–50% of cases of IE occurs systemic embolization [1–4] and up to 65% of EEs involves the central nervous system which are associated with a higher mortality rate. The incidence of embolic complications is higher in IE located on aortic and mitral valve and in IE due to *Staphylococcus aureus*, Candida species, HACEK and Abiotrophia organisms. The highest rate of embolic events is seen within the first 2–4 weeks of antimicrobial therapy [5], and it drops dramatically during the first 2 weeks of successful antibiotic therapy, from 13 to <1.2 embolic events per 1000 patient-days. Prediction of individual patient risk for embolization has proven extremely difficult. Echocardiography is the main investigation used in a lot of studies to identify a high-risk subset of patients with IE who might benefit from early surgery in order to avoid embolization. Higher embolic rates revealed by several studies using transthoracic echocardiography (TTE) and TEE were seen with the increase of the VEG dimensions [6]. Vegetation mobility has not been shown to be an independent risk factor for embolic events, probably because it is strongly correlated with VEG size [5]. In other studies, the embolic complications were by the infecting organism and the number of VEG, the number of valves involved and VEG characteristics.

That is why the first objective of our study was to identify the echographic parameters which were associated with the presence of an EE in patients with IE. Using these variables we tried to define the echographic parameters which can help in defining the high-risk groups for EE in IE patients and to evaluate the real value of the TEE for the EE prediction in these patients. Finally, we examined the relationship between the incidence of an EE occurrence during the antibiotic treatment and the type of antibiotherapy and the echographic predictors for a new EE during antibiotherapy.

2. Materials and method

A prospective study was performed on 236 consecutive patients diagnosed with IE according to Duke criteria [7] in our institute. The study protocol was approved by the institute management and Ethics Committee. All patients included in the trial gave written, informed consent. The study was in accordance with the Declaration of Helsinki regarding the human rights. The follow-up period was extended 3 years after randomization or until cardiac surgery whatever occurred the first and included clinical and echocardiographic examination for each visit.

The study protocol was completed with demographic data, the clinical status of the patient, VEG echographic parameters, EE occurrence, the antibiotic treatment efficacity and duration. The main echographic parameters measured on the VEG were: the maximum length (L), the maximum (tmax) and minimum (tmin) thickness, the narrowest diameter, the presence of the neck and its dimensions (lneck) and the mobility defined as the angle of displacement of long axis of vegetation throughout the cardiac cycle (**Figure 1**). The data base was done using Visual Fox Pro program.

The main prediction variables used were: NYHA class for heart failure, Duke criteria used for IE diagnosis (fever, new regurgitation murmur, blood cultures, inflammatory tests, leukocytosis, anemia), type of IE (on native valve or prosthetic) and the type of the surgical intervention. The main outcome variables were: the presence and the type of EE, death occurrence and its causes.

The characteristics of the studied group were as follows:

- 58% male, the mean age was 47.8 ± 6 years;

- 77.12% of the patients were in NYHA class III;

- 86.96% of the patients had fever >38°C;

- a significant regurgitation murmur was present on 56.78% patients;

- 69.91% of the patients presented positive blood cultures (24.58% with *Staphylococcus aureus*);

- 38.14% of the patients presented anemia;

- 2.12% of the patients had prosthesis endocarditis;

- cardiac surgery was performed on 96.16% patients.

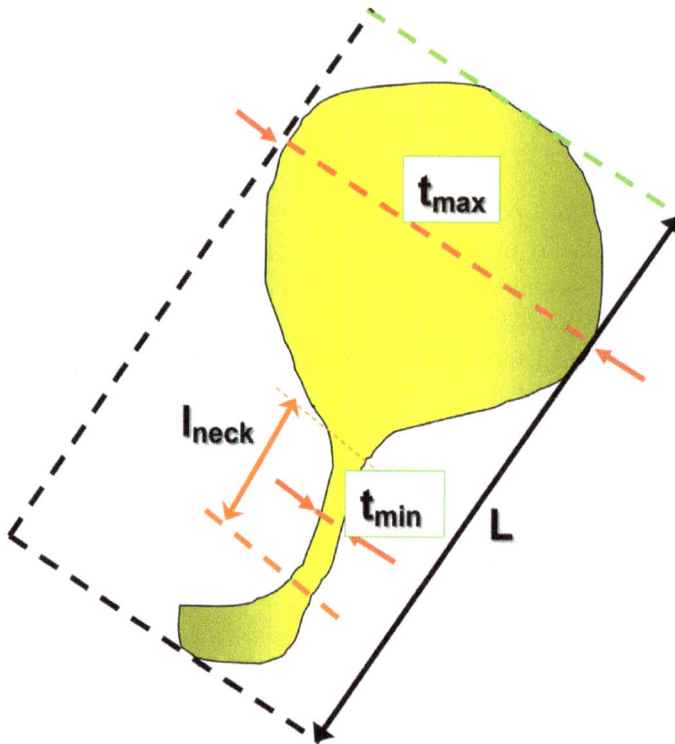

Figure 1. The echographic parameters measured on the vegetations.

The data collected represented the fields of a database in the Visual Fox Pro program. Data were processed using the Excel, Epi Info, Systat and SPSS programs for measurement of the power association between the prediction and outcome variables using the following tests:

a. for qualitative variables CHI square test or Fischer exact test (if expected cell size was less than 5)

b. for quantitative variables: T test (Student test), ANOVA test or U test depending on the samples volumes and Kruskal Wallis nonparametric tests.

The main methods of statistical correlation used in the study were the following:

- For quantitative variables analysis of simple linear and multivariate regression and correlation coefficient calculation;

- Relative risk calculation and the 95% confidence interval;

- Calculation of the positive and negative predictive value.

No sample size assumptions have been made. No confirmatory statistical hypothesis was pre-specified, but a detailed analysis plan was defined before the database was locked. Continuous data are expressed as mean ± SD. Discrete variables are expressed as counts (percentages).

According to the exposure level to the risk factors, data were grouped on the presence of an EE and the type of the treatment (surgical intervention or medical therapy). For each exposure level, there were introduced the number of patients with an EE (cases) and the number of patients without an EE (controls). The confounders were controlled by stratification.

Data interpretation was performed taking into account the following hypothesis:

- a relative risk >1 was considered unfavorable; for these patients, the occurrence of an EE was increased due to the presence of the group characteristic by the RR value;

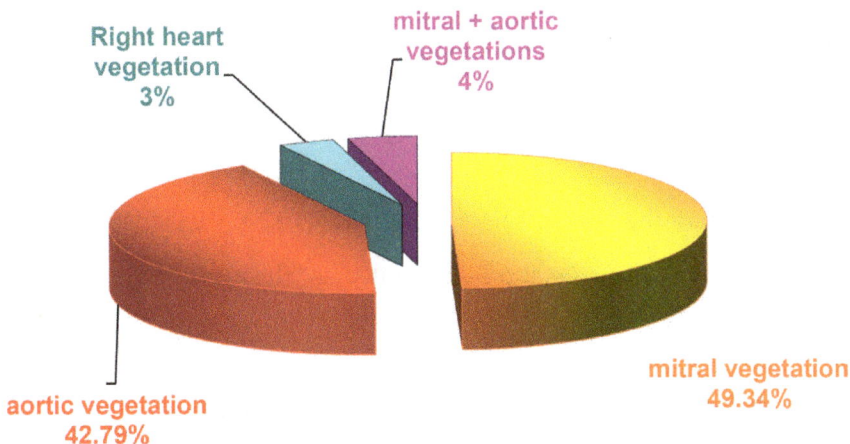

Figure 2. Patient distribution by vegetations site (229 patients).

- a relative risk = 1 included the patients subgroups classified as with no effect of the presence of group characteristic;

- a relative risk < 1 was considered favorable; for these patients, the occurrence of an EE was decreased due to the presence of the group characteristic by the RR value.

The patients were divided into two groups depending on the occurrence of the EE: group A—121 patients without an EE and group B—115 patients with an EE.

Depending on the VEG site, most of the patients (49.34%) had VEG on mitral valve, 42.79% on aortic valve, 4% both on mitral and aortic valve and 3% had right heart endocarditis (**Figure 2**).

3. Results

1. The incidence of the EE in patients with IE (diagnosed on Duke criteria) was 51.27% (121 patients). There were no significant differences for the occurrence of EE according to sex, age, fever presence, anemia, vegetation site or the presence of a significant regurgitation murmur (**Figure 3**).

2. The univariate analysis has shown a significant correlation between the EE presence and IE with staphylococcus, IE of the right heart, the length and mobility of vegetation. The only independent predictors for the EE revealed by the multivariate regression analysis were: the maximum length > 15 mm (RR = 4.92, p = 0.0001) and the increased mobility of the VEG with the maximal angle > 60.7 degree ± 12 (RR = 8.2, p = 0.003) (**Figure 4**). The univariate regression analysis has shown a significant correlation between the presence of an EE and the following parameters:

- IE with Staphylococcus (R^2 = 0.71, p < 0.0001);

- right heart IE (R^2 = 0.43, p < 0.0001);

- the maximum length of the vegetation (R^2 = 0.921, p < 0.01);

- the mobility of the vegetation (R^2 = 0.48, p < 0.001).

The multivariate regression analysis showed that the only echographic independent predictors of the EE were:

- the maximum length of the vegetation > 15 mm (RR = 4.92, p = 0.0001);

- the increased mobility of the vegetation—estimated as "the maximal angle of displacement of long axis of the vegetation throughout the cardiac cycle" more than 60.70 ± 12 (RR = 8.2, p = 0.003).

The maximum length of the VEG more than 15 mm increased the embolic risk by 4.92 times and its value between 10 mm and 15 mm by 1.84 times. Values less than 10 mm of the maximum length of the VEG turned out to be protective for EE, the associated RR being 0.92.

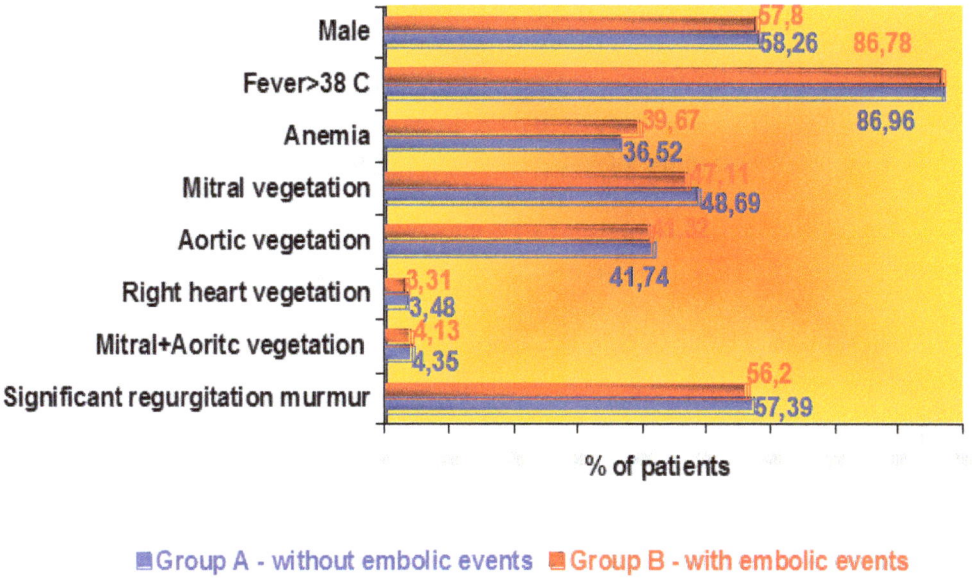

Figure 3. The occurrence of an embolic event depending on clinical parameters. Mean age: group A—48.7 ± 5 years; group B—46.9 ± 6 years.

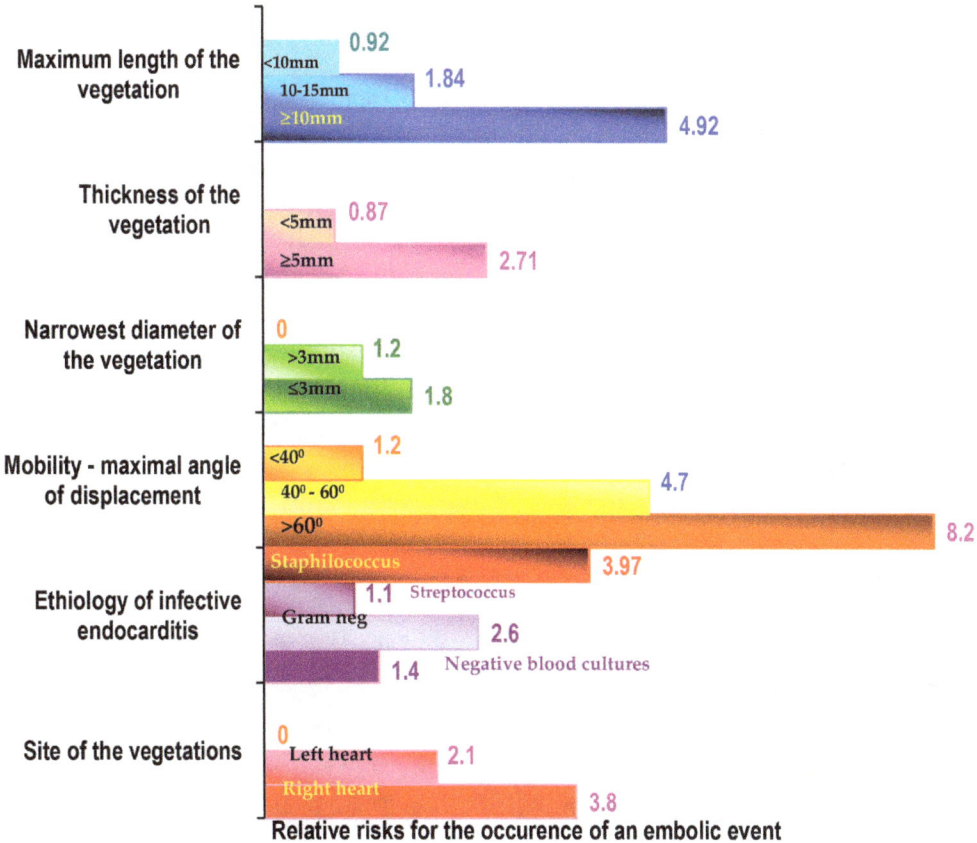

Figure 4. The relative risks for the occurrence of an EE depending on different echo parameters.

Values more than 5 mm of the maximum thickness of the VEG have increased the risk of the EE occurrence among our patients by 2.71 times. For thinner VEG, under 5 mm, the risk for EE was significantly reduced. The narrowest diameter (respectively the neck thickness—l_{neck}) less than 3 mm increased the risk for EE by 1.8 times. Regarding the mobility of the VEG, it significantly influenced the frequency of EE occurrence. Thus, the maximal angle of the VEG displacement between 400 and 600 increased by 4.7 times the risk for EE and for its values more than 600, by 8.2 times. The analysis by etiologic agent of IE showed a higher risk of EE in IE with *Staphylococcus aureus* and with Gram-negative bacteria. As other studies also showed, the likelihood of EE occurrence is higher in IE on right heart, the presence of infectious process on the tricuspid valve increasing the risk for EE by 3.8 times.

3. The differences between the patients with and without EE according to echocardiographic parameters of VEG are shown in **Table 1**.

Thus, the maximum length of the VEG was nearly twice in patients who suffered an EE compared with patients without an EE (about 12.6 mm and respectively about 6.2 mm).

In addition, the maximum thickness of the VEG measured by TEE was higher with about 3.3 mm in patients in group B. The ratio between the thickness of the VEG neck and the maximum thickness of the VEG was higher in patients without an EE (0.78 in group A respectively 0.42 in group B). In the same way, the VEG mobility (which was estimated by the measurement of the maximal angle of displacement of the vegetation was about three times bigger in patients who suffered an EE (25.1 degrees in group A and respectively 71.8 degrees in group B).

4. The rate of the EE occurred after starting the antibiotic treatment was 23.14% (28 patients) and simple linear and multivariate regression analysis found only in two independent predictors. These independent predictors for the occurrence of the EE, once antibiotic treatment has been started were the length of the VEG more than 15 mm and a high mobility of the VEG with maximal angle of displacement of long axis during the cardiac cycle >65 degrees (**Figure 5**). Thus, the maximum length of the VEG more than 15 mm increased the risk for EE occurrence by 7.1 times, the maximum width more than 5 mm increased the EE risk by 3.2 times and a neck/thickness ratio < 0.5 increased the EE risk by 3.5 times. Regarding the VEG mobility, the maximal angle of displacement values between 40 and 60 degrees increased the risk of the EE occurrence by 4.1 times and for its values >650, by 9.2 times. The IE due to a staphylococcal infection was associated with a more frequent EE occurrence, but the VEG localization on the right or left heart do not influence at the same level the EE risk as before the beginning the antibiotic treatment.

Echographic parameters	Embolic event		p value
	No	Yes	
Maximum length (mm)	6.2 ± 0.03	12.6 ± 0.04	<0.001
Maximum thickness (mm)	3.9 ± 0.01	7.2 ± 0.02	<0.003
Neck/thickness ratio	0.78 ± 0.2	0.42 ± 0.2	<0.001
Maximal angle of displacement of the vegetation	25.1 ± 10	71.8 ± 14	<0.0001

Table 1. Echographic differences between patients with IE who suffered or without EE.

Parameters

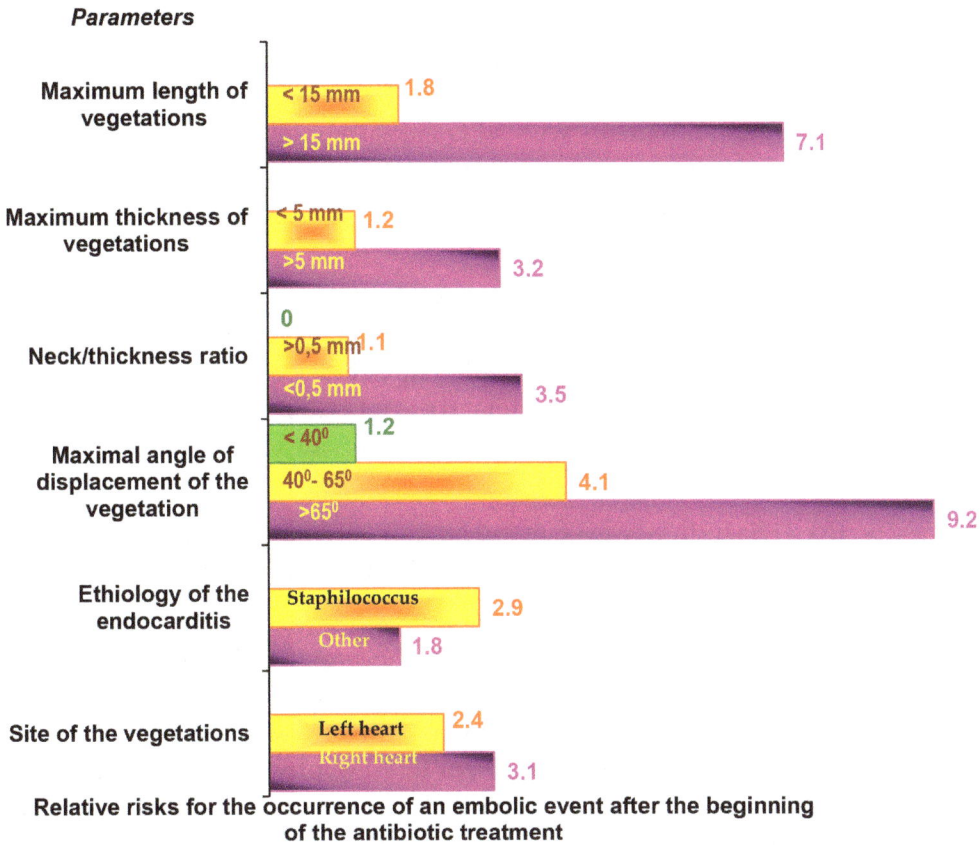

Relative risks for the occurrence of an embolic event after the beginning
of the antibiotic treatment

Figure 5. Correlation between clinical and echo parameters and the appearance of the embolic events after the antibiotic treatment has been started.

4. Discussions

The prediction of individual patient risk for embolization has proven extremely difficult. Many studies have attempted to use echocardiography to identify a high-risk subset of IE patients who might benefit from early surgery to avoid embolization [5, 6, 8–16]. In several studies using TTE was shown a trend toward higher embolic rates with VEG more than 1 cm in diameter located on the left heart [6]. In our study, the VEG dimension associated with a higher EE rate was about 15 mm probably because of a more precise measurement by TEE. Regarding the VEG diameter, in another study based on TEE, mitral VEG diameter more than 1 cm was associated with the highest incidence of embolism [6]. The association was strengthened when analysis was limited to those patients who had not yet experienced a clinical EE. Among such patients, the predictive accuracy for embolism with large mitral VEG was nearly 100% and in our study that value was about 94%. Mugge et al. had found particularly for patients with mitral valve IE, a VEG diameter greater than 10 mm was highly sensitive in identifying patients at risk for EE. On the other hand, VEG size was not significantly different in patients with and without severe heart failure or in patients surviving or dying during acute IE. In addition, no significant correlation was found between VEG size and IE location or type of infective organism. VEG with a maximal diameter of >10 mm were associated with a 50% incidence of EE, compared with a 42% incidence of emboli in patients with VEG measuring less or equal to 10 mm. Inter observer variability was higher with respect to vegetation shape, mobility, and attachment characteristics. Echocardiographic VEG characteristics were not helpful in defining the risk of embolic complications in patients with IE [5].

Heinle et al. found that patients with a maximum VEG diameter > 10 mm had a significantly higher incidence of EE than those with < or = 10 mm (p < 0.05). There were no significant differences in the frequency of emergent valve replacement between patients with aortic value and mitral valve IE. The maximum size and total score reflecting mobility, extent and consistency of VEG using two-dimensional echocardiography provide useful information to predict the occurrence of EE in patients with IE [6].

Another prospective TEE study, however, found no clear correlation of VEG size with embolization, and transthoracic and TEE characteristics of VEG were not helpful in defining embolic risk in patients with IE [8].

De Castro used multivariate analysis and identified echocardiographic accessible risk factors for subsequent embolism a VEG size of more than 10 mm and mitral valve involvement [8]. Risk factors associated with in-hospital increased mortality rate were embolism, a vegetation size of more than 10 mm, and *Staphylococcus aureus* IE. Also, precise echocardiographic visualization of VEG helps to stratify patients into a high-risk sub-group, needing early prophylactic surgical intervention.

Overall, these data are compatible with previous observations that in general, mitral VEG, regardless their size, are associated with higher rates of embolization (25%) than aortic VEG (10%) [10]. On the other hand, the highest embolic rate (37%) has been seen in the subset of patients with mitral VEG attached to the anterior rather than the posterior mitral leaflet. In particular, mobile VEG attached to the mitral valve with a maximal diameter > 10 mm may be prone to EE [10]. In a retrospective study, Deprele et al. analyzed the risk factors for systemic emboli in IE [13]. They found that the risk of emboli was 57% when the VEG measured >10 mm and only 22% when it was <10 mm (p = 0.003). The mobility of the VEG was also a risk factor: 48% if the vegetation was mobile; and 9% if fixed (p = 0.003). Sex, age, pathogen, antibiotic treatment, type of valve and the number and position of the VEG were not found to be risk factors. With multivariate analysis, only mobility was identified as a risk factor.

The effect of VEG size on embolic potential was specific to the infecting organism, with large VEG independently predicting EE only in the setting of streptococcal IE [13, 17–19]. In contrast, staphylococcal or fungal IE appears to carry a high risk of embolization that is independent of the VEG size.

The evolution of VEG size revealed by TEE appears to predict EE; however an increase in VEG size revealed by TEE over 4–8 weeks of antibiotic therapy. In patients with IE and increasing VEG size, the EE rate among was twice that of patients with static or decreasing VEG size. In addition, a second peak of late EE occurred at 15–30 weeks after diagnosis of IE, and it was associated with failure of a VEG to stabilize or diminish in size as defined by echocardiography [5, 6].

Because of the known decrease in embolic risk over the first 2 weeks of antibiotic therapy, the benefit of surgery in avoiding catastrophic embolic events is the greatest early in the course of the IE. Early surgical intervention may preclude a primary or recurrent major EE but exposes the patient to both the immediate and the life-long risks of valve replacement. That is why, the strategy for surgical intervention to avoid systemic embolization in IE still remains specific to the individual patient, benefit being the greatest in the early phase of IE when embolic rates are the highest and when other predictors of a complicated course are present (i.e., recurrent embolization, congestive heart failure aggressive, antibiotic-resistant organisms or prosthetic-valve IE). Surgical options must be considered when large VEG are detected on the mitral valve, particularly the anterior leaflet. Failure of a VEG to stabilize or diminish in size on TEE during clinically adequate therapy may also predict later EE.

5. Conclusions

1. The unfavorable prognostic in IE is predicted by the VEG dimension and mobility measured by TEE and is correlated with the EE.

2. The most important echographic predictors of the EE occurrence were: VEG length > 15 mm, neck/thickness fraction > 0.69, maximal angle of displacement of VEG throughout of the cardiac cycle > 60.7 degrees.

3. During the antibiotic treatment, the embolic risk depends only on the VEG mobility and dimension, and it does not depend on infectious agent and on the VEG site.

4. Early TEE in IE can identify the patients with high risk for an EE and who are candidates for the early surgical treatment (patients with very mobile VEG and with VEG length > 15 mm).

Conflict of interest

There is no conflict of interest.

Author details

Luminita Iliuta[+]

Address all correspondence to: luminitailiuta@yahoo.com

University of Medicine and Pharmacy "Carol Davila", Bucharest, Romania

[+]Fellow of the European Society of Cardiology.

References

[1]   Bayer AS. Infective endocarditis. Clinical Infectious Diseases. 1993;**17**:313-320

[2]   Francioli P. Central nervous system complications of infective endocarditis. In: Scheld WM, Whiteley RJ, Durack DT, editors. Infections of the Central Nervous System. New York, NY: Raven Press; 1991. pp. 515-559

[3]   Lerner P. Neurologic complications of infective endocarditis. The Medical Clinics of North America. 1985;**69**:385-398

[4]   Steckelberg JM, Murphy JG, Ballard D, Bailey K, Tajik AJ, Taliercio CP, Giuliani ER, Wilson WR. Emboli in infective endocarditis: The prognostic value of echocardiography. Annals of Internal Medicine. 1991;**114**:635-640

[5]   Mugge A, Daniel WG, Frank G, Lichtlen PR. Echocardiography in infective endocarditis: Reassessment of prognostic implications of vegetation size determined by the transthoracic and the transesophageal approach. Journal of the American College of Cardiology. 1989 Sep;**14**(3):631-638

[6]   Heinle S, Wilderman N, Harrison JK, Waugh R, Bashore T, Nicely LM, Durack D, Kisslo J. Value of transthoracic echocardiography in predicting embolic events in active infective endocarditis. Duke Endocarditis Service. American Journal of Cardiology. 1994;**74**(8):799-801

[7]   Durack DT, Lukes AS, Bright DK. New criteria for diagnosis of infective endocarditis: Utilization of specific echocardiographic findings. Duke Endocarditis Service. The American Journal of Medicine. 1994;**96**:200-209

[8]   Koie S, Iwase M, Hasegawa K, Matsuyama H, Yamamoto H, Takeda K, Kato C, Kimura M, Hishida H, Kamiya H, Ohno M. Echocardiographic prediction of risk for embolism in patients with infective endocarditis. Journal of Cardiology. 1997;**29**(Suppl 2):117-122

[9]   De Castro S, Magni G, Beni S, Cartoni D, Fiorelli M, Venditti M, Schwartz SL, Fedele F, Pandian NG. Role of transthoracic and transesophageal echocardiography in predicting embolic events in patients with active infective endocarditis involving native cardiac valves. The American Journal of Cardiology. 1997;**80**(8):1030-1034

[10] Rohmann S, Erbel R, Gorge G, Makowski T, Mohr-Kahaly S, Nixdorff U, Drexler M, Meyer J. Clinical relevance of vegetation localization by transoesophageal echocardiography in infective endocarditis. European Heart Journal. 1992;**13**(4):446-452

[11] Mugge A, Daniel WG. Echocardiographic assessment of vegetations in patients with infective endocarditis: Prognostic implications. Echocardiography. 1995;**12**(6):651-661

[12] Daniel WG, Mugge A, Grote J, Hausmann D, Nikutta P, Laas J, Lichtlen PR, Martin RP. Comparison of transthoracic and transesophageal echocardiography for detection of abnormalities of prosthetic and bioprosthetic valves in the mitral and aortic positions. The American Journal of Cardiology. 1993;**71**:210-215

[13] Deprele C, Berthelot P, Lemetayer F, Comtet C, Fresard A, Cazorla C, Fascia P, Cathebras P, Chaumentin G, Convert G, Isaaz K, Barral X, Lucht F. Risk factors for systemic emboli in infective endocarditis. Clinical Microbiology and Infection. 2004;**10**(1):46-53

[14] Shively BK, Gurule FT, Roldan CA, Leggett JH, Schiller NB. Diagnostic value of transesophageal compared with transthoracic echocardiography in infective endocarditis. Journal of the American College of Cardiology. 1991;**18**:391-397

[15] Lutas EM, Roberts RB, Devereux RB, Prieto LM. Relation between the presence of echocardiographic vegetations and the complication rate in infective endocarditis. American Heart Journal. 1986;**112**:107-113

[16] Sanfilippo AJ, Picard MH, Newell JB, Rosas E, Davidoff R, Thomas JD, Weyman AE. Echocardiographic assessment of patients with infectious endocarditis: Prediction of risk for complications. Journal of the American College of Cardiology. 1991;**18**:1191-1199

[17] Fowler VG Jr, Li J, Corey GR, Boley J, Marr KA, Gopal AK, Kong LK, Gottlieb G, Donovan CL, Sexton DJ, Ryan T. Role of echocardiography in evaluation of patients with Staphylococcus aureus bacteremia: Experience in 103 patients. Journal of the American College of Cardiology. 1997;**30**:1072-1078

[18] Fowler VG, Sanders LL, Kong LK, et al. Infective endocarditis due to Staphylococcus aureus. Clinical Infectious Diseases. 1994;**28**:106-114

[19] Bayer AS, Lam K, Ginzton L, Norman DC, Chiu CY, Ward JI. Staphylococcus aureus bacteremia: Clinical, serologic and echocardiographic findings in patients with and without endocarditis. Archives of Internal Medicine. 1987;**147**:457-462

12

Culture Negative Endocarditis: Advances in Diagnosis and Treatment

Marion J. Skalweit

Abstract

Culture-negative endocarditis (CNE) is a challenging clinical entity, both diagnostically and therapeutically. In this chapter, the changed epidemiology and microbiology of CNE are reviewed with cases highlighting typical pathogens in patients pre-treated with antibiotics, less common fastidious pathogens such as bacteria of the HACEK group, nutritionally deficient bacteria, *Legionella* spp. and Mycobacteria, "quintessential" CNE pathogens such as *Bartonella* spp., *Coxiella burnetti* and *Tropheryma* whipplei, as well as fungal CNE. Contemporary diagnostic methods are reviewed including polymerase chain reaction-based pathogen 16s RNA amplification coupled with electrospray ionization mass spectrometry (PCR/ESI-MS). Finally, treatment options per the recently updated 2015 American Heart Association and European Society for Cardiology guideline are presented.

Keywords: culture-negative endocarditis, *Bartonella* spp., *Coxiella burnetti* and *Tropheryma whipplei*, PCR/ESI-MS

1. Introduction

Culture-negative endocarditis (CNE) is one of the most challenging infectious diseases clinical syndromes both diagnostically and therapeutically. The prevalence of CNE varies widely in various modern series: it is estimated that on average, in 20% (range 5–71%) of echocardiographically evident endocarditis, both native and prosthetic valve, blood cultures do not yield a specific pathogen [1–7]. The morbidity but not necessarily mortality associated with CNE is higher than in instances where a specific pathogen is found, primarily due to the increased burden of diagnostic testing, delays in administration of antibiotics and the extended use of broad spectrum anti-microbial agents [8]. This chapter will review the epidemiology and likely microbiology of CNE, as well as enhanced diagnostic methods and treatment recommendations.

A useful definition of CNE has been put forth by Tattevin et al. [9] wherein one can think of this entity as (1) true bacterial endocarditis with blood cultures sterilized by previous receipt of antimicrobials; (2) CNE caused by fastidious or unusual organisms such as the bacteria known as the "HACEK" group, nutritionally deficient *Streptococci*, *Pasturella* spp., *Helicobacter* spp., Mycobacteria and fungal organisms and (3) "true" CNE involving intracellular organisms that are detectable via serology or polymerase chain reaction (PCR) of valvular tissue, e.g. *Bartonella quintana*, *Coxiella burnetti* and *Tropheryma whipplei*. In addition, there are non-infectious causes of endocarditis, e.g. murantic that will not be covered in this chapter.

2. Epidemiology of CNE

The epidemiology of infective endocarditis, and hence CNE, has changed over the last five decades [5, 10]. Patients are generally older and male, with greater numbers of hospital associated cases, and with indwelling devices such as catheters, pacemakers and prosthetic valves. Accordingly the numbers of cases of infective endocarditis with *Staphylococcus aureus*, coagulase-negative *Staphylococci* and *Enterococci* have increased. With the advent of novel diagnostic methods (PCR-based testing), the prevalence of CNE may have decreased to 14.2% [5] in the last decade, but other reviews indicate otherwise [10]. Specific aspects of the patient's medical history may provide "epidemiological clues" (Table 6 in Ref. [1]) to the microbiological cause. Military personnel have some higher risk of CNE due to *C. burnetti* for example [11].

3. Microbiology of CNE

The microbiology of CNE is varied and depends on host and environmental factors that predispose to one type of pathogen versus another [1]. As per the classification of Tattevin et al. [9], the microbiologic discussion will follow this paradigm.

3.1. CNE due to pre-treatment of typical bacterial endocarditis

According to one of the largest surveys of infective endocarditis recently performed, in the last decade, 29.7% of IE were due to *S. aureus*, 17.6% were due to oral *Streptococci*, 10% were due to coagulase-negative *Staphylococci* and 10% were due to *Enterococci*. Approximately, 16% of IE cases were thus due to Gram-negative bacteria, fungi and mycobacteria that could be cultured from blood. Because the presentation of infective endocarditis can be non-specific and is often associated with clinical sepsis, patients receive empiric broad spectrum anti-bacterials before sufficient numbers of blood cultures can be obtained. In one contemporary survey, antibiotics were used before blood cultures 74% of the time, with many patients coming from outside hospitals before a diagnosis of endocarditis was established [4]. The distribution of bacterial etiologies in these cases should represent what is seen generally when blood cultures are obtained prior to initiation of antibiotics. PCR of valve tissue in the cases where pretreatment occurred showed a predominance of *Streptococcus oralis* (54%), *Streptococcus aureus* (7.7%) and *Streptococcus gallolyticus* (formerly known as *Streptococcus bovis*) 5.1%. This likely reflects the ability of these organisms to attach to endovascular epithelium and be detectable by PCR methods.

3.2. CNE due to fastidious micro-organisms

3.2.1. HACEK group

Much of the early literature regarding CNE focused on infections with so-called "fastidious" organisms that were traditionally difficult to grow in blood culture, due to specific nutritional requirements of these organisms. These included a number of oral Gram-negative bacteria (*Haemophilus* species, *Aggregatibacter* species, *Cardiobacterium hominis*, *Eikenella corrodens* and *Kingella* species) that came to be known by the acronym "HACEK" (reviewed in [12]). Automated blood culture methodology involved the use of media that lacked particular nutrients like hemin, and extended incubation of 3 weeks was recommended in order to isolate HACEK group and other fastidious Gram negatives (ref). However, as early as 1993, it was evident that extended incubation was no longer necessary in order to isolate these bacteria [13, 14]. Standard 5–7 day incubation was sufficient to recover an organism in most instances.

HACEK organisms are rarely the cause of infective endocarditis, and because of the improved ability to isolate these organisms from standard blood culture specimens, even more rarely the cause of CNE. In a recent series, four out of 77 patients with HACEK IE had negative blood cultures [15]. Of these, three had previously received antibiotics. Diagnosis was made by culture of devices, and in one patient, by PCR of valvular tissue. *Cardiobacterium valvarum* has been described as an unusual *Cardiobacterium* spp. associated with endocarditis, in this case, an infected aortic graft in a middle-aged man with gingivitis and a sub-acute bacterial endocarditis presentation. In this case, the organism grew in blood culture but could not be identified by routine microbiological examination. 16S rRNA analysis revealed the species.

Pediatric populations, especially young children between the ages of 6 months and four years, appear to be particularly vulnerable to infections with *Kingella kingae* [16]. *K. kingae* is present in the oropharynx and respiratory tract of young children and can be transmitted person-to-person with resulting outbreaks of infection. *K. kingae* has a variety of colonization and virulence factors such as pili that allows the organism to anchor itself to human mucosal epithelium, polysaccharide capsule that decreases opsonization by complement, the ability to produce exopolysaccharide and biofilm that is an important factor in the formation of endovascular vegetations and RTX toxin, a potent cytotoxin that targets macrophages and respiratory epithelium [17]. Fortunately, bacteremia and endocarditis are relatively rare syndromes associated with this organism [16], causing 7.1–7.8% of pediatric endocarditis cases [18, 19]. The presentation can be dramatic as illustrated in a child with mycotic aneurysm of the aorta and cerebral infarcts [20].

3.2.2. Non HACEK group organisms

Other fastidious bacteria causing CNE include *Pasturella multocida* and other *Pasturella* spp. which constitute part of the normal oral flora of dogs and cats in particular [21]. While bite wounds are obviously a portal of entry for *Pasturella* spp., in immunocompromised patients, more superficial contact especially with cat fur, minor cat scratches and cat saliva can lead to bacteremia and subsequent endocarditis [22]. Culture-negative endocarditis caused by *Abiotrophia defectiva* and *Granulicatella* spp.—so-called nutritionally deficient *Streptococci* [23] —can also be associated with infected intracranial aneurysms and may be difficult to isolate in routine blood cultures [24]. Special consideration for length of therapy must be given and is covered below. *Clostridia* and other anaerobic organisms [25] may be difficult to recover in routine blood cultures if specimens are not handled appropriately. These organisms are likely a rare cause of CNE, but true prevalence is unknown. *Gemella* spp. have been described rarely as a cause of CNE [9, 21] including *Gemella burgeri* tricuspid valve endocarditis [26] and *Gemella hemolysans* prosthetic valve endocarditits identified by PCR of prosthetic valve material and requiring implantation of a total artificial heart as a bridge to transplantation [27]. *Brucella mellitensis* is another unusual pathogen associated with culture-negative endocarditis [2], especially in regions of the world where consumption of unpasteurized milk (cow, goat and sheep) occurs. In one series of six patients subsequently found to have *Brucella* endocarditis, only two patients had blood cultures that revealed the diagnosis [28]. Several different *Legionella* spp. have been reported as causes of culture-negative endocarditis, both in native valves and prosthetic valves. These include cases of *Legionella pneumophila* in an immunocompromised patient with pneumonitis, a positive BAL fluid *Legionella* antigen, and subsequent BAL fluid and blood isolation of the organism when subcultured onto buffered charcoal yeast extract agar (BCYE agar) [29]. Another CNE case with *L. pneumophila* was identified when the patient presented with septic arthritis and the organism was identified from synovial fluid by 16s rDNA PCR and was subsequently found to have a new murmur and a mitral vegetation [30]. Mycobacteria are another rare cause of CNE, especially in association with porcine bioprosthetic valves [31]. This study from a reference laboratory conducted between 2010 and 2013 found PCR evidence of Mycobacterial infection in six out of 370 valve samples submitted from patients with suspected CN [31] with five cases of *Mycobacterium chelonae* and one case of *M. lentiflavum****. While typically associated with immunodeficiency states, mycobacterial infections have also been reported in immunocompetent hosts as in the case of a patient with disseminated *M. chelonae* infection and resulting pacemaker CNE [32]. Special stains and cultures for acid fast bacilli should be considered in patients with device-related CNE [33]. Finally there are also rare reports with unusual causes of endovascular infections such as CNE in an immunocompromised patient on high dose corticosteroids [34] and infected aortic aneurysm in an immunocompetent patient [35] with *Helicobacter cinaedi*.

3.3. CNE due to *Bartonella* spp., *C. burnetti* and *T. whipplei*

This section deals with CNE attributable to organisms that are not typically identified with blood cultures but are responsible for a significant portion of cases of culture-negative infective endocarditis [36].

Bartonella endocarditis has been described as the "quintessential culture-negative endocarditis" [37]. *Bartonella* species were first described as a cause of infectious endocarditis in 1993 (reviewed in [38]). A recent study in Brazil estimated that 19.6% of CNE cases were due to *Bartonella* spp. [36]. There are currently 23 different species of *Bartonella* reported; the most common etiology of CNE, however, is the result of louse transmitted *B. quintana* especially in homeless persons, or infection with *Bartonella henselae* transmitted by contact with young cats. *B. henselae* is more often associated with immunocompromised hosts and prosthetic valve endocarditis [39–41]. Diagnosis of *Bartonella* CNE is typically made via serologies and/or PCR of valvular material. Further modifications to the modified Duke diagnostic criteria for endocarditis have been proposed to incorporate positive PCR, Western blot or serum IgG titer ≥800 as major criteria [38]. Unusual clinical presentations with severe renal impairment have been described with *Bartonella* CNE where there is a delay in diagnosis including anti-neutrophil cytoplasmic antibody (ANCA) positive necrotizing glomerulonephritis [42], C3 predominant glomerulonephritis [39] and proliferative glomerulonephritis (GN) with erythroblastopenia [43]. One case of *B. henselae* tricuspid valve CNE was diagnosed after the patient presented with chronic pulmonary emboli [44]. In this patient, the source was felt to be a tick bite rather than exposure to cats.

C. burnetti is a rickettsial like organism associated with true CNE [9, 21]. In Brazil, it was estimated that the prevalence of *C. burnetti* as a cause of CNE was 7.9% [36] by PCR and serologic methods. In France, in the 1990s, annual incidence was estimated at 1 per million or <5% of all cases of endocarditis [45]. Acquisition in humans is usually through exposure to parturient animals such as sheep [21]. Presentation can be quite severe especially in immuno-compromised persons, pregnant women and in persons with prosthetic valves or native valvular heart disease [46]. A new genotype, MST 54 [47] was recently described in a child with CNE secondary to congenital heart disease from an area endemic for *C. burnetti*.

T. whipplei is an *Actinomycete* bacterium found in the stool and environment [48]. Stool carriage in uninfected humans can be detected in the range of wards of 4–31%. An infectious cause of lipodystrophia intestinalis, later known as Whipple's disease, was first proposed by George Whipple in 1907 based on the presence of lipid laden foamy macrophages in the lamina propria of the small intestine. Clinical manifestations are protean, but generally patients present with diarrhea, weight loss, fever and malabsorption. *T. whipplei* is a known cause of CNE, and its true prevalence may be underestimated. When associated with arthralgia in middle-age men, it is almost pathognomonic for *T. whipplei* as the etiologic agent [49, 50]. While the organism can be cultured in fibroblasts [48], diagnosis of CNE typically requires PCR analysis of valvular tissue [51].

3.4. CNE due to fungal pathogens

Invasive mold infections are another cause of CNE, due to the difficulty in isolating these organisms from routine blood cultures. They are an important cause especially of early culture-negative prosthetic valve endocarditis [52] but can cause late prosethetic valve, pacemaker associated as well as native valve endocarditis. Among cases in the recent literature, infections with *Aspergillus* spp. [53–55], *Histoplasma capsulatum* [56–58] and *Trichosporin* spp. [59,

60] are the most widely reported. Commercial tests that detect fungal wall antigens such as galactomannan [2, 61, 62] and β-1,3-D-glucan [62] can show good sensitivity and specificity in diagnosis of fungal CNE. Jinno et al. [56] reported negative urine *Histoplasma* antigen results in their patient with *H. capsulatum* CNE, with diagnosis based on valvular pathology and tissue culture.

4. Diagnostic methods

Our understanding of the etiology of CNE and our ability to offer more targeted treatment to patients with CNE have been dramatically affected by the large number of novel diagnostic tests now available to add to our investigative armamentarium. The following discussion will focus on methods that allow diagnosis without removal of infected valves or cardiac devices (prosthetic valves, endovascular grafts, pacemaker and defibrillator leads, ventricular assist devices, etc.) versus methods that require removal of tissue or a device for diagnostic and therapeutic reasons.

4.1. Non-invasive methods

Imaging using positron emission tomography (PET) scanning has been utilized to diagnose a case of *T. whipplei* endocarditis [63]. The infected prosthetic valve was subsequently removed providing material for PCR-based methods to confirm the diagnosis, but the impetus to remove the valve came from the PET scan. Four-dimensional cardiac MRI was used to better define valvular damage and diagnose aortic valve endocarditis in a case of *C. burnetti* CNE in a patient with exposure to domesticated buffalos and positive serologies [64]. PCR combined with electrospray ionization mass spectrometry (PCR/ESI-MS) methods have been applied to detect pathogens in blood cultures in patients already receiving antibiotics and made a diagnosis in 41 out of 410 cases, although not specifically in persons with CNE [65]. Broad range PCR on blood culture specimens has also been utilized [2]. Serum galactomannan and β-1,3-D-glucan have already been mentioned as serum diagnostic tests for fungal CNE [2, 61, 62].

4.2. Invasive methods

Methodologies to increase numbers of planktonic organisms that can be cultured from devices have been devised, using sonication of the devices [66, 67]. Metagenomic analysis of the results of next generation sequencing has been used to diagnose *A. defectiva* CNE [68]. A universal PCR/sequencing test has been applied to diagnose CNE on blood and valvular tissue [69]. Immunofluorescent antibody detection, Western blot analysis and real time-PCR of 16s RNA have been used to diagnose CNE due to *Bartonella* spp. [38]. PCR/ESI-MS has been utilized on valve tissue to diagnose CNE [70, 71].

5. Treatment of CNE

There are some distinct differences in the management of infective endocarditis according to the United States [1] versus European guidelines [72] updated in 2015. These are reviewed in Tattevin et al. [73]. However, in regard to treatment of the following etiologic agents of CNE, there is good agreement in general.

5.1. Empiric therapy for CNE

For patients with acute clinical presentations of native valve endocarditis, according to the US guidelines, empiric coverage for *S. aureus*, β-hemolytic *Streptococci* and aerobic Gram-negative bacilli is provided. Such regimens should include vancomycin and cefepime at the beginning. For patients with a subacute presentation of native valve endocarditis, additional empirical coverage of viridans *Streptococci*, HACEK and *Enterococci* is added. Vancomycin and ampicillin-sulbactam is a suggested regimen. If blood cultures eventually become positive for a typical pathogen, empiric treatment can be tailored accordingly. For patients with early (<1 year) culture-negative prosthetic valve endocarditis, empiric coverage for *Staphylococci*, *Streptococci*, *Enterococci* and Gram-negative bacilli is appropriate. Vancomycin, rifampin, gentamicin and cefepime are offered as options. For late prosthetic valve endocarditis, antibiotic therapy to cover viridans *Streptococci*, *Staphylococci* and *Enterococci* such as vancomycin and ceftriaxone is suggested. Empiric antibiotics can be narrowed based on specific pathogens that are subsequently identified. Surgical source control and removal of infected devices are required more often with the pathogens associated with CNE.

5.2. *A. defectiva, Granulicatella* spp.

As summarized in the European guidelines, these nutritionally deficient bacteria produce endocarditis with a protracted course which is associated with large vegetations (≥10 mm), higher rates of complications and valve replacement (around 50%), possibly due to delayed diagnosis and treatment. Antibiotic recommendations include penicillin G, ceftriaxone or vancomycin for 6 weeks, combined with an aminoglycoside for at least the first 2 weeks.

6. HACEK

Per the US and European guidelines, microbiologic susceptibility testing might be difficult to perform on HACEK microorganisms, and they should be considered ampicillin resistant secondary to β-lactamase production. Penicillin and ampicillin should not be used for the treatment of patients with endocarditis. Ceftriaxone should be used unless the patient has a severe β-lactam allergy. The duration of therapy for HACEK native valve endocarditis is 4 weeks; for prosthetic valve infections, duration of therapy is 6 weeks or longer. Gentamicin is not recommended in the US guidelines because of its nephrotoxicity risks but is an option in the European guidelines. A fluoroquinolone (ciprofloxacin, levofloxacin, ormoxifloxacin) can be used in patients with a β-lactam allergy. Ampicillin-sulbactam is also a treatment option.

Bartonella spp.	Doxycycline 100 mg/12 h orally for 4 weeks
	plus gentamicin (3 mg/24 h) i.v. for 2 weeks
Brucella spp.	Doxycycline (200 mg/24 h)
	plus cotrimoxazole (960 mg/12 h)
	plus rifampin (300–600/24 h)
	for ≥3–6 months orally
Coxiella burnetti	Doxycycline (200 mg/24 h)
	plus hydroxychloroquine (200–600 mg/24 h) orally
	(>18 months of treatment)
Legionella spp.	Levofloxacin (500 mg/12 h) i.v. or orally for ≥6 weeks
	or clarithromycin (500 mg/12 h) i.v. for 2 weeks, then
	orally for 4 weeks
	plus rifampin (300–1200 mg/24 h)
T. whipplei	Doxycycline (200 mg/24 h)
	plus hydroxychloroquine (200–600 mg/24 h)c orally for
	≥18 months

Treatment of the following unusual pathogens in CNE is best summarized in the European guidelines and in Broqui et al. [21].

7. Fungal CNE

Per the European guidelines, for *Aspergillus* infections, voriconazole is the drug of choice, and some experts recommend the addition of an echinocandin or amphotericin B. Surgery is generally required, and prolonged suppressive therapy is recommended. For *H. capsulatum*, surgical management followed by 6 weeks of amphotericin B and additional suppressive oral itraconazole is recommended. Most agents have poor activity against other mold species like *Trichosporon* spp. The mainstay of therapy is surgical.

Author details

Marion J. Skalweit

Address all correspondence to: msh5@case.edu

Louis Stokes Cleveland Department of Veterans Affairs Medical Center and Case Western Reserve University School of Medicine, Departments of Medicine and Biochemistry, Division of Infectious Diseases, Ohio, USA

References

[1] Baddour LM, Wilson WR, Bayer AS, Fowler VG, Jr., Tleyjeh IM, Rybak MJ, et al. Infective endocarditis in adults: diagnosis, antimicrobial therapy, and management of complications: a scientific statement for healthcare professionals from the American Heart Association. Circulation. 2015 Oct 13;132(15):1435–86. PubMed PMID: 26373316.

[2] El-Kholy AA, El-Rachidi NG, El-Enany MG, AbdulRahman EM, Mohamed RM, Rizk HH. Impact of serology and molecular methods on improving the microbiologic diagnosis of infective endocarditis in Egypt. Infection. 2015 Oct;43(5):523–9. PubMed PMID: 25808262.

[3] Hase R, Otsuka Y, Yoshida K, Hosokawa N. Profile of infective endocarditis at a tertiary-care hospital in Japan over a 14-year period: characteristics, outcome and predictors for in-hospital mortality. Int J Infect Dis. 2015 Apr;33:62–6. PubMed PMID: 25576825.

[4] Lamas CC, Fournier PE, Zappa M, Brandao TJ, Januario-da-Silva CA, Correia MG, et al. Diagnosis of blood culture-negative endocarditis and clinical comparison between blood culture-negative and blood culture-positive cases. Infection. 2015 Dec 15 44(4): 459–66. PubMed PMID: 26670038.

[5] Slipczuk L, Codolosa JN, Davila CD, Romero-Corral A, Yun J, Pressman GS, et al. Infective endocarditis epidemiology over five decades: a systematic review. PLoS One. 2013;8(12):e82665. PubMed PMID: 24349331. Pubmed Central PMCID: 3857279.

[6] Topan A, Carstina D, Slavcovici A, Rancea R, Capalneanu R, Lupse M. Assesment of the Duke criteria for the diagnosis of infective endocarditis after twenty-years. An analysis of 241 cases. Clujul Med. 2015;88(3):321–6. PubMed PMID: 26609264. Pubmed Central PMCID: 4632890.

[7] Wang LW, Noel B, Descloux E, Baron DW. Antiphospholipid syndrome: an important differential diagnosis for culture-negative endocarditis. Am J Med. 2015 Mar;128(3): 250–3. PubMed PMID: 25433300.

[8] Siciliano RF, Mansur AJ, Castelli JB, Arias V, Grinberg M, Levison ME, et al. Community-acquired culture-negative endocarditis: clinical characteristics and risk factors for mortality. Int J Infect Dis. 2014 Aug;25:191–5. PubMed PMID: 24971520.

[9] Tattevin P, Watt G, Revest M, Arvieux C, Fournier PE. Update on blood culture-negative endocarditis. Med Mal Infect. 2015 Jan–Feb;45(1–2):1–8. PubMed PMID: 25480453.

[10] Vogkou CT, Vlachogiannis NI, Palaiodimos L, Kousoulis AA. The causative agents in infective endocarditis: a systematic review comprising 33,214 cases. European Journal of Clinical Microbiology & Infectious Diseases: Official Publication of the European Society of Clinical Microbiology. 2016 May 11 35(8):1227–45. PubMed PMID: 27170145.

[11] Gough A, Clay K, Williams A, Jackson S, Prendergast B. Infective endocarditis in the military patient. J R Army Med Corps. 2015 Sep;161(3):283–7. PubMed PMID: 26243804.

[12] Revest M, Egmann G, Cattoir V, Tattevin P. HACEK endocarditis: state-of-the-art. Expert Rev Anti Infect Ther. 2016 May;14(5):523–30. PubMed PMID: 26953488.

[13] Baron EJ, Scott JD, Tompkins LS. Prolonged incubation and extensive subculturing do not increase recovery of clinically significant microorganisms from standard automated blood cultures. Clin Infect Dis. 2005 Dec 1;41(11):1677–80. PubMed PMID: 16267743.

[14] Doern GV, Davaro R, George M, Campognone P. Lack of requirement for prolonged incubation of Septi-Chek blood culture bottles in patients with bacteremia due to fastidious bacteria. Diagn Microbiol Infect Dis. 1996 Mar;24(3):141–3. PubMed PMID: 8724399.

[15] Chambers ST, Murdoch D, Morris A, Holland D, Pappas P, Almela M, et al. HACEK infective endocarditis: characteristics and outcomes from a large, multi-national cohort. PLoS One. 2013;8(5):e63181. PubMed PMID: 23690995. Pubmed Central PMCID: 3656887.

[16] Principi N, Esposito S. *Kingella kingae* infections in children. BMC infectious diseases. 2015;15:260. PubMed PMID: 26148872. Pubmed Central PMCID: 4494779.

[17] Yagupsky P. Kingella kingae: carriage, transmission, and disease. Clin Microbiol Rev. 2015 Jan;28(1):54–79. PubMed PMID: 25567222. Pubmed Central PMCID: 4284298.

[18] Marom D, Levy I, Gutwein O, Birk E, Ashkenazi S. Healthcare-associated versus community-associated infective endocarditis in children. The Pediatric infectious disease journal. 2011 Jul;30(7):585–8. PubMed PMID: 21289530.

[19] Webb R, Voss L, Roberts S, Hornung T, Rumball E, Lennon D. Infective endocarditis in New Zealand children 1994–2012. The Pediatric infectious disease journal. 2014 May; 33(5):437–42. PubMed PMID: 24378941.

[20] Feldman LF, Hersh Z, Birk E, Amir G, Wertheimer G. [Mycotic aneurysm of the ascending aorta and cerebral infarcts in a 17-month old child with *Kingella kingae* endocarditis]. Harefuah. 2015 Jun;154(6):369–72, 405. PubMed PMID: 26281080.

[21] Brouqui P, Raoult D. Endocarditis due to rare and fastidious bacteria. Clin Microbiol Rev. 2001 Jan;14(1):177–207. PubMed PMID: 11148009. Pubmed Central PMCID: 88969.

[22] Wilkie IW, Harper M, Boyce JD, Adler B. *Pasteurella multocida*: diseases and pathogenesis. Curr Top Microbiol Immunol. 2012;361:1–22. PubMed PMID: 22643916.

[23] Rhodes HM, Hirigoyen D, Shabnam L, Williams DN, Hansen GT. Infective endocarditis due to *Abiotrophia defectiva* and Granulicatella sp. complicated by infectious intracranial cerebral aneurysms: a report of 3 cases and review of the literature. J Med Microbiol. 2016 Apr 5 65(6):493–9. PubMed PMID: 27046228.

[24] Carleo MA, Del Giudice A, Viglietti R, Rosario P, Esposito V. Aortic valve endocarditis caused by *Abiotrophia defectiva*: case report and literature overview. In Vivo. 2015 Sep–Oct;29(5):515–8. PubMed PMID: 26359407.

[25] Brook I. Infective endocarditis caused by anaerobic bacteria. Arch Cardiovasc Dis. 2008 Oct;101(10):665–76. PubMed PMID: 19056073.

[26] Pachirat O, Watt G, Pussadhamma B. First case of tricuspid valve endocarditis caused by Gemella bergeri. Case Rep Med. 2015;2015:704785. PubMed PMID: 26294915. Pubmed Central PMCID: 4534595.

[27] Ramchandani MS, Rakita RM, Freeman RV, Levy WC, Von Homeyer P, Mokadam NA. Total artificial heart as bridge to transplantation for severe culture-negative prosthetic valve endocarditis due to Gemella haemolysans. ASAIO J. 2014 Jul–Aug;60(4):479–81. PubMed PMID: 24727539. Pubmed Central PMCID: 4375059.

[28] Gunes Y, Tuncer M, Guntekin U, Akdag S, Ali Gumrukcuoglu H, Karahocagil M, et al. Clinical characteristics and outcome of Brucella endocarditis. Trop Doct. 2009 Apr; 39(2):85–8. PubMed PMID: 19299289.

[29] Samuel V, Bajwa AA, Cury JD. First case of *Legionella pneumophila* native valve endocarditis. Int J Infect Dis. 2011 Aug;15(8):e576–7. PubMed PMID: 21641261.

[30] Thurneysen C, Boggian K. *Legionella pneumophila* serogroup 1 septic arthritis with probable endocarditis in an immunodeficient patient. J Clin Rheumatol. 2014 Aug; 20(5):297–8. PubMed PMID: 25057741.

[31] Bouchiat C, Saison J, Boisset S, Flandrois JP, Issartel B, Dauwalder O, et al. Nontuberculous mycobacteria: an underestimated cause of bioprosthetic valve infective endocarditis. Open forum infectious diseases. 2015 Apr;2(2):ofv047. PubMed PMID: 26213691. Pubmed Central PMCID: 4511745.

[32] Hooda A, Pati PK, John B, George PV, Michael JS. Disseminated *Mycobacterium chelonae* infection causing pacemaker lead endocarditis in an immunocompetent host. BMJ Case Reports. 2014;2014. PubMed PMID: 25535221.

[33] McMullen AR, Mattar C, Kirmani N, Burnham CA. Brown-pigmented Mycobacterium mageritense as a cause of prosthetic valve endocarditis and bloodstream infection. Journal of clinical microbiology. 2015 Aug;53(8):2777–80. PubMed PMID: 26063854. Pubmed Central PMCID: 4508415.

[34] Bartels H, Goldenberger D, Reuthebuch O, Vosbeck J, Weisser M, Frei R, et al. First case of infective endocarditis caused by *Helicobacter cinaedi*. BMC infectious diseases. 2014;14:586. PubMed PMID: 25403102. Pubmed Central PMCID: 4243372.

[35] Nishida K, Iwasawa T, Tamura A, Lefor AT. Infected abdominal aortic aneurysm with *Helicobacter cinaedi*. Case reports in surgery. 2016;2016:1396568. PubMed PMID: 26885430. Pubmed Central PMCID: 4739218.

[36] Siciliano RF, Castelli JB, Mansur AJ, Pereira dos Santos F, Colombo S, do Nascimento EM, et al. *Bartonella* spp. and *Coxiella burnetii* associated with community-acquired, culture-negative endocarditis, Brazil. Emerging Infectious Diseases. 2015 Aug;21(8): 1429–32. PubMed PMID: 26197233. Pubmed Central PMCID: 4517744.

[37] Keynan Y, MacKenzie L, Lagace-Wiens P. Quintessential culture-negative endocarditis. The Canadian Journal of Cardiology. 2016 Mar;32(3):395 e9–e10. PubMed PMID: 26342845.

[38] Edouard S, Nabet C, Lepidi H, Fournier PE, Raoult D. Bartonella, a common cause of endocarditis: a report on 106 cases and review. Journal of Clinical Microbiology. 2015 Mar;53(3):824–9. PubMed PMID: 25540398. Pubmed Central PMCID: 4390654.

[39] Georgievskaya Z, Nowalk AJ, Randhawa P, Picarsic J. *Bartonella henselae* endocarditis and glomerulonephritis with dominant C3 deposition in a 21-year-old male with a Melody transcatheter pulmonary valve: case report and review of the literature. Pediatric and Developmental Pathology: the Official Journal of the Society for Pediatric Pathology and the Paediatric Pathology Society. 2014 Jul–Aug;17(4):312–20. PubMed PMID: 24896298.

[40] Sosa T, Goldstein B, Cnota J, Bryant R, Frenck R, Washam M, et al. Melody valve *Bartonella henselae* endocarditis in an afebrile teen: a case report. Pediatrics. 2016 Jan; 137(1). PubMed PMID: 26659816.

[41] Sumatani I, Kagiyama N, Saito C, Makanae M, Kanetsuna H, Ahn K, et al. Infective endocarditis with negative blood culture and negative echocardiographic findings. Journal of Echocardiography. 2015 Jun;13(2):66–8. PubMed PMID: 26184640.

[42] Van Haare Heijmeijer S, Wilmes D, Aydin S, Clerckx C, Labriola L. Necrotizing ANCA-positive glomerulonephritis secondary to culture-negative endocarditis. Case Reports in Nephrology. 2015;2015:649763. PubMed PMID: 26819786. Pubmed Central PMCID: 4706874.

[43] Lemoine M, Edet S, Francois A, Bessin C, Guerrot D. Proliferative glomerulonephritis and erythroblastopenia associated with *Bartonella quintana* endocarditis [Glomerulo-nephrite proliferative et erythroblastopenie associees a une endocardite a *Bartonella quintana*]. Nephrologie & Therapeutique. 2015 Dec;11(7):569–72. PubMed PMID: 26404944.

[44] Verdier-Watts F, Peloni JM, Piegay F, Gerome P, Aussoleil A, Durand-de-Gevigney G, et al. An exceptional case of tricuspid infective endocarditis due to Bartonella henseale revealed by an old pulmonary embolism [Un cas exceptionnel d'endocardite infectieuse tricuspide a *Bartonella henselae* revelee par une embolie pulmonaire]. Annales de Cardiologie et d'angeiologie. 2016 Feb;65(1):48–50. PubMed PMID: 25869466.

[45] Raoult D, Tissot-Dupont H, Foucault C, Gouvernet J, Fournier PE, Bernit E, et al. Q fever 1985–1998. Clinical and epidemiologic features of 1,383 infections. Medicine. 2000 Mar;79(2):109–23. PubMed PMID: 10771709.

[46] Ngatchou W, Stefanidis C, Ramadan AS, De Canniere D. Recurrent endocarditis of a bicuspid aortic valve due to Q fever. Interactive cardiovascular and thoracic surgery. 2007 Dec;6(6):815–7. PubMed PMID: 17693439.

[47] Briggs BJ, Raoult D, Hijazi ZM, Edouard S, Angelakis E, Logan LK. Coxiella burnetii endocarditis in a child caused by a new genotype. The Pediatric Infectious Disease Journal. 2016 Feb;35(2):213–4. PubMed PMID: 26535879.

[48] Marth T, Moos V, Muller C, Biagi F, Schneider T. *Tropheryma whipplei* infection and Whipple's disease. The Lancet Infectious Diseases. 2016 Mar;16(3):e13–22. PubMed PMID: 26856775.

[49] Alozie A, Zimpfer A, Koller K, Westphal B, Obliers A, Erbersdobler A, et al. Arthralgia and blood culture-negative endocarditis in middle age men suggest *Tropheryma whipplei* infection: report of two cases and review of the literature. BMC Infectious Diseases. 2015;15:339. PubMed PMID: 26282628. Pubmed Central PMCID: 4539700.

[50] Gruber JR, Sarro R, Delaloye J, Surmely JF, Siniscalchi G, Tozzi P, et al. *Tropheryma whipplei* bivalvular endocarditis and polyarthralgia: a case report. Journal of Medical Case Reports. 2015;9:259. PubMed PMID: 26577283. Pubmed Central PMCID: 4650277.

[51] Herrmann MD, Neumayr A, Essig A, Spiess J, Merk J, Moller P, et al. Isolated Whipple's endocarditis: an underestimated diagnosis that requires molecular analysis of surgical material. The Annals of Thoracic Surgery. 2014 Jul;98(1):e1–3. PubMed PMID: 24996742.

[52] Thuny F, Fournier PE, Casalta JP, Gouriet F, Lepidi H, Riberi A, et al. Investigation of blood culture-negative early prosthetic valve endocarditis reveals high prevalence of fungi. Heart. 2010 May;96(10):743–7. PubMed PMID: 19910288.

[53] Kalokhe AS, Rouphael N, El Chami MF, Workowski KA, Ganesh G, Jacob JT. Aspergillus endocarditis: a review of the literature. International Journal of Infectious Diseases: IJID: Official Publication of the International Society for Infectious Diseases. 2010 Dec;14(12):e1040–7. PubMed PMID: 21036091.

[54] Kodali A, Khalighi K. A case of late implantable cardiac device infection with Aspergillus in an immunocompetent host. The American Journal of Case Reports. 2015;16:520–3. PubMed PMID: 26250569. Pubmed Central PMCID: 4530982.

[55] Rao U, O'Sullivan M. Lesson of the month (2). An unique presentation of infective endocarditis. Clinical Medicine. 2011 Dec;11(6):625–6. PubMed PMID: 22268325.

[56] Jinno S, Gripshover BM, Lemonovich TL, Anderson JM, Jacobs MR. *Histoplasma capsulatum* prosthetic valve endocarditis with negative fungal blood cultures and negative histoplasma antigen assay in an immunocompetent patient. Journal of Clinical Microbiology. 2010 Dec;48(12):4664–6. PubMed PMID: 20926709. Pubmed Central PMCID: 3008473.

[57] Ledtke C, Rehm SJ, Fraser TG, Shrestha NK, Tan CD, Rodriguez ER, et al. Endovascular infections caused by *Histoplasma capsulatum*: a case series and review of the literature. Archives of pathology & laboratory medicine. 2012 Jun;136(6):640–5. PubMed PMID: 22646271.

[58] Lorchirachonkul N, Foongladda S, Ruangchira-Urai R, Chayakulkeeree M. Prosthetic valve endocarditis caused by *Histoplasma capsulatum*: the first case report in Thailand.

Journal of the Medical Association of Thailand = Chotmaihet thangphaet. 2013 Feb;96 Suppl 2:S262–5. PubMed PMID: 23590052.

[59] Izumi K, Hisata Y, Hazama S. A rare case of infective endocarditis complicated by Trichosporon asahii fungemia treated by surgery. Annals of Thoracic and Cardiovascular Surgery: Official Journal of the Association of Thoracic and Cardiovascular Surgeons of Asia. 2009 Oct;15(5):350–3. PubMed PMID: 19901894.

[60] Rath PC, Purohit BV, Agrawal B, Reddy K, Nutankavala L, Narreddy S, et al. Pacemaker lead endocarditis due to Trichosporon species. The Journal of the Association of Physicians of India. 2015 Apr;63(4):66–8. PubMed PMID: 26591175.

[61] Badiee P, Amirghofran AA, Ghazi Nour M. Evaluation of noninvasive methods for the diagnosis of fungal endocarditis. Medical Mycology. 2014 Jul;52(5):530–6. PubMed PMID: 24915853.

[62] Tattevin P, Revest M, Lefort A, Michelet C, Lortholary O. Fungal endocarditis: current challenges. International Journal of Antimicrobial Agents. 2014 Oct;44(4):290–4. PubMed PMID: 25178919.

[63] Jos SL, Angelakis E, Caus T, Raoult D. Positron emission tomography in the diagnosis of Whipple's endocarditis: a case report. BMC Research Notes. 2015;8:56. PubMed PMID: 25889155. Pubmed Central PMCID: 4345011.

[64] Thadani SR, Dyverfeldt P, Gin A, Chitsaz S, Rao RK, Hope MD. Comprehensive evaluation of culture-negative endocarditis with use of cardiac and 4-dimensional-flow magnetic resonance imaging. Texas Heart Institute journal/from the Texas Heart Institute of St Luke's Episcopal Hospital, Texas Children's Hospital. 2014 Jun;41(3):351– 2. PubMed PMID: 24955064. Pubmed Central PMCID: 4060342.

[65] Jordana-Lluch E, Gimenez M, Quesada MD, Rivaya B, Marco C, Dominguez MJ, et al. Evaluation of the broad-range PCR/ESI-MS technology in blood specimens for the molecular diagnosis of bloodstream infections. PloS One. 2015;10(10):e0140865. PubMed PMID: 26474394. Pubmed Central PMCID: 4608784.

[66] Inacio RC, Klautau GB, Murca MA, da Silva CB, Nigro S, Rivetti LA, et al. Microbial diagnosis of infection and colonization of cardiac implantable electronic devices by use of sonication. International Journal of Infectious Diseases: IJID: Official Publication of the International Society for Infectious Diseases. 2015 Sep;38:54–9. PubMed PMID: 26216762.

[67] Rohacek M, Erne P, Kobza R, Pfyffer GE, Frei R, Weisser M. Infection of cardiovascular implantable electronic devices: detection with sonication, swab cultures, and blood cultures. Pacing and clinical electrophysiology: PACE. 2015 Feb;38(2):247–53. PubMed PMID: 25377386.

[68] Fukui Y, Aoki K, Okuma S, Sato T, Ishii Y, Tateda K. Metagenomic analysis for detecting pathogens in culture-negative infective endocarditis. Journal of Infection and Chemo-

therapy: Official Journal of the Japan Society of Chemotherapy. 2015 Dec;21(12):882–4. PubMed PMID: 26360016.

[69] Haag H, Locher F, Nolte O. Molecular diagnosis of microbial aetiologies using SepsiTest in the daily routine of a diagnostic laboratory. Diagnostic Microbiology and Infectious Disease. 2013 Aug;76(4):413–8. PubMed PMID: 23747029.

[70] Brinkman CL, Vergidis P, Uhl JR, Pritt BS, Cockerill FR, Steckelberg JM, et al. PCR-electrospray ionization mass spectrometry for direct detection of pathogens and antimicrobial resistance from heart valves in patients with infective endocarditis. Journal of Clinical Microbiology. 2013 Jul;51(7):2040–6. PubMed PMID: 23596241. Pubmed Central PMCID: 3697732.

[71] Wallet F, Herwegh S, Decoene C, Courcol RJ. PCR-electrospray ionization time-of-flight mass spectrometry: a new tool for the diagnosis of infective endocarditis from heart valves. Diagnostic Microbiology and Infectious Disease. 2013 Jun;76(2):125–8. PubMed PMID: 23523601.

[72] Habib G, Lancellotti P, Antunes MJ, Bongiorni MG, Casalta JP, Del Zotti F, et al. 2015 ESC Guidelines for the management of infective endocarditis: The Task Force for the Management of Infective Endocarditis of the European Society of Cardiology (ESC). Endorsed by: European Association for Cardio-Thoracic Surgery (EACTS), the European Association of Nuclear Medicine (EANM). European Heart Journal. 2015 Nov 21;36(44):3075–128. PubMed PMID: 26320109.

[73] Tattevin P, Mainardi JL. Analysis of the 2015 American and European guidelines for the management of infective endocarditis. Med Mal Infect. 2016 Jun 10. pii: S0399-077X(16)30049-X. doi: 10.1016/j.medmal.2016.05.008. [Epub ahead of print] Review. PMID:27297743.

13

Infective Endocarditis in End-Stage Renal Disease Patients in Developing Countries: What is the Real Problem?

Díaz-García Héctor Rafael,

Contreras-de la Torre Nancy Anabel,

Alemán-Villalobos Alfonso,

Carrillo-Galindo María de Jesús,

Gómez-Jiménez Olivia Berenice,

Esparza-Beléndez Edgar,

Ramírez-Rosales Gladys Eloísa,

Portilla-d Buen Eliseo and Arreola-Torres Ramón

Abstract

The epidemiology of infective endocarditis (IE) has changed over the last decades, due to various factors. This chapter focuses on IE in patients with end-stage renal disease. Then it reviews the most relevant reports published in the last decade worldwide; the different scenarios in developing countries versus developed countries; different microorganisms, treatment times, and outcomes; and also our own experience in these patients. Finally, it mentions the recommendations that have helped some developed countries to reduce more than 50% of bacteremia in catheter patients and how to make them possible in developing countries.

Keywords: end-stage renal disease (ESRD), developing countries, hemodialysis (HD), infective endocarditis (IE), catheter-related bacteremia (CRB), rheumatic heart disease (RHD)

1. Introduction

The epidemiology of infectious endocarditis (IE) has changed over the past five decades, with many contributing factors for the increasing incidence. The survival rate of chronically ill patients with nephropathy and cardiac patients has increased by transplanting or immuno-suppressing, which is a consequence of medical advances. All risk factors in certain subgroups of patients are associated with the use of intracardiac or intravascular devices, prosthetic implants or catheters, and immunosuppressive drugs, causing increased health care-related infections. Despite advances in medicine, in-hospital mortality rate of IE remains high with no significant decrease observed since the 1960s [1].

Despite many scientific efforts that have been made to realize the magnitude of this problem in different regions of the world, assessing its incidence is difficult because of the few epide-miological studies that currently exist globally; the incidence of endocarditis may vary from one country to another, between 1.5 and 11.6 per 100,000 inhabitants. Apart from its incidence, it is recognizing that this is a condition that involves high morbidity and mortality [2].

Infective endocarditis (IE) in patients with end-stage renal disease (ESRD) is a problem that continues *in crescendo* worldwide, with high morbidity and mortality, but in developing countries, the problem is more alarming due to various factors such as underdevelopment, economic inequality, and limitations in health care systems. The treatment has not changed in recent decades and instead epidemiological characteristics show very specific changes that vary from the developed countries to developing countries [3, 4].

Some authors have proposed modifications in the IE classification to address hemodialysis (HD) patients in a different category, because they represent a crescent population of IE patients and diagnostic and treatment challenge for clinicians and surgeons [5].

This chapter highlights some identified differences as well as some regional differences between developed and developing countries, and provides strategies to reduce IE in HD patients, which can be performed in any health care facility.

2. Epidemiology

The precise incidence of IE is difficult to ascertain because case definition has varied over time between authors and clinical centers [6].

IE varies according to the region. Limited data suggest that the characteristics of IE in low-income countries differ from those in industrialized countries. It is estimated that over 33,700 rheumatic heart disease (RHD)-related IE cases arise each year in developing countries and that this leads to over 8400 deaths [7].

Many literature reports and a few retrospective series have been presented on infective endocarditis in the hemodialysis population. The true incidence of IE in HD patients is, at best, an underestimate in retrospective studies. It is reported that it occurs in 6% of HD patients.

The incidence of IE in HD patients is estimated to be 308/100,000 patient-years, which is 50- to 180-fold higher than 1.7–6.2 cases per 100,000 patient-years reported for the general population [8].

In a recent retrospective cohort study in Taiwan undertaken to determine IE and the mortality risk factors among HD patients, the prevalence of IE of 6.9% was reported. The overall mortality in HD patients with IE was 60.0% [9]. The mortality rate is also higher (30–77.8%) in HD patients than in IE patients in the general population (17%) [4]. There is a high postoperative mortality 11–80% in HD patients which requires surgical intervention for IE [10].

3. The ESRD patients in dialysis

The main risk factors for HD patients to get IE are recurrent bacteremia, uremia, immune-system damage, and premature degeneration of the heart valves caused by abnormalities in calcium and phosphorus homeostasis and chronic inflammation [8].

In 2006 the National Kidney Foundation established their guideline recommendations to select and place the access of HD being first choice arteriovenous fistula followed by fistula with synthetic graft leaving tunneled catheters and nontunneled as an alternative only when you do not have any of the first two options. Despite the goal since these guidelines were made in 2006 to have 50% of HD in AVF, this percentage has been achieved only in some European countries, but in North America, it has less percentage than what the guidelines suggest [11].

Mechanical and infectious complications most frequently limit the use of a central venous catheter (CVC). Infection is the most common cause of morbidity and the second cause of death after cardiovascular disease in HD patients. The incidence of catheter-related bacteremia (CRB) in HD patients depends on the type and location of the CVC, the characteristics of the population, insertion techniques and safety measures, and manipulation of HD catheters in each center. The CRB rate in nontunneled CVC is between 3.8 and 6.6 episodes/1000 days of the use of CVC and between 1.6 and 5.5 episodes/1000 days of the use of tunneled CVC. The use of a tunneled CVC carries an increased risk of bacteremia 7 to 20 times compared to the arteriovenous fistulas (AVF) [12].

The International Collaboration on Endocarditis Prospective Cohort Study conducted a prospective cohort study with 2781 adults diagnosed with infective endocarditis in 58 hospitals in 25 countries from June 2000 to September 2005, which reported an IE incidence of 21% in chronic HD patients (more than 90 days) and 25% chronic IV access in North America; 8% in chronic HD patients and 5% chronic IV access in South America; and 4% in chronic HD patients and 5% chronic IV access in Europe [13].

The above statistics differ from those reported by other authors from different parts of the world; UK presents a lower incidence of reported cases of endocarditis; and Doulton Timothy et al. reported a series of 28 cases of IE using the Duke criteria, at St. Thomas' Hospital (1980–1995), Guy's (1995–2002), and King's College Hospitals (1996–2002). Of this

28 patients, 27 patients were on chronic HD and 1 in peritoneal dialysis (PD) patient. 40% of the HD patients were treated with AVF's and the AVF was the definite or suspected site of entry for the causative organism in eight cases of IE representing the 26.6% of the total of patients with IE. The presumption that the AVF was the source of bacteremia in these episodes is supported by the fact that the causative organism in seven episodes was commensal skin pathogens *Staphylococcus aureus* (*S. aureus*) in six patients and *Staphylococcus epidermidis* (*S. epidermidis*) in one patient [3]. In contrast, Jones et al. conducted a retrospective study between the years 1998 and 2011. Forty-two patients were identified with developed IE out of a total incident dialysis population of 1500 over 13 years. Ninety-five percent of patients (40/42) were on long-term HD and five percent (2/42) on PD. Mean patient age was 55.2 years (IQR: 43–69), and the mean duration of HD prior to IE was 57.4 months. Primary HD access at the time of diagnosis was an AVF in 35% (14/40), a dual-lumen tunneled catheter (DLTC) in 55% (22/40), and a dual-lumen nontunneled catheter (DLNTC) in 10% (4/40). *S. aureus*, including methicillin-resistant *S. aureus* (MRSA), was present in 57.1% (24/42) [14, 15].

4. IE risk factors in dialysis patients

Dialysis is a well-established risk factor for IE. Mylonakis et al. reported that end-stage renal disease in HD patients has a higher rate of morbidity and mortality compared to general population. Infections are the major cause of morbidity and mortality and are the second leading cause of death in HD patients surpassed only by cardiovascular disease. And these occur in about 12–22% of ESRD patients [15–17].

The mortality rate in patients with IE ranges from 30 to 56% in one year and in-hospital mortality is twice more frequent than the general population with IE.

4.1. HD-related bacteremia

One of the factors that increase the risk of developing IE in HD patients is bacteremia, which are exposed to repetitive vascular access through an arteriovenous fistula (AVF), polytetrafluoroethylene (PTFE) grafts or percutaneous catheters for HD, or cuffed or noncuffed dual lumen catheter.

The incidence of bacteremia is related to vascular access type, ranging from 1.6 to 7.7 per 1000 days with percutaneous catheters and 0.2 to 0.5 per 1000 days with AVF, according to the reference.

The use of catheters during HD is the leading cause of bacteremia in HD patients [4, 8, 15, 18].

A hierarchy of bacteremia risk exists among various types of HD vascular access; it is less common in patients with native arteriovenous fistulae, while synthetic grafts, cuffed catheters, and uncuffed catheters yield a progressively increasing risk.

These episodes of bacteremia during HD are relatively common. They can be endogenous or exogenous: through the microorganism flora found in the patient (endogenous) or through the pathogen from another source such as might occur through hands or contaminated instruments (exogenous) [5].

There are three points where the pathogens can enter the bloodstream (BS):

(a) Product contamination of the infusion.

Contamination of parenteral fluids is exceptional at the present time due to the rigorous control sterility and subject to quick degradation once the expiration date is reached. In these cases, bacteremia usually caused by Gram-negative bacteria (Enterobacteriaceae or nonfermenting Gram-negative bacilli) particularly serious and epidemic type may occur.

(b) Contamination of connection and intraluminal space.

Contamination of the connection point of vascular catheters is the second most common cause of arrival of microorganisms to the bloodstream (after related to the place of insertion) and the most common involved in intravascular devices longer than 2 weeks. It is, therefore, the usual way of colonization of CVC, whether or not tunneled, when it occurs after 2 weeks from implantation. In this way, microorganism colonizations progress through the intraluminal surface of catheters, forming biofilm colonization all the way from the outside end to the intravascular end.

(c) Contamination adjacent to the site of insertion and extraluminal surface skin.

Access to microorganisms from the skin adjacent the insertion site of the catheter is the most common for colonization and subsequent infection-related pathogenic mechanism. This is the only way for a microorganism to get into the bloodstream in the first 8 days (in the absence of product contamination infusion). Microorganisms on the skin through the insertion point enter the extraluminal surface of catheters and form the biofilm at that level to the intravascular end.

Another option of extraluminal contamination of a vascular catheter colonization can be by hematogenous spread of a microorganism originated in a distant focus, which is very rare, observed mainly in critically ill patients with long-term catheters or in patients with intestinal diseases [19].

4.2. Degenerative heart valve disease (DHVD)

Patients with ESRD have increased incidence of degenerative disease of the heart valves, which is one of the major risks of IE. The calcific aortic stenosis and mitral annular calcification with consequent failure are the most common diseases. It has been found that this condition occurs prematurely in this group of patients 10–20 years prior to the general population. Degenerative heart valve disease is caused due to disorders of calcium and phosphorus homeostasis, in the setting of secondary hyperparathyroidism, and due to the chronic micro-inflammatory milieu of uremia associated with ESRD [5].

4.3. Rheumatic heart disease (RHD)

The RHD, which was the leading cause of IE in the preantibiotics era, is now rare in developed countries. However, it remains a highly prevalent disease in developing countries. More developed areas, such as Hong Kong and Thailand, still have a case of IE in 18 and 12%, respectively.

Chou et al. in their study compared 68,426 adult patients with ESRD in HD with two groups: with IE and without IE. They found that 1.2% without IE and 4.4% with IE, respectively, had the RHD, having a statistical significance $p < 0.001$, relative to RHD and IE in HD patients [16]. The same study shows the differences in incidence among Asian countries and the western countries. However, many western countries, such as in the case of Mexico and parts of South America, are still considered to be endemic for this disease. Simsek-Yavuz et al. in their study in Turkey also noted the difference in incidence among the developed countries and found low incidence of RHD compared with developing countries. They presented their work in 325 patients with IE that 33% had RHD.

Although this study is not specifically for HD patients, it demonstrates a high prevalence of RHD in IE [20].

4.4. Chronic degenerative diseases (CDD)

• *Diabetes*

There is a close relationship between HD patients and diabetes, with the incidence of IE.

There are studies that have an incidence of 33–59.4% of patients having statistical significance compared with HD patients with DM without IE, $p < 0.001$ [15, 16].

• *Systemic hypertension*

This condition is related to ESRD patients with HD and IE having an incidence of up 89.9% [15].

• *Coronary artery disease (CAD)*

Kamalakannan et al. in their study with 69 patients showed an incidence of 24.6% of CAD in HD patients with IE. Chou et al. found $p < 0.001$ between HD patients with IE versus the HD patient without IE. This disease is considered to be a potential cause of death in the short and long term in these patients [8, 15, 16].

• *Congestive heart failure (CHF)*

Kamalakannan et al. in their study with 69 patients showed an incidence of 18.8% of CHF in this group of patients. Chou et al. compared CHF in HD patients with IE versus HD patients without IE and found significant differences $p < 0.001$, being the HD patients with IE, the group with more CHF, which also indicates the direct cause of death in these patients in the short term [8, 15, 16].

4.5. Preexisiting cardiac abnormalities

These account for 13.5–33.3% of the causes associated with IE in HD patients, and include the presence of valve prostheses, previous valvular heart disease, heart transplantation, pericarditis, myocarditis, and intracardiac devices.

The incidence of cardiac device infective endocarditis (CDIE) has been reported between 0.06 and 0.6% per year or 1.14 per 1000 device-years [15, 16, 21].

4.6. Intravenous drug users

Although it is a rare case of IE in HD patients, Kamalakannan et al. reported an incidence of 11.6% representing eight patients of the study [8]. Also in some countries such as Finland they found an increase in IV drug abuse as a risk factor for IE patients being 0% in the 1980s and mid-1990s to 20% in 2000–2004 [22].

4.7. Elderly patients

A relationship has been found between the advanced ages of the patient with ESRD on HD; some authors considered ≥ 65 years and others ≥ 70 years with IE. Nori et al. reported a frequency of IE 27%, the highest among age groups for patients ≥ 70 years. Chou et al. reported 48% of HD patients with IE ≥ 65 years. The ages of the Patients in HD with IE were 62.12 ± 13.09 years versus 60.11 ± 14.06 years in HD patients without IE, resulting in a $p < 0.001$, confirming that the advanced age is a risk factor for IE. Watt et al. presented a comparison of patients treated in Rennes, France, versus patients treated in Khon Kaen, Thailand (from rural areas in Thailand), finding a statistical difference in the age with an average of 70 versus 47 years, respectively.

Also elderly patients are considered to have a poor prognostic factor in IE in HD patients.

Also older age is a determinant of the clinical features in IE. Fewer patients can go to surgical treatment and mortality is higher than in younger patients [7, 13, 15, 16, 23].

4.8. Methicillin-susceptible *Staphylococcus aureus* (MSSA) and methicillin-resistant *Staphylococcus aureus* (MRSA) infection

Staphylococcus aureus represents the primary pathogen in IE in HD patients causing up to 80% of the IE. This pathogen is much more frequent than in the general population with IE. This can be explained that more than 50% of patients in dialysis are carriers of *S. aureus*; nose as a reservoir has shown an increased risk of subsequent infections. It is also important to consider that this pathogen by the fact is responsible for a high number of septic complications compared with other microorganisms. Finally, recent studies have shown that as much as 50% of *S. aureus* IE is MRSA. These strains in particular are more difficult to eradicate and are associated with a worse prognosis than methicillin-susceptible *S. aureus*. In general, patients with MRSA got it as an in-hospital infection; however, studies have shown the existence of community-acquired strains, which are microbiologically different from those acquired during hospitalization. Those strains are called community-acquired *Staphylococcus aureus* methicillin-resistant (CA-MRSA). It is a predisposing factor in these patients and a challenge for physicians involved with patients with MRSA IE [1, 5, 24].

4.9. Other microorganisms

Streptococcus viridans is currently considered to be the second cause of IE after *S. aureus*. Other pathogens such as *Enterococci* occupy the third place. The relevance of the latter is that its incidence has been increasing, plus it is more associated with nosocomial infection compared with *Streptococcus*. These pathogens if presented in prosthetic valves are more likely to cause intracardiac abscesses and less likely to have detectable vegetations on echocardiography than those presented in IE in native valves [1].

4.10. Immunosuppression

In patients with ESRD, there is a malfunction in polymorphonuclear and mobility of granulocytes, which reduce defense of the patient's cells, thus failing to remove bacteria from the bloodstream properly [5].

5. Heart valves with IE in HD

As mentioned earlier the incidence of IE in HD patients is higher than in general population and it is caused by multiple factors. But it is closely related to frequent episodes of bacteremia related to dialysis access and the predisposition of these patients to present premature degeneration of the heart valves eventually causing bacterial implantation in the valves. This is an issue of major public health presenting a very poor prognosis in short and long term, with 23.5% in-hospital mortality and 61.6% mortality in 1 year.

Despite the high rates of IE and poor prognosis for these patients, there has not been a substantial change in mortality over the past two decades. This can be the result of not having important changes in the therapeutic armamentarium [25]. Reports of multiple studies have shown that left valves with IE in HD patients are affected twice the time compared to the right valves; as well as the mitral valve is affected in more patients than the aortic valve. It is theorized that the thickening of these valves, which is common in this group of patients, can lead to increased susceptibility to acquire IE because of alterations in the laminar flow. Mitral annular calcification, which is also common in ESRD, has also shown increased susceptibility to IE [8].

5.1. Transthoracic echocardiogram (TTE) versus transesophageal echocardiogram (TEE)

TTE as a first-line diagnostic tool can work, but Kamalakannan et al. reported only 55.3% positive for vegetations in IE in HD and after using TEE 92.5% were positive for vegetations [8].

5.2. Medical treatment

Medical treatment for IE in HD patients, if considering the current guidelines for IE in general population, must have some important considerations in this group of patients.

Vancomycin should not be used in IE with MSSA, because of two reasons: (1) its low bactericidal activity when compared with oxacillin or cefazolin and (2) its main role in strains of *S. aureus* with reduced glycopeptides and vancomycin-resistant *Enterococci* sensitivity. Conversely, when dealing with a patient with IE with MRSA, vancomycin (possibly in combination with rifampicin) remains the drug of choice, if it is possible to obtain and maintain plasma levels between 15 and 20 mg/L without toxicity [5].

5.3. Surgical treatment

You can repair a valve anytime with a TEE confirmation of good valve function, which is better than replacement.

Valve replacement is a key part of therapy in patients with IE [25]. A large retrospective study by Rankin et al. used the Society of Thoracic Surgeons national database to analyze 1862 valve surgery operations in dialysis patients with endocarditis from 1994 to 2003 and reported an operative mortality of 24.4%. In this study, several risk factors for hospital mortality were proposed in HD patients with IE, including (salvage surgery/shock, surgery on both valves, elderly, affected mitral valve, high BMI, arrhythmias, active endocarditis, and female gender) [26]. A more recent study of Leither et al. found lower mortality in patients who underwent surgery of left-sided surgery compared to those reported by Ranki et al.

Current indications for surgery in a patient with IE (general population) according to the guidelines are valve disease causing CHF, recurrent emboli, persistent despite appropriate antibiotic treatment infection, and mobile and large vegetation formation of myocardial abscesses. However, these recommendations are made for IE general population; currently, there are no specific guidelines for IE in HD patients, taking into account that this indication may be debatable for these patients. Dialysis patients have a higher risk for mortality in the context of IE, lower life expectancy, high surgical risk, and often other associated morbidities [25]. In this context, there are some studies with very different results: Spies et al. reported 73% mortality and Kamalakannan et al. reported 80% survival in patients undergoing surgery, in in-hospital survival and only 43% survival with medical treatment. However, in the study of Kamalakannan et al. 12 of the 15 patients (80%) survived, but 24 of the 69 patients had indication for surgery according to the guidelines of IE for the general population, indicating that selection bias likely strongly influenced the outcomes reported in these studies [8, 25, 27].

About surgical treatment in this group of patients, there has always been controversy over what type of prosthesis to be used: biological or mechanical. These controversies started from two studies from the 1970s that were case series (*n* = 4 patients) in dialysis, where accelerated calcification of biological valves was documented. Now there are enough studies that compare the use of mechanical versus. bioprosthesis with no significant differences. Thourani et al., in 2011, demonstrated a in HD patients with IE patients undergoing valve replacement of 18.1%, with no difference between mechanical and bioprosthetic after 10 years [28]. Other studies have shown a higher incidence of bleeding and cerebrovascular events in patients with mechanical valves compared with bioprosthesis. In addition to oral anticoagulants, which are problematic in ESRD patients, most patients are prone to bleeding.

Since no significant differences are found between the types of valve prosthesis to be placed in HD patients with IE, it is recommended to individualize each case. But as a general rule, bioprosthesis is placed in most HD patients with IE, especially in patients with increased risk of bleeding associated with anticoagulation, leaving mechanical prostheses for young patients without other morbidity in whom life expectancy is longer than the bioprosthesis and also, for young patients who are candidates for renal transplantation in the future [25].

6. IE in HD patients in western Mexico

Our group works at a reference center, in the Mexican Institute of Social Security (IMSS for its acronym in Spanish) and takes care of all cardiothoracic surgical patients in the west of Mexico that are affiliated to IMSS. This means that more than 10 states represent more than 8.5 million affiliated people and possible patients. There are other hospitals in western Mexico that deal with endocarditis patients, but a patient who has surgical indication or who is seriously ill is sent to our center.

We retrospectively analyzed the last 5 year cases of IE in our center. There were 173 cases of which 77 (44.5%) were surgically treated. In these 77 patients, 33 (42.85%) patient where in HD. We used the IE in general population guidelines for the decision of medical or surgical treatment in all our patients.

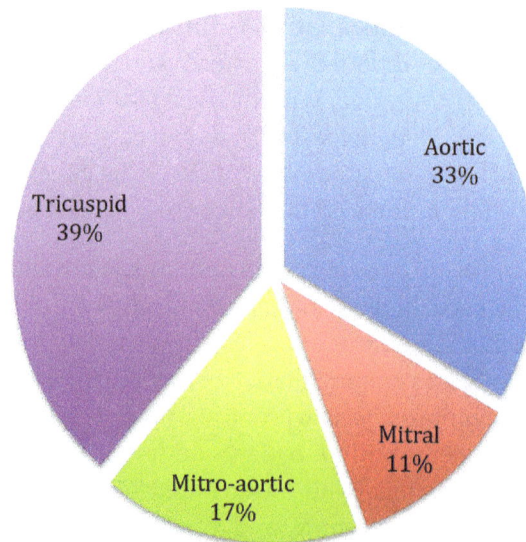

Figure 1. Affected valves in HD patients (IMSS 2011–2015).

In contrast to what previous publications have described regarding IE in HD patients, the most commonly infected valve in our surgical population was the tricuspid valve (**Figure 1**). Also, having a mean age of 38.5 years ranging between 19 and 76 years, which is significantly lower than previous reports. We consider that this can be related to the long mean time of nontunneled HD catheters observed in our patients and also for not having proper safety protocols for the prevention of bacteremia in the HD facilities. This also could be caused by Mexico's overpopulation in public health services and the long-lasting waiting list for AVFs or kidney transplantation, causing good transplant candidates to end up as chronic dialysis patients and making them more susceptible to bacteremia and infections. Even though our hospital is the leading center for kidney transplantation in all Latin America, the waiting list is affected by the overpopulation commented before.

7. Differences between case series of IE in ESRD patients

The following tables summarizes some of the most representative contemporary case series of IE in ESRD patients published in the last decade. The percentage of HD patients with IE who are undergoing cardiac surgery ranges from 7.8 to 53% in different regions of the world and also the associated pathologies are listed in **Table 1**. *S. aureus* is the microorganism most frequently involved in all series (**Table 1**). The valves involve with IE in previous studies involved most frequently the left side valves (**Table 2**). There are significant differences in the percentage of ESRD patients with AVFs in different regions, the highest being in Europe (**Table 3**). And morbidity and mortality also differ between regions (**Table 4**).

Authors	Doulton T, Sabharwal N, Cairns H, et al.	Jones D, McGill L, Rathod K, et al.	Nori U, Manoharan A, Thornby J, et al.	Kamalakannan D, Manohara R, Johnson L, et al.	Chou M, Wang J, Wu W, et al.	Chang C, Kuo B, Chen T, et al.	Baroudi S, Qazi R, Lentine K, et al.
Journal	Kidney International, 2003; 64: 720-727	Nephron Clinical Practice, 2013; 123: 151–156	Nephrology Dialysis Transplantation 2006; 21: 2184–2190	Annals of Thoracic Surgery 2007; 83: 2081–2086	International Journal of Cardiology 2015; 179: 465–469	Journal of Nephrology 2004; 17:228-235	NDT PLUS Nephrology Dialysis Transplantation
Year	2003	2013	2006	2007	2015	2004	2008
Country	UK	UK	USA	USA	Taiwan	Taiwan	USA
Years of the study	22	13	5	15	9	15	16

	1980–1995, 1995–2002, 1996–2002	1998–2011	1999–2004	1990–2004	1999–2007	1988–2002	1990–2006
Years in which the study was conducted							
Participant centers	St. Thomas H. Guy's H. King's College H. (London)	Royal London Hospital. (London)	Columbus, Ohio Detroit, Michigan Houston, Texas	St. John Hospital and Medical Center. Detroit, Michigan.	National	Taipei Veterans General Hospital.	Saint Louis University Hospital.
IE patients (n)	28 pts.	42 pts.	52 pts.	69 pts.	502 (39 surgical)-7.8	20 pts.	59 pts.
Cardiac surgery	53% (15/28 pts.)	21% (9/42 pts.)	24% (13/52 pts.)	34% (24/69 pts.)	7.8% (39 pts.)	*(20 /20 pts.)	12% (7/59 pts.)
Male patients	60.7% (17 pts.)	52.2% (22 pts.)	52%	45% (31 pts.)	35.9% (14 pts.)	(13 pts.)	47% (28 pts.)
Mean age	54.1 (22-81)	55.2 (43-69)	60 (36-82)	56 +-13	52.6 +- 11.7	64.6+-12.9	57.3 +- 13.8
Diabetic%	8	33.3% (14 pts.)	42% (22 pts.)	37.7% (26 pts.)	46.2% (18 pts.)	45% (9 pts.)	59% (35)
Hypertension %	*	66.6% (28 pts.)	79% (41 pts.)	89.9% (62 pts.)	NR	75% (15 pts.)	93% (55)
Immuno suppression %	*	9.5% (4 pts.)	*	(3 pts.)	NR	*	5% (3 pts.)
Staphylococcus aureus	63.3% MRSA	57.1% (24/42 pts.)	20% (11 pts.)	*	*	*	45% (27 pts.)

* For the type of stratification of patients in the publication, the data are present but not reported in this table. NR: not reported.

Table 1. Infective endocarditis publications in ESRD patients in dialysis surgical treatment: demographic information.

Authors	Doulton T, Sabharwal N, Cairns H, et al.	Jones D, McGill L, Rathod K, et al.	Nori U, Manoharan A, Thornby J, et al.	Kamalakannan D, Manohara R, Johnson L, et al.	Chou M, Wang J, Wu W, et al.	Chang C, Kuo B, Chen T, et al.	Baroudi S, Qazi R, Lentine K, et al.
Journal	Kidney International, 2003; 64: 720-727	Nephron Clinical Practice, 2013; 123:151–156	Nephrology Dialysis Transplantation 2006; 21: 2184–2190	Annals of Thoracic Surgery 2007; 83: 2081–2086	International Journal of Cardiology 2015; 179:465 –469	Journal of Nephrology 2004; 17: 228–235	NDT PLUS Nephrology Dialysis Transplantation

Year	2003	2013	2006	2007	2015	2004	2008
Country	UK	UK	USA	USA	Taiwan	Taiwan	USA
Involved heart valve%							
Mitral	41.4%	30.9% (13/42 pts.)	50% (27 pts.)	*	*	64%	63% (37 pts.)
Aortic	37.9%	42.8% (18/42 pts.)	43% (23 pts.)	*	*	18%	17% (10 pts.)
Tricuspid	NR	5 pts.	19% (10 pts.)	*	*	9%	*
Mitral and aortic	17.2%	9.5% (4/42 pts.)	*	*	*	9%	*
Previous valve lesions	13 pts. (51.7%)	33.3% (14 pts.)	*	10.1% (7 pts.)	*	*	*
Previous valvular prosthesis	2 pts	9.5% (4 pts.)	13% (7 pts.)	4.3% (3 pts.)	*	*	*

* For the type of stratification of patients in the publication, the data are present but not reported in this table. NR: not reported.

Table 2. Infective endocarditis publications in ESRD patients in dialysis surgical treatment: involved heart valves.

Authors	Doulton T, Sabharwal N, Cairns H, et al.	Jones D, McGill L, Rathod K, et al.	Nori U, Manoharan A, Thornby J, et al.	Kamalakannan D, Manohara R, Johnson L, et al.	Chou M, Wang J, Wu W, et al.	Chang C, Kuo B, Chen T, et al.	Baroudi S, Qazi R, Lentine K, et al.
Journal	Kidney International, 2003; 64: 720–727	Nephron Clinical Practice, 2013; 123:151–156	Nephrology Dialysis Transplantation 2006; 21: 2184–2190	Annals of Thoracic Surgery 2007; 83: 2081–2086	International Journal of Cardiology 2015; 179: 465–469	Journal of Nephrology 2004; 17: 228–235	NDT PLUS Nephrology Dialysis Transplantation
Year	2003	2013	2006	2007	2015	2004	2008
Country	UK	UK	USA	USA	Taiwan	Taiwan	USA
Dialysis access route%							
PTFE graft	10.8%	NR	13% (7 pts.)	21.7% (15 pts.)	*	15% (3 pts.)	44.1% (26 pts.)
AVF	41.3%	35% (14/40 pts.)	4% (2 pts.)	11.6% (8 pts.)	*	25% (5 pts.)	5.1% (3 pts.)
Tunneled catheter DL	37.9%	55% (22/40 pts.)	72% (39 pts.)	66.7% (46 pts.)	*	5% (1 pt.)	26 pts.

Nontunneled catheter	3.4%	10% (4/40 pts.)	2% (1 pt.)	0 (0%)	*	55% (11 pts.)	2 pts.
Peritoneal dialysis	3.4% (1)	5% (2/42 pts.)	NR	0 (0%)	*		
Mean time of HD before IE	46.3 (1.5-180)	57.4 (9.7 -85.5)	*	37+-32	*	12.9+-19.1	52.9 +- 58

* For the type of stratification of patients in the publication, the data are present but not reported in this table. NR: not reported.

Table 3. Infective endocarditis publications in ESRD patients in dialysis surgical treatment: dialysis access route.

Authors	Doulton T, Sabharwal N, Cairns H, et al.	Jones D, McGill L, Rathod K, et al.	Nori U, Manoharan A, Thornby J, et al.	Kamalakannan D, Manohara R, Johnson L, et al.	Chou M, Wang J, Wu W, et al.	Chang C, Kuo B, Chen T, et al.	Baroudi S, Qazi R, Lentine K, et al.
Journal	Kidney International, 2003; 64: 720–727	Nephron Clinical Practice, 2013; 123:151–156	Nephrology Dialysis Transplantation 2006; 21: 2184–2190	Annals of Thoracic Surgery 2007; 83: 2081–2086	International Journal of Cardiology 2015; 179: 465–469	Journal of Nephrology 2004; 17: 228–235	NDT PLUS Nephrology Dialysis Transplantation
Year	2003	2013	2006	2007	2015	2004	2008
Country	UK	UK	USA	USA	Taiwan	Taiwan	USA
Survival to discharge after surgery	14 pts (93.3%)	88.8% (8 pts.)	*	*	*	*	*
Survival 3 months after surgery	*	86.9%	*	*	66.5%	*	*
Survival 1 year after surgery	*	77%	*	*	58.4%	*	*
In-hospital mortality% nonsurgical patients	*	14.3%	19 pts. (37%).	*	23.5%	*	*
In-hospital mortality% surgical patients	1 pt. (6.9%)	11.1%	*	*	25.9%	*	*
Subsequent mortality	>50% 1 year survival	29.2% - 1 month	32.7% - 3 months	13 pts. Follow-up	*	*	*

* For the type of stratification of patients in the publication, the data are present but not reported in this table. NR: not reported.

Table 4. Infective endocarditis publications in ESRD patients in dialysis surgical treatment: survival, in-hospital mortality, and overall mortality.

8. Prevention and future considerations

After analyzing the literature of IE in different regions of the world, we found different pathogens depending on the endemic regions for some pathologies, for example, RHD, usage of antibiotic treatment before having a diagnosis, endemic zones for rare pathogens such as *Brucella* spp. in Turkey or even zoonosis reported by Watt et al. [7, 16, 20].

One of the recommendations for developing countries must be an adequate treatment and follow-up for group A beta-hemolytic streptococcus to prevent rheumatic fever and its cardiac complications, which is one of the most common causes of IE in general population and in HD 19 patients in developing countries [16].

There are many different scenarios between developed and developing countries, but we think that the security measures for prevention of bacteremia in HD can be achieved in any health care unit using HD program regardless of the place. Reducing bacteremia in HD patients will reduce their incidence of IE [16].

Pronovost et al. in their study made in 103 UCIs in Michigan used basic changes in their practice of catheter implantation and management. An evidence-based intervention resulted in a large and sustained reduction (up to 66%) in rates of catheter-related bloodstream infection that was maintained throughout the 18-month study period [29].

8.1. Michigan and bacteremia zero recommendations

1. Wash your hands

Wash your hands before inserting a central venous catheter (CVC). Bottom Line: Proper hand hygiene is required before and after palpating catheter insertion sites, as well as before and after inserting, replacing, accessing, repairing, or dressing an intravascular catheter. In addition, the use of gloves does not obviate the need for hand hygiene. Category IA: Proper hand hygiene procedures can be achieved through the use of either a waterless, alcohol-based product or an antibacterial soap and water with adequate rinsing.

2. Clean the skin with chlorhexidine

Bottom Line: Disinfect clean skin with an appropriate antiseptic before catheter insertion and during dressing changes. A 2% chlorhexidine-based preparation is the preferred solution, Category IA [29].

Chaiyakunapruk et al., in their meta-analysis compared chlorhexidine versus povidone-iodine solution for vascular catheter site care, finding that the use of chlorhexidine reduces the risk for catheter-related bloodstream infection by 49% [30]. The same authors in another study, published one year later, concluded that the use of chlorhexidine, rather than povidone, for central catheter site care resulted in a 1.6% decrease in the incidence of catheter-related bloodstream infection, a 0.23% decrease in the incidence of death, and savings of $113 per catheter used [31].

3. Use of full-barrier precautions during CVC insertion

Bottom Line: Maintain aseptic technique for the insertion of intravascular catheters. Category IA: Maximal sterile barrier precautions (e.g., cap, mask, sterile gown, sterile gloves, and large sterile drape) during the insertion of CVCs substantially reduce the incidence of catheter-related bloodstream infection (CR-BSI) compared with standard precautions (e.g., sterile gloves and small drapes) [29].

4. Avoid the femoral site

Bottom Line: A subclavian site is preferred for infection control purposes, although other factors (e.g., the potential for noninfectious and catheter-operator skill) should be considered for deciding where to place the catheter. Category IA: The site at which a catheter is placed influences the subsequent risk for catheter-related infection and phlebitis. For adults, lower extremity insertion sites are associated with a higher risk of infection than upper extremity sites. As a result, authorities recommend that CVCs be placed in the subclavian site instead of a jugular or femoral site to reduce the risk for infection [29].

5. Remove unnecessary central venous catheters

Bottom Line: Promptly remove any intravascular catheter that is no longer essential. Category IA: One of the most effective strategies for preventing CR-BSIs is to eliminate, or at least reduce, exposure to central venous catheters. The decision regarding the need for a catheter, however, is complex and therefore difficult to standardize into a practice guideline. Nonetheless, to reduce exposure to central venous catheters, the ICU team should adopt a strategy to system-atically evaluate daily whether any catheters or tubes can be removed [29].

6. Hygienic management of catheters

Minimize the manipulation of the connections and clean the injection sites of the catheter with isopropyl alcohol 70° before its use. Category IA: Another characteristic of this study was that the people in charge of the catheters needed to do an auto-test online, assist to safety meetings before they can be part of the study [32]. This study was performed in 68% of all ICUs in Spain, with a reduction of 50% in the bacteremia related to catheter in a two-year period [19].

In addition to the intervention to reduce the rate of catheter-related bloodstream infection, the ICUs implemented the use of a daily goal to improve clinician-to-clinician communication within the ICU, an intervention to reduce the incidence of ventilator-associated pneumonia, and a comprehensive unit-based safety program to improve the safety culture. The period necessary for the implementation of each intervention was estimated to be 3 months [29].

8.2. Our recommendations for developing countries

After analyzing the literature and the results in the different countries and our own experience, we made some recommendations that could help any HD program in developing countries for reducing their bacteremia incidence, and thus reducing the risk of IE.

1. Form a HD team

They should be the only people involved in the HD process. This can be achieved by online auto-test of the use of catheters and the safety recommendations for it. This team must have a leader, who has to be in constant training through conferences and workshops. This must be transmitted to the whole group, also by training and evaluations. Having a checklist for every procedure could also help reduce errors or omissions in the process. The personnel involved in this HD team must be able to teach all the safety measures for the patient and their family members to avoid infection of any HD access. They must provide standardized knowledge about topics such as vascular access care, hand hygiene, risks related to catheter use, recognizing signs of infection, and instructions for access management when away from the dialysis unit.

2. Cardiac screening for all ESRD patients

An ESRD patient who is going to start HD treatment should have a cardiac screening to rule out previous cardiac pathology. A patient with a heart disease should be considered for closer monitoring.

3. Respect hierarchy in vascular access for HD

Before HD, always consider that the hierarchy of bacteremia risk exists among various types of HD vascular access; it is less common in patients with native arteriovenous fistulae, while synthetic grafts, cuffed catheters, and uncuffed catheters yield a progressively increasing risk.

4. Respect hierarchy in vascular access when using catheters for HD

In the case of using catheters, the hierarchy of bacteremia risk is less common in subclavian catheters, jugular catheters, and femoral catheters, progressively increasing risk.

5. Use the Michigan and bacteremia zero recommendations when using catheters

When using a catheter for HD, always take the six recommendations given above from Pronovost et al. made in ICUs in Michigan and Bacteremia Zero from Spain, which reduce more than 50% of catheter-related bacteremia.

6. Nasal cultures for all ESRD patients

Nasal cultures for *S. aureus* for new patients and serial cultures for chronic patients and use of nasal mupirocin are recommended.

7. Inspect and clean catheter exit sites

Exit sites should be routinely inspected for infection at every dialysis session, and subjected to swabbing and bacterial culture whenever infection is suspected.

8. Suspicion of IE in HD patients? Always use TEE

TTE if not conclusive TEE to rule out or confirm the diagnosis; if TTE conclusive, use TEE to rule out other cardiac lesions or unidentified vegetations in other valves.

9. Vancomycin not as prophylactic

Confirm IE in HD patients; do not use prophylactic vancomycin if you suspect any pathogen different from MRSA.

10. Mechanical prosthesis not the only option for IE in HD patients

Biological prosthesis is a good option for these patients; the heart team must individualize each case; and consider the benefits or disadvantages of mechanical or biological prosthesis.

9. Conclusion

Here we have addressed the different protocols and outcomes among developed countries due to ESRD patients' population, economy and health care differences in each country. This means that the recommendations of different associations and foundations have not been completely followed up by all HD systems even in developed countries.

So to answer the question: what is the problem in developing countries? There are many answers.

Late ESRD diagnosis or any risk factors can end in ESRD, due to not having a routine checkup in primary health care service.

Incomplete protocols, as already stated, are common in developing countries, making changes to these protocols based on "saving" money only or to provide more medical care to a large number of patients, giving them suboptimal care due to inadequate time for each patient. Because health care providers in developing countries have too many patients, it is not possible to offer optimal service quality.

Unavailability of the adequate equipment.

Not having the right timing between dialysis treatments, and especially between diagnosis and definitive treatment with kidney transplant.

Long waiting lists due to fewer transplant centers for kidney transplantation.

In developing countries, most of the patients are uneducated, or they do not have accurate information about their diseases or their HD route.

In the recommendations given in this chapter, after analyzing the literature and the guidelines for preventing IE in ESRD patients, we summarized the prevention strategies and sought to apply them in any developing country for having less incidence of IE in ESRD patients.

Being part of a health care institution in a developing country, you have to learn how to manage this and other related difficulties. The only method to give a solution to this problem is by analyzing the procedure of other hospitals, either from your region or from other countries, which will give you good arguments for requesting anything missing in your program to provide quality care to their patients. In other words, you have to demonstrate that is cost-effective and it will benefit the patient and the hospital.

Author details

Díaz-García Héctor Rafael[1*], Contreras-de la Torre Nancy Anabel[1],
Alemán-Villalobos Alfonso[1], Carrillo-Galindo María de Jesús[1],
Gómez-Jiménez Olivia Berenice[1], Esparza-Beléndez Edgar[1], Ramírez-Rosales Gladys Eloísa[2],
Portilla-d Buen Eliseo[3] and Arreola-Torres Ramón[1,2,3]

*Address all correspondence to: heradiga@hotmail.com

1 Cardiac Surgery Service, Centro Médico Nacional de Occidente Instituto Mexicano del Seguro Social, Mexico

2 Immunology Laboratory, University Center of Health Sciences, Universidad de Guadalajara, Mexico

3 Surgical Research Division, Biomedical Research Center, Centro Médico Nacional de Occidente Instituto Mexicano del Seguro Social, Mexico

References

[1] Slipczuk L, Codolosa JN, Davila CD, Romero-Corral A, Yun J, Pressman GS, et al. Infective endocarditis epidemiology over five decades: a systematic review. PLoS One. 2013;8(12):e82665.

[2] Bin Abdulhak AA, Baddour LM, Erwin PJ, Hoen B, Chu VH, Mensah GA, et al. Global and regional burden of infective endocarditis, 1990–2010. Global Heart. 2014;9(1):131–143.

[3] Doulton T, Sabharwal N, Cairns HS, Schelenz S, Eykyn S, O'Donnell P, et al. Infective endocarditis in dialysis patients: new challenges and old. Kidney International. 2003;64(2):720–727.

[4] Chang C-F, Kuo BI-T, Chen T-L, Yang W-C, Lee S-D, Lin C-C. Infective endocarditis in maintenance hemodialysis patients: fifteen years' experience in one medical center. Journal of Nephrology. 2004;17(2):228–235.

[5]   Nucifora G, Badano LP, Viale P, Gianfagna P, Allocca G, Montanaro D, et al. Infective endocarditis in chronic haemodialysis patients: an increasing clinical challenge. European Heart Journal. 2007;28(19):23072312.

[6]   Tleyjeh IM, Abdel-Latif A, Rahbi H, Scott CG, Bailey KR, Steckelberg JM, et al. A systematic review of population-based studies of infective endocarditis. CHEST Journal. 2007;132(3):1025–1035.

[7]   Watt G, Lacroix A, Pachirat O, Baggett HC, Raoult D, Fournier P-E, et al. Prospective comparison of infective endocarditis in Khon Kaen, Thailand and Rennes, France. The American Journal of Tropical Medicine and Hygiene. 2015;92(4):871–874.

[8]   Kamalakannan D, Pai RM, Johnson LB, Gardin JM, Saravolatz LD. Epidemiology and clinical outcomes of infective endocarditis in hemodialysis patients. The Annals of Thoracic Surgery. 2007;83(6):2081–2086.

[9]   Saxena AK, Panhotra BR. Haemodialysis catheter-related bloodstream infections: current treatment options and strategies for prevention. Swiss Medical Weekly. 2005;135(9-10):127–138.

[10]   Omoto T, Aoki A, Maruta K, Masuda T. Surgical outcome in hemodialysis patients with active-phase infective endocarditis. Annals of Thoracic and Cardiovascular Surgery. 2016; 22(3):181–185.

[11]   Gilmore J. KDOQI clinical practice guidelines and clinical practice recommendations-2006 updates. Nephrology Nursing Journal. 2006;33(5):487.

[12]   Hoen B, Paul-Dauphin A, Hestin D, Kessler M. EPIBACDIAL: a multicenter prospective study of risk factors for bacteremia in chronic hemodialysis patients. Journal of the American Society of Nephrology. 1998;9(5):869–876.

[13]   Durante-Mangoni E, Bradley S, Selton-Suty C, Tripodi M-F, Barsic B, Bouza E, et al. Current features of infective endocarditis in elderly patients: results of the international collaboration on endocarditis prospective cohort study. Archives of Internal Medicine. 2008;168(19):2095–2103.

[14]   Pisoni RL, Young EW, Dykstra DM, Greenwood RN, Hecking E, Gillespie B, et al. Vascular access use in Europe and the United States: results from the DOPPS. Kidney International. 2002;61(1):305–316.

[15]   Jones DA, McGill L-A, Rathod KS, Matthews K, Gallagher S, Uppal R, et al. Characteristics and outcomes of dialysis patients with infective endocarditis. Nephron Clinical Practice. 2013;123(3-4):151–156.

[16]   Chou M-T, Wang J-J, Wu W-S, Weng S-F, Ho C-H, Lin Z-Z, et al. Epidemiologic features and long-term outcome of dialysis patients with infective endocarditis in Taiwan. International Journal of Cardiology. 2015;179:465–469.

[17] Mylonakis E, Calderwood SB. Infective endocarditis in adults. New England Journal of Medicine. 2001;345(18):1318–1330.

[18] Hoen B. Infective endocarditis: a frequent disease in dialysis patients. Nephrology Dialysis Transplantation. 2004;19(6):1360–1362.

[19] Ferrer C, Almirante B. Venous catheter-related infections. Enferm Infecc Microbiol Clin. 2014;32(2):115–124.

[20] Şimşek-Yavuz S, Şensoy A, Kaşıkçıoğlu H, Çeken S, Deniz D, Yavuz A, et al. Infective endocarditis in Turkey: aetiology, clinical features, and analysis of risk factors for mortality in 325 cases. International Journal of Infectious Diseases. 2015;30:106–114.

[21] Athan E, Chu VH, Tattevin P, Selton-Suty C, Jones P, Naber C, et al. Clinical characteristics and outcome of infective endocarditis involving implantable cardiac devices. JAMA. 2012;307(16):1727–1735.

[22] Heiro M, Helenius H, Mäkilä S, Hohenthal U, Savunen T, Engblom E, et al. Infective endocarditis in a Finnish teaching hospital: a study on 326 episodes treated during 1980–2004. Heart. 2006;92(10):1457–1462.

[23] Nori US, Manoharan A, Thornby JI, Yee J, Parasuraman R, Ramanathan V. Mortality risk factors in chronic haemodialysis patients with infective endocarditis. Nephrology Dialysis Transplantation. 2006;21(8):2184–2190.

[24] Kuo C, Lin J-C, Peng M-Y, Wang N-C, Chang F-Y. Endocarditis: impact of methicillin-resistant *Staphylococcus aureus* in hemodialysis patients and community-acquired infection. Journal of Microbiology, Immunology, and Infection. 2007;40(4):317–324.

[25] Leither MD, Shroff GR, Ding S, Gilbertson DT, Herzog CA. Long-term survival of dialysis patients with bacterial endocarditis undergoing valvular replacement surgery in the United States. Circulation. 2013;128(4):344–351.

[26] Rankin JS, Milford-Beland S, O'Brien SM, Edwards FH, Peterson ED, Glower DD, et al. The risk of valve surgery for endocarditis in patients with dialysis-dependent renal failure. The Journal of Heart Valve Disease. 2007;16(6):617–122; discussion 22.

[27] Spies C, Madison JR, Schatz IJ. Infective endocarditis in patients with end-stage renal disease: clinical presentation and outcome. Archives of Internal Medicine. 2004;164(1):71–75.

[28] Thourani VH, Sarin EL, Keeling WB, Kilgo PD, Guyton RA, Dara AB, et al. Long-term survival for patients with preoperative renal failure undergoing bioprosthetic or mechanical valve replacement. The Annals of Thoracic Surgery. 2011;91(4):1127–1134.

[29] Pronovost P, Needham D, Berenholtz S, Sinopoli D, Chu H, Cosgrove S, et al. An intervention to decrease catheter-related bloodstream infections in the ICU. New England Journal of Medicine. 2006;355(26):2725–2732.

[30] Chaiyakunapruk N, Veenstra DL, Lipsky BA, Saint S. Chlorhexidine compared with povidone-iodine solution for vascular catheter–site care: a meta-analysis. Annals of Internal Medicine. 2002;136(11):792–801.

[31] Chaiyakunapruk N, Veenstra DL, Lipsky BA, Sullivan SD, Saint S. Vascular catheter site care: the clinical and economic benefits of chlorhexidine gluconate compared with povidone iodine. Clinical Infectious Diseases. 2003;37(6):764–771.

[32] Martínez MP, Lerma FÁ, Badía MR, Gil CL, Pueyo ML, Tobajas CD, et al. Prevention of bacteremia related with ICU catheters by multifactorial intervention: A report of the pilot study. Med Intensiva. 2010;34(9):581–589.

Permissions

The contributors of this book come from diverse backgrounds, making this book a truly international effort. This book will bring forth new frontiers with its revolutionizing research information and detailed analysis of the nascent developments around the world.

We would like to thank all the contributing authors for lending their expertise to make the book truly unique. They have played a crucial role in the development of this book. Without their invaluable contributions this book wouldn't have been possible. They have made vital efforts to compile up to date information on the varied aspects of this subject to make this book a valuable addition to the collection of many professionals and students.

This book was conceptualized with the vision of imparting up-to-date information and advanced data in this field. To ensure the same, a matchless editorial board was set up. Every individual on the board went through rigorous rounds of assessment to prove their worth. After which they invested a large part of their time researching and compiling the most relevant data for our readers.

The editorial board has been involved in producing this book since its inception. They have spent rigorous hours researching and exploring the diverse topics which have resulted in the successful publishing of this book. They have passed on their knowledge of decades through this book. To expedite this challenging task, the publisher supported the team at every step. A small team of assistant editors was also appointed to further simplify the editing procedure and attain best results for the readers.

Apart from the editorial board, the designing team has also invested a significant amount of their time in understanding the subject and creating the most relevant covers. They scrutinized every image to scout for the most suitable representation of the subject and create an appropriate cover for the book.

The publishing team has been an ardent support to the editorial, designing and production team. Their endless efforts to recruit the best for this project, has resulted in the accomplishment of this book. They are a veteran in the field of academics and their pool of knowledge is as vast as their experience in printing. Their expertise and guidance has proved useful at every step. Their uncompromising quality standards have made this book an exceptional effort. Their encouragement from time to time has been an inspiration for everyone.

The publisher and the editorial board hope that this book will prove to be a valuable piece of knowledge for researchers, students, practitioners and scholars across the globe.

List of Contributors

Fabian Andres Giraldo Vallejo
Instituto del Corazón de Bucaramanga, Bucaramanga, Colombia

Cheima Wathek and Riadh Rannen
Military Hospital of Tunis, Ophthalmology Department, Faculty of Medicine of Tunis, Tunis El Manar University, Tunis, Tunisia

Takashi Murashita
Heart and Vascular Institute, West Virginia University, Morgantown, WV, USA

Julie M. Aultman, Emanuela Peshel and Cyril Harfouche
Northeast Ohio Medical University, Rootstown, Ohio, United States

Michael S. Firstenberg
Northeast Ohio Medical University, Rootstown, Ohio, United States
The Medical Center of Aurora, Aurora, CO, United States

Ahmed Fayaz and Medhat Reda Nashy
King Fahd Hospital of University, Khobar, Saudi Arabia

Sarah Eapen
Summa Akron City Hospital, Akron, Ohio, United States

Michael S. Firstenberg
The Medical Center of Aurora, Aurora, Colorado, United States
Northeast Ohio Medical Universities, Rootstown, Ohio, United States

Miguel Castro, Javier Álvarez, Javier F. Feijoo, Marcio Diniz, Lucía García-Caballero, Pedro Diz and Jacobo Limeres
Special Needs Unit and OMEQUI Research Group, School of Medicine and Dentistry, Santiago

de Compostela University, Santiago de Compostela, Spain

John F. Sedgwick and Gregory M. Scalia
Department of Echocardiography, Cardiology Program, The Prince Charles Hospital, Brisbane, Australia
The University of Queensland, Brisbane, Australia

Vikas Yellapu and Stanislaw P. Stawicki
Department of Research and Innovation, St. Luke's University Health Network, Bethlehem, Pennsylvania, USA

Daniel Ackerman
Center for Neurosciences, St. Luke's University Health Network, Bethlehem, Pennsylvania, USA

Santo Longo
Department of Pathology, St. Luke's University Health Network, Bethlehem, Pennsylvania, USA

Mio Ebato
Division of Cardiology, Showa University Fujigaoka Hospital, Yokohama, Kanagawa, Japan

Luminita Iliuta
University of Medicine and Pharmacy "Carol Davila", Bucharest, Romania

Marion J. Skalweit
Louis Stokes Cleveland Department of Veterans Affairs Medical Center and Case Western Reserve University School of Medicine, Departments of Medicine and Biochemistry, Division of Infectious Diseases, Ohio, USA

Díaz-García Héctor Rafael, Contreras-de la Torre Nancy Anabel, Alemán-Villalobos Alfonso, Carrillo-Galindo María de Jesús, Gómez-Jiménez Olivia Berenice and Esparza-Beléndez Edgar
Cardiac Surgery Service, Centro Médico Nacional de Occidente Instituto Mexicano del Seguro Social, Mexico

Arreola-Torres Ramón
Cardiac Surgery Service, Centro Médico Nacional de Occidente Instituto Mexicano del Seguro Social, Mexico
Immunology Laboratory, University Center of Health Sciences, Universidad de Guadalajara, Mexico

Surgical Research Division, Biomedical Research Center, Centro Médico Nacional de Occidente Instituto Mexicano del Seguro Social, Mexico

Ramírez-Rosales Gladys Eloísa
Immunology Laboratory, University Center of Health Sciences, Universidad de Guadalajara, Mexico

Portilla-d Buen Eliseo
Surgical Research Division, Biomedical Research Center, Centro Médico Nacional de Occidente Instituto Mexicano del Seguro Social, Mexico

Index

www.ingramcontent.com/pod-product-compliance
Lightning Source LLC
Chambersburg PA
CBHW061954190326
41458CB00009B/2868